What Families Who Are Dealing With a Brain Tumor Have to Say About Brain Tumor Series

…explains the complex issues of brain tumors in a manner that the general public can understand - without 'talking down' to us… the tone is crisp and reads well… Ray G, Albany NY

Written well from the beginning… you can … see this book is not like a Physician's Desk Reference. Patty A, a survivor in NJ

I was struck by how much I did not know even though I have been researching brain mets on behalf of several friends with melanoma and breast cancer brain mets. Helen S, NY

…a roadmap through what is complicated and scary to the lay reader. The Checklist To Assess My Team & Care is empowering, challenging and clear ….and will piss off lots of doctors! … in a good way. Shira G, TV writer, CA

Inspiringly hopeful…so admirable - coming from a physician instead of an on-line bulletin board or support group. Katie C, UCLA, Los Angeles

I have wished for this book. The chapter on the Team is probably the best thing I have read on this… ever! "… successful patients not only learn how to 'work the system' but they also learn how to live in this foreign land." This book shows you how. Loice, Philadelphia, PA

You can take comfort in having Dr. Zeltzer with you during your brain tumor journey. Naomi Berkowitz, Executive Director, American Brain Tumor Association, Chicago, IL

D1469484

MORE COMMENTS FROM READERS WHO ARE DEALING WITH A BRAIN TUMOR AND WHAT THEY HAVE TO SAY

The personal e-mail comments express familiar situations I'm sure will strike a vote with all those who read the book...it connects on a personal level. Christine D, Austin, TX

A "how to" book when your world is falling apart... you're a person... not a patient or a statistic. A lot of great information how to get to the right place. Alan A, Newberry Park , CA

We really like the conversational tone. The subject is so serious...it is so nice to read something that is not too technical, not condescending. '...this was written for me.' Lindsay F, Los Angeles, CA

...an excellent resource for brain tumor patients in North America... valuable to health care professionals with a special interest in brain tumors...adds significantly to the current available literature. Dr. Rolando Del Maestro, Clinical Director, Brain Tumour Research Centre, Montreal, Canada

...an important resource for patients. Keith Black M.D., Director, Maxine Dunitz Neurosurgical Institute, Los Angeles, CA

...Zeltzer empowers patients stressing the importance of becoming informed, being unafraid to ask questions, getting a second opinion, and doing research ...helpful chapters deal with children's brain tumors and the navigation of the healthcare system (HMOs, Medicare and Medicaid, Social Security Disability). ... ...search words provide readers with ... focused terminology. Recommended for public and consumer health libraries, especially those that own Zeltzer's earlier book. Beth Hill, Univ. of Idaho Library (Library Journal 2006]

BRAIN TUMORS – FINDING THE ARK

MEETING THE CHALLENGES OF TREATMENT CHOICES, SIDE EFFECTS, CHILDREN'S
UNIQUE NEEDS, HEALTHCARE COSTS & LONG TERM ADJUSTMENT

BY PAUL M. ZELTZER MD

Shilysca Press
Encino, California

Connetquot Public Library
760 Ocean Avenue
Bohemia, NY 11716

Zeltzer, Paul M. 1942-

Brain Tumors – Finding the Ark: Meeting the Challenges of Treatment Choices, Side Effects, Children's Unique Needs, Healthcare Costs & Long Term Adjustment

1. Health   2. Illness   3. Brain Tumors   4. New Age Metaphysics

Library of Congress Control Number: 2005924365
ISBN: 0-9760171-1-3

Copyright © 2006 by Paul M. Zeltzer. All rights reserved.
Copyright © 2006 all illustrations and graphics by Paul M. Zeltzer

Layout and design: Apron Strings Design & Katja Loesch

Cover picture: The Ark, Item: #794561 from ArtToday Inc., a wholly owned subsidiary of Jupiter-media Corporation, doing business as JupiterImages and/or Clipart.com.

This book may not be reproduced in whole or part in any manner including Internet use, without express permission, except in case of brief quotation embodied in critical articles and reviews.

Printed in Canada on acid-free paper.

Published by

Shilysca Press
Encino, California

Shilysca Press (a Division of Shilysca, Inc.)
5041 Valjean Avenue
Encino, California 91436

Website: www.survivingbraincancer.com
E-mail address: info@survivingbraincancer.com

Questions about the book contents: Go to the Q and A section at www.survivingbraincancer.com or e-mail your specific question to the author at info@survivingbraincancer.com

DEDICATION

To Lonnie: for your support, indulgence, love and affection in my calling to write the book,

To my daughters: Shira, for helping me find the voice to tell the story; Alysa, for comments and critique; Carin, for helpful comments, tabular organization, and acting as my agent.

Finally to my high school English teacher, Phyllis Bartine Clemens, who opened my mind to think about the power and meanings of words.

IMPORTANT NOTE:

The information in this book is intended to supplement, not substitute for, the expertise and judgment of your physician, pharmacist or other healthcare professional. It should not be understood to indicate that use of any drug or any other therapy is safe, appropriate, or effective for you.

Consult your healthcare professional before proceeding with any advice from this book.

ACKNOWLEDGMENTS

This book series would not have been possible without those who saw the vision of the project in its initial stages: George Diaz, Mary Naughton, and Lucy Gonda. Al Musella also provided constructive criticism and support. Ken Johnson at Neopharm and Guilford Pharmaceuticals also supported this work. Rick Sontag, Kay Verble, and The Sontag Foundation enabled distribution of the book in a major way.

My writing plan included editorial input from people affected by and committed to the subject – the group to whom this book is directed. Many of my lay colleagues are people I've met on the Internet or talked with on the phone. Others have been my patients or we have talked at National meetings. I am indebted for both kind words and harsh yet deserved critique: Patty Adorno, Thijs H. Aaftink, Kathleen Davis, Stephen Duffy, David Edge, Antonia Ithurralde-Hicks, Dennis Kilroy, Neal Levitan, Ed Martin, Pamela Mathers, Dani McCauley, Murray and Lenore Neidorf, Jan O'Brien, Stina O'Leary, John Ott, Sheryl Shetsky, Helen Sloniker, Maria Sansalone, and Phill Weissman.

My professional colleagues gave unselfishly of their time to make insightful commentary and point out inaccuracies: Brian Pikul, Moise Danielpour, Susan Panullo, and Larry Seigler, Michele Burnison, Melvin Deutsch, Victor Levin , Minesh Mehta (Chapter 17); Marsha Drozdoff, Deana Luchs, Cynthia Meyers, Evan Ross, Jean Wallace (Chapter 18); Pat McGrath (Chapter 20); Carrie Fisher, Dan von Hoff (Chapter 21); Leland Albright, Archie Bleyer, Finn Bretnach, Juda Carter, Leah Ellenberg, Mark Greenberg, Mark Hauber, Tania Maher-Shiminski, Loice Swisher (Chapters 22A, 22B); Ruth Hoffman and Grace Monaco-Powers of CandeLighters, Ted Schreck (chapters 23A,23B) Scott Pomeroy and Ian Pollack (Chapter 24); Bill Duke, (Chapter 25). I thank Jon Finlay, Valerie and Victor Ostrower, Rochelle Simmons, and Jacob Zighelboim for helpful conversations and insights.

I have been blessed with wonderful editors. Ping Ho, my content editor, provided critique on language and organization. Writing for the public was more difficult compared with my previous science writing. Caryn Freeman, undertook the daunting task of correcting my non-parallel constructions. Kristin Loberg completed the editing and provided insightful commentary. Julie Beenhower-Macht provided layout counsel and developed a meaningful theme and cover design. Katja Loesch completed the layout and added original line art and drawings.

The book outline was developed in part from answering the "unanswered questions" about brain tumors posted on websites or in e-mail communications over a seven-year period. Most quotations were made anonymous and I have tried to remain true to their content. I am indebted to you whose words expressed, in such pristine ways, the complex medical and emotional issues. You are my heroes.

SHORT TABLE OF CONTENTS

CONTENTS

CHAPTER 19
CANCER-FIGHTING DRUGS – CHEMOTHERAPY, ANTIBIOTICS, MARROW STIMULANTS AND THEIR SIDE EFFECTS   93

CHAPTER 22B
CHILDREN AND BRAIN TUMORS – LONGER TERM PSYCHOLOGICAL AND SOCIAL ISSUES *217*

CHAPTER 23A
HEALTH CARE COVERAGE SYSTEMS AT-A-GLANCE – WHAT A BRAIN TUMOR PATIENT MUST KNOW   *239*

PREFACE TO FINDING THE ARK

I have been a physician for children and adults with brain tumors since 1978. I always found it so interesting how one family could "work the system," seek and find useful information, not be intimidated by the doctors and nurses, and be *successful* patients. Others seemed more dependent on the doctors and did not seem to know which questions to ask. It was not necessarily lack of education or being rich versus poor. I wanted all my patients to be *successful* and get the best care available.

I wrote the first book for the person who recently learned that they have a brain tumor. Brain Tumors: Leaving the Garden of Eden: A Survival Guide To Diagnosis, Learning the Basics, Getting Organized and Finding your Medical Team contains the basics of getting organized, surfing the internet, your Team, facts about your specific brain tumor, ensuring your correct diagnosis, medications you may be taking, obtaining second opinions, and the referral medical center.

This book contains information you need after diagnosis. It has action-oriented, problem-solving tools for making therapy decisions, life-saving details about medications and their side effects, two chapters on healthcare and insurance, clinical trials, inherited aspects of brain tumors, and two chapters on Children: special considerations.

The book is organized consistently between chapters. My graphics consultant, Julie Macht-Beenhower, chose text and fonts of a size and quality most helpful for those with visual problems. The dimensions of the book and special flat binding were chosen with your usage in mind.

The diagnosis of cancer or "brain tumor" is similar to the events in the Garden of Eden. So many of my patients tell me about seeing their lives as divided into before a brain tumor (Eden) and afterward (The Fall) as their punishment and pain. "What did I do so wrong for my child or myself to deserve this?" they often ask. I maintain that you are the CEO of your body. You can work with and understand those feelings, so that you receive the best care, are aware of the choices and alternatives, and do not feel punished.

We physicians try to get patients to tell their stories in terms of MRI scans, blood counts, and symptoms – all things familiar to *us*. But each *individual* is changed in unique ways that do not fit our medical model. You, the patient and family, need to be treated and appreciated for your uniqueness. Your personal story is both a Legacy (Chapter 25) and a narrative. It is something important to share with family and loved ones. It can be part of your recovery and healing process too. With these books, I hope to provide you with some tools to understand…and tell your story.

Paul Zeltzer MD
June 7, 2005.

CHAPTER 17

Traditional Approaches to Treatment

There was no collective opinion or single new treatment. Rather, I encountered vast disagreement about my disease and the proper course of action to defeat it! This was at first, very unnerving!

Neal Levitan, Executive Director, Brain Tumor Society

Key search words

- treatment
- neurosurgery
- radiosurgery
- gliadel
- intrathecal chemotherapy

- metastasis
- neurooncology
- clinical trial
- gliasite
- quality of life

- medical specialist
- radiation therapy
- chemotherapy
- brachytherapy

OVERVIEW

This chapter takes the broad overview – the big picture if you will – about the major therapies offered to most patients. Here I outline treatments and some controversies about their use. The chapter follows the order in Table 17-1. You also might want to review Chapter 8, Diagnosis, in the companion book,[1] to clarify that you are secure with your diagnosis and are prepared for a deeper understanding about treatment choices.

Table 17-1 Major Approaches & Options for Treatment
Surgery
Radiation Therapy
Chemotherapy (FDA-approved or useful)
Chemotherapy in active trials (Chapters 19, 21)
Newer experimental approaches (Chapter 21)

The e-mail below typifies the concern, mystery and desperation that many people feel when someone close is receiving therapy. It points out that important questions cannot be answered *unless* we know the specifics of diagnosis.

> *I just found out that my younger brother (21years old) has an inoperable brain tumor. All I can remember was that it was a frontal, temporal "something" tumor. He said that the worst-case scenario is he has six years to live. I know that he is getting some radiation (sounds like stereo-something). I know it is benign. He told me that the procedure was to see if they could "shrink it." Two weeks after the procedure, they will do another MRI to see where they stand. It was the size of a quarter. Could you tell me whether inoperable really means inoperable and what is the mortality rate if it is inoperable?*
>
> Steve, Missoula, MT

How should you understand Steve's predicament?
1. Inoperable is an opinion – not a fact!
2. Benign tumors rarely receive radiation.
3. Mortality *rates* do not apply to individuals.
4. Steve needs much more specific information.
5. No doctor can predict how long any patient will live.

Bottom Line Your insurance company can deny your primary care physician and specialist's treatment recommendations.

THERAPY – WHO MAKES THE CHOICE?

Traditional treatments for most brain tumors have included surgery, external beam radiation and sometimes chemotherapy. With these therapies, there has been notable progress over the last seven decades (Figure 17-1). Despite our successes, neurooncologists and other researchers continue to work on developing newer, less toxic treatments with better survival rates and quality of life.

How does this affect you? A primary brain lymphoma or glioma, a metastasis to the brain from a tumor elsewhere, or a diffuse coating of tumor along the spine called *leptomeningeal* spread, represent complex problems. One of medicine's secrets is that most oncologists have had little training or experience with these challenges. Many physicians do not believe that treatments offer any benefits. You need to know about your oncologist's core beliefs. His or her attitude can affect the choices offered to you (see Table 17-2). Moreover, this could influence your outcome. This is another reason why my advice is to have a neurooncologist on your team.

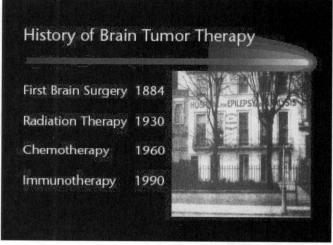

Figure 17-1 History of brain tumor therapies. Maida Vale Hospital, London, England, site of first successful brain surgery, 1884.

Table 17-2 Factors That Affect Your Treatment Choices
1. Known treatment options for your type of tumor.
2. Knowledge, attitude, and competency of your oncologist.
3. HMO or insurance company policies.
4. Available clinical trials
5. Your knowledge of the options
6. Your own prejudices, personal needs and desires.

To make matters more complicated, your care and treatment options may actually be determined solely on a cost basis by an insurance company clerk

Bottom Line Your oncologist's core beliefs and attitude can affect your outcome.

or administrator. Access to physical therapy and rehabilitation, home visits and equipment – even surgery or approved medications for nausea–prevention like Zofran or chemotherapies like Temodar or Gliadel – can be denied by your insurance company, despite recommendations of your primary care physician or specialist (Chapter 23: Managing Costs, Benefits and Your Healthcare With Insurance, HMOs And More…).

As with any type of serious illness, a time may come when the good fight is over and the tumor appears to be winning. When is it time to say, "Enough! I want to spend more time with family, rather than with medical personnel and institutions?" That is an individual decision that should be based on the best available *information*, rather than on assumptions. (See Chapter 25: Your Legacy.) This book shows you how to obtain this information.

SURGERY

WHAT ARE THE GOALS OF SURGERY?

While the goals of surgery may sound straightforward, the skills to perform the procedures are anything but simple (see Table 17-3). Brain function and quality of life depend upon the ability of the neurosurgeon to remove the tumor without touching the brain.

Table 17-3 The Major Goals of Surgery
1. Preserve or improve your neurological function.
2. Obtain a piece of the tumor to confirm the diagnosis (biopsy).
3. Remove the tumor completely or partially.
4. Insert a shunt, if needed, to drain fluid or relieve pressure on the brain.
5. Implant chemotherapy wafers when needed.

Dr. Steven Brem of the Moffitt Cancer Center, University of South Florida College of Medicine often says, "We really should be called tumor surgeons, rather than brain surgeons, since we want to avoid the brain most of the time!" The expertise and skills to look for in a neurosurgeon and the questions for you to ask before, and after, surgery are in Chapters 10-15 for your tumor type and in Chapter 5, Doctors and other Team members.[1] You can visit web sites that show the skull and brain anatomy as well as answers about "awake" craniotomies and functional mapping (see Table 17-10). Descriptions of open and closed stereotactic biopsies are discussed in Chapter 8: Traditional Approaches to Initial Diagnosis. Major choices that you and your neurosurgeon must make about surgery are summarized (see Table 17-4).

Table 17-4 Major Neurosurgical Approaches & Treatment Options
1. Biopsy
2. Partial removal (debulking)
3. Total resection
4. Awake craniotomy
5. Pre-op Functional MRI
6. Intra-operative brain mapping
7. Intra-operative MRI

"INOPERABLE" – WHAT DOES THAT MEAN?

What is *inoperable* to one neurosurgeon can be considered *definitely operable* by a more experienced surgeon. This is another reason to get second opinions about your particular case. Obviously, there are some tumors deep within the brain or in critical areas of the brain stem that even the most skilled surgeon cannot remove. Likewise, a *glioblastoma multiforme* that has crossed over the middle to the other side usually cannot be removed entirely. However, there are many other situations where the sheer skill and experience of the neurosurgeon determine how much tumor can be removed. Technical developments such as computer-assisted navigational devices, functional MRI, and mapping of critical motor and sensory areas during surgery have allowed the neurosurgeon to be more aggressive in removing tumor while not endangering brain function.[2]

Inoperable is an opinion – not a fact.

HOW DOES CHOICE OF NEUROSURGEON AFFECT YOUR SURVIVAL CHANCES?

Many studies have shown that the more tumor tissue that is removed, the better the survival rate, and sometimes quality of life.[3] This is true for both newly diagnosed and recurrent tumors. Dr Leland Albright of the University of Pittsburgh and I studied the effect of the surgeon's skill in leaving more or less than 1.5 cc (¼ teaspoon) of tumor. We found that patients with medulloblastoma who had less than ¼ teaspoon of tumor remaining had 25 percent better survival, even five years later! This means that perseverance in getting the last bit of tumor has long lasting significance.[4,5] See the adjoining summary of results with different tumors with greater or lesser (complete) surgical resections in children (Table 17-5).

Table 17-5 Effect of Tumor Resection on Survival for 5+ Years Without Return of Tumor		
Tumor type	Complete Resection	Incomplete Resection
Medulloblastoma	75%	50%
Anaplastic Astrocytoma	42%	14%
Glioblastoma	27%	4%

ARE ALL NEUROSURGEONS SKILLED AT REMOVING TUMORS?

A neurosurgeon's skills can be defined as a "numbers game." What do I mean by this? Let's do the math. There are about 30,000 primary brain tumors diagnosed yearly in the United States, and there are about 4,500 active neurosurgeons. This means that, if all things were equal, the average neurosurgeon would operate on six to seven patients per year. But we know that each of the 20 largest centers in North America operate on more than 200 primary brain tumors annually. Thus, the majority see far fewer than six to seven cases each year. Therefore most neurosurgeons have limited experience. How does this pertain to you?

> Not all neurosurgeons are equally skilled in removing brain tumors.

Survival time and quality of life for people undergoing neurosurgery in high volume centers were dramatically better in centers having 50 or more surgeries per year.[6] A study from the Johns Hopkins Hospital found that the death rate was 2.5 percent at high-volume centers and 4.9 percent at low-volume hospitals.[7] For this reason, I encourage anyone with a brain tumor to go to the neurosurgeon (center) who has the most experience. (See Chapter 7 for tables listing these centers.[1])

> Centers performing 50+ surgeries a year have better survivals and fewer deaths.

It is often difficult for a neurosurgeon to know whether or not he/she can perform a maximal resection *before* surgery. So it is up to the patient, after the first surgery, to obtain second and third opinions in order to know that the maximal amount of tumor, which can be safely removed, was removed. Reviewing the pre- and post-operative scans with your doctor is a good first step.

WHICH MEDICATIONS OR PROCEDURES WILL I RECEIVE BEFORE OR DURING SURGERY?

A *steroid* (strong type of cortisone called dexamethasone, Decadron) is given to most patients for at least 48 hours before surgery, and longer if the primary doctor or neurosurgeon observes significant brain swelling (edema). Often this is started before the patient sees the neurosurgeon. After surgery, steroids are tapered off over days to weeks, depending upon the degree of edema.

Anti-seizure medication is commonly given before or during surgery, if the tumor is in the front or top part of the brain. If the patient has had a seizure, these medications may be continued for six months or longer. There is a debate among professionals about which class of seizure medications to use. Dilantin (phenytoin) has been used for more than 30 years; however, it "revs up" liver enzymes, which in turn inactivate some of the newer chemotherapy agents. Check with your doctor. It is usually not recommended to give an anticonvulsant if there has been no seizure.[8] Some newer clinical chemotherapy trials require patients to be on non-"enzyme-inducing anticonvulsants" (EIACs) that do not affect the levels of chemotherapy (see Table 17-10).

Table 17-6 Common Medications and Preparations with Neurosurgery	
Steroids	Navigational frame
Anti-seizure medication	Central venous line
Intravenous antibiotics	Urinary catheter
Diuretic (water pill)	Shunts (tubes)

Intravenous antibiotics may be given before an operation and for 24 hours afterward to protect against post-operative brain and skin infections.

A *diuretic* (a medication that releases water through the kidneys called furosemide or Lasix) and another, called mannitol, may be given to reduce brain swelling.

A *stereotactic (navigational, "Stealth") frame* identifies tumor location by incorporating the MRI picture into the neurosurgeon's view through a microscope. The frame is attached with navigation screws or "buttons" that are stuck on the scalp before an MRI scan to set up three-dimensional coordinates. This process is similar to setting up a stereotactic biopsy or stereotactic radiation therapy. The

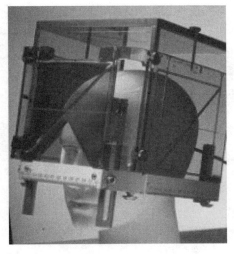

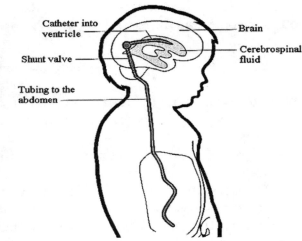

Figure 17-2 Stereotactic set up. Department of Neurosurgery, University of Pittsburgh, 2003. (Courtesy Dr. Mel Deutsch)

Figure 17-3 Shunt draining fluid from ventricles into abdomen

neurosurgeon then *navigates* during surgery comparing the MRI picture with what he actually sees (Figure 17-2).

A *central venous line* (plastic catheter in the arm or leg vein) may be placed, if your head will be elevated during surgery. This prevents air from reaching and harming blood vessels in the brain.

A *catheter* is inserted into the bladder to drain urine, after anesthesia is started.

Shunts (tubes) are implanted to divert spinal fluid from the brain when there is too much pressure inside the head (see Figure 17-3). See Table 17-10 for more information.

See also Chapter 9: Medications for Pain, Fatigue, Seizures and Brain Swelling.[1]

WHAT HAPPENS IMMEDIATELY AFTER SURGERY?

Patients are often placed in an intensive care unit for the initial 12 to 24 hours, depending upon their condition. It can be longer if you are unstable with fluctuating blood pressure, delayed awakening, labored breathing, or swelling of or increased pressure within the brain. Details of

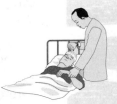

the post-operative procedures, timing of follow-up visits, should be discussed with your surgeon *before* surgery.

What Are Your Neurosurgeon's Responsibilities?

The following are your neurosurgeon's responsibilities after your surgery:
- To show you pre- and post-operative scans demonstrating the exact results of surgery;
- To explain how much tumor was removed, why, and any complications of surgery;
- To discuss the results of the biopsy;
- To care for you until you have recovered from surgery. This includes your time in the ICU until your incisions have healed and you are free from infection;
- To assist in a referrals such as rehabilitation, if needed.

The neurosurgeon will often discontinue being an active participant in your care, once you have recovered fully from the effects of surgery.

What Should You Ask the Neurosurgeon Before He Signs Off Your Case?

Questions to ask your neurosurgeon before you are finished with him/ her are:
- Which other team members will you recommend that I see after surgery?
- May I have a copy of the surgery and MRI scan reports for my notebook?
- Who will monitor my steroid dosage?
- See additional questions in Chapter 5: Doctors and Other Team Members.[1]

RADIATION

How Did It Come to Be Used for Cancer Treatment?

Radiation therapy is often the next step after surgery, although this can vary based on your individual tumor type. In the late 1890s three major discoveries occurred:
- Henri Becquerel discovered radioactive energy particles from uranium and called them "x-rays," because they were unlike any known energy.
- Madame Curie discovered the green glow of Radium in the process of refining uranium; for 75 years, it was used to illuminate watch hands so we could tell time in the dark.

- Wilhelm Roentgen made his accidental discovery while investigating energy emissions from a glass vacuum tube with electrodes at either end (like a large fluorescent light tube). The medical student, who built the device, developed a red rash (the first case of radiation dermatitis) on his hands after long hours of exposure to the x-rays. He subsequently spoke with his professors about his belief that this reaction might harm cancer. This led doctors to treat the first breast cancer patient with a one-hour exposure of a few *roentgens*, the new unit of radioactivity. By 1915, many physicians were treating gliomas and pituitary tumors using radiation therapy.

The x-ray or high-energy particles (electron, proton, and neutron) cause unrepairable damage to the DNA of the brain tumor cell so that it can not divide. Over the past 50 years, technical advances have made radiation more precise, more powerful, and less harmful to surrounding tissues. The newest "beams" have a high energy that passes through skin and targets the tumor below the surface.

Are the Rumors about Radiation Therapy True?

By the time you begin thinking about radiation therapy, you are undoubtedly feeling better. The anxiety over the anticipation of surgery has abated; you have recovered from the after-effects of anesthesia. You are ready to fight this invader and get started on the next phase in your treatment.

Most people have not had personal experience with radiation and it has an element of mystery and fear about it. Unlike light (color waves), radiation waves cannot be seen. Unlike heat waves, they cannot be felt; yet, their effects are powerful. Many of my patients have heard horror stories:

> *Radiation is the next step before dying.*
> *Your hair will fall out.*
> *You can become sterile.*
> *It can mess you up.*

It is important to remember that radiation therapy is another type of powerful therapy designed to harm the tumor cells more than the normal cells. It is potent and effective. If used for the right reasons – at the right time and in the right place – its benefits should outweigh any harm. This section tells you about its major uses and side effects of which to be aware.

WHAT ARE THE DIFFERENT TYPES OF RADIATION THERAPY?

There are two major forms of radiotherapy for treating brain tumors: External beam and Internal beam ("brachytherapy"). Each has advantages and disadvantages. Your radiotherapist should discuss with you the pros and cons specific to your particular tumor (see Table 17-7).

Table 17-7 Major Radiation Therapy Approaches & Treatment Options
External Beam
1. Whole brain radiation
2. Conformal 3-D radiation   Shaped beam radiation: IMRT

3. Stereotactic Radiosurgery (SRS)
    Fractionated stereotactic Radiosurgery:
    Gamma knife / X-Knife / CyberKnife

4. Proton beam Radiation
Internal Beam
1. Brachytherapy
2. Gliasite

External beam therapy is the most common type of radiation treatment in the United States. Rays from a distance are aimed through metal tubes to hit the tumor, plus an extra margin of normal brain tissue. For tumors that travel in the spinal fluid, the whole spine must be treated. Whole brain, GammaKnife Radiosurgery (single dose), stereotactic radiation (multiple dose) are examples.

Internal beam therapy uses a radioactive source (such as iodine or radium) that is placed inside or around the tumor cavity. It delivers very high doses of radiation directly into the tumor, sparing normal skin, bone, and brain tissue.

EXTERNAL BEAM

Up to 10 years ago, it was common to "shape" the energy beam with lead blocks (shielding normal tissues from the path) and aim it from two opposite directions. While, theoretically, this avoided exposure to normal brain areas, the actual scatter to normal brain and thyroid gland in the neck was great. In modern radiotherapy units, computer-assisted techniques use metal "leaves" or shields that can shape the effective beam to any design. One type is called Intensity Modulated Radiation Therapy (IMRT) or conformal-shaped field technique.

External beam radiation is usually given four to five days per week for five to six weeks. Chances for immediate complications are low, but damage can still occur to the normal brain surrounding the tumor. Care must be taken with treatment, especially near the optic nerves and brainstem. Long-term side effects will be discussed later and in Chapter 20.

There are four special types of external beam radiation therapy, in addition to standard opposed-beam techniques:

- Radiosurgery
- Stereotactic fractionated
- Stereotactic hyperfractionated
- Proton beam
- Opposed beam technique (standard)

The actual energy for these treatments is generated from three sources: radioactive cobalt (Gamma rays); linear accelerator (electrons and x-rays); and cyclotron (neutrons and protons); the latter hurls and smashes atoms, allowing them to release their energy.

Radiosurgery

This technique uses a "cobalt gamma unit" (GammaKnife) and delivers very high, one-time doses of radiation to a small area through a helmet containing 201 tiny holes that can be opened or closed to create any shape. The 201 beams at different angles are focused on the target like a magnifying glass focuses the rays of the sun. They converge or meet at the point of the tumor. This procedure has a low complication rate (2 percent) and minimizes injury to normal brain tissue. Radiosurgery was originally designed by Dr. Lars Leksell in Sweden to treat abnormal collections of blood vessels called arteriovenous malformations (AVMs). Its use has been economically driven because it can be performed on an outpatient basis in hours, rather than days. Radiosurgery is reserved for tumors less than 3 cm (about 1.5 inches) because of the risk of severe brain swelling.

Radiosurgery has been used successfully to treat acoustic neuromas and meningiomas that are difficult to reach by surgery. Recently, a single radiosurgical *boost* has been given upon completion of a traditional radiation therapy for glioblastomas,[10] other gliomas, meningiomas, and metastases. Development of necrosis (dead tissue) within the tumor or normal brain areas is a side effect.

◻**Bottom Line** ➤ Radiosurgery is NOT surgery. It is a powerful form of Radiation Therapy.

Stereotactic Radiation Therapy (SRT)

Fractionated or divided stereotactic radiation, SRT differs from Radiosurgery. It is delivered over multiple treatment sessions (one or two per week for up to 10 weeks), rather than one session. When boosting previously radiated areas, daily or frequent treatments are given over one to three weeks. Radiosurgery and SRT require the head or spine to be in a special frame or device that allows precise, accurate delivery of the radiation beams from different angles (see Figure 17-2). Unlike radiosurgery, there are no tumor size limits, as acute side effects are less severe.

Ordinary radiation followed by SRT boosts has increased survival of patients with *glioblastoma multiforme* tumors.[9,10] The machines are made by different manufacturers with brand names such as X-Knife, CyberKnife, Clinac and others. These latter machines are not dedicated to treatment only for the brain, but now can be utilized throughout the body and spine.

Hyperfractionated Radiation Therapy

With this therapy a dose of radiation is divided or fractionated into two or more doses per day. This method was used in the 1980s and 1990s on the premise that more radiation could be delivered, since normal tissue would recover faster than tumor cells.

Hyperfractionated radiation therapy was used for glioblastomas and diffuse brain stem gliomas. There is no convincing evidence that this approach produces superior results.[11] In the case of brain stem gliomas, additional toxicity and serious infections were noted. Hyperfractionated radiation therapy should be administered under research conditions as a clinical trial, but it is *not* accepted as standard therapy.

Proton Beam

This form of radiation therapy is delivered through a powerful accelerating device (cyclotron) that smashes atoms, releasing protons and neutrons with high energies. There are only two units in the United States: one in Boston and the other in Loma Linda, California. Experience with proton beam irradiation has been limited, and it has not yet shown any clear advantage for most brain tumors, except possibly chordomas. The particles have such high energy that they not only kill tumor cells, but also can cause necrosis by damaging blood vessels and other tissues (see also Table 17-10).

"Internal Beam" (Brachytherapy)

Brachytherapy has been studied for more than 30 years, with many clinical trials coming from the University of California, San Francisco; it has been successful in prolonging life. Its strength is also its greatest limitation, however. Most gliomas extend beyond the main tumor; thus, the radiation does not reach far enough. In these cases, SRT provides a better alternative, as it shares many of the same advantages.

GliaSite is an FDA-approved form of brachytherapy, approved for treatment of newly diagnosed and recurrent malignant brain tumors and metastases. A small balloon, with a catheter leading out from beneath the skin, is inserted into the tumor cavity by the neurosurgeon at the time of tumor removal. The balloon is injected with radioactive liquid iodine (later removed) that stays for three to seven days and cooks the tumor from within. This technique was reported to prolong life[12] (see Tables 17-10).

> Brachytherapy is radiation directly in contact with the tumor.

Radioactivity in Injectable Liquids

Radioactive Phosphorus and Yttrium have been injected into inoperable cysts of benign and malignant tumors and craniopharyngiomas for the past 40 years to reduce fluid formation. This therapy is best used when the cyst can contain the radioactive liquid so it does not leak out and become diluted, or touch the brain surface.

Antibodies are proteins, or immune molecules, that can target cancer cells. In this procedure, antibodies attached to radioactive atoms are injected into a vein or directly into the tumor. Using this latter technique, brain tumors shrank in patients with recurrent disease. It is not yet known whether or not this is more effective than other methods.[13,14] Tumor-seeking antibodies with radioactive compounds also have been injected directly into the blood stream with some good responses.

Will Radiation Therapy Offer Me any Benefit?

The answer is: Yes...and no. Radiation therapy is the most extensively used treatment for all brain tumors, including metastases. The major debate among radiation therapists is which type of radiation to give and over what time interval to give it. Though most people with brain tumors will benefit from radiation, some will not. Sometimes the downside of the therapy could be greater than the benefit. This is true for infants and very young children in whom the radiation to the developing brain can cause severe and permanent developmental and neurological damage. Patients older than 70 also are at risk.[15] For other tumors like lymphomas and germinomas, it may be better to give chemotherapy first and treat with radiation later.

WHY DO I NEED TO KNOW ABOUT THE DIFFERENT TYPES OF RADIATION THERAPY?

Most radiation therapists are knowledgeable about what type of radiation therapy to give and when to give it. Others have commercial business attachments to a particular treatment modality, such as GammaKnife, or to a particular Radiosurgery center, a situation that could pose a conflict of interest. You need to be certain that you are in the hands of an expert who is giving you an *unbiased* recommendation. The choice can influence your survival, quality of life, or both. The safety of radiation therapy should be a concern to patients, as expressed in the following submission to the www.virtualtrials.com web site:

> *My grandmother-in-law is home after having radiation done on the top of her brain. She wants to know about the side effects and if they are going to last forever or if they go away eventually.*

> Robert, Joplin, MO

Clearly, if this patient had radiation, which can cause dementia and poor quality of life as a possible side effect, she seems not to have been informed. This underscores the importance of family and friends in helping older people make decisions and cut through hospital, insurance, and administrative bureaucracy.

Let me give you two more scenarios related to radiation therapy that I have experienced with patients who have had a medulloblastoma and *glioblastoma multiforme* respectively:

> **Example 1:** Roger, a 28-year-old mechanic, had a partially removed medullo-blastoma. He was given no chemotherapy option and received radiation only to his head. Six months later, after surfing the Internet, he found additional treatment options to increase the odds of longer survival.

The standard treatment for this *childhood* tumor is radiation to the entire brain *and* spine (because cells from the tumor travel in the spinal fluid throughout the nervous system) plus chemotherapy. However, Roger's options are now limited, because while adding spinal radiation and chemotherapy after-the-fact are feasible, additional radiation to the brain will probably lead to brain damage. Roger should have been given his options before treatment began. A second opinion after surgery would have helped him tremendously.

Example 2: Sara is a 59-year-old homemaker who had a glioblastoma completely removed from her temporal lobe (the part of the brain associated with seizures and word/speech recognition) after having had her first seizure. She and her husband had no questions for the radiation oncologist. After a standard course of radiation, she received a single Radiosurgery boost.

Sara's daughter submitted the following e-mail to an Internet brain tumor support group:

Question: *I was wondering if anyone could tell me their experience with after effects following one stereotactic radiosurgery session. My mom had been doing so well with a GBM, after she had surgery in July 2002 and had received regular radiation. She suffered no neurological deficits at all and came through it with flying colors. In November 2002, her MRI showed that the original tumor was gone, but there was a very small "lesion" to the right of her original tumor site in the left temporal lobe. So...they suggested Radiosurgery to "zap" it.*

Ever since the Radiosurgery and being on Depakote [anti-seizure medication], she just doesn't seem like herself and has really slowed down. She can't remember conversations that just happened; she seems in a daze a lot of the time. Right now, I am thinking that I wish we had not done it. I know we make the best decisions we can. I am trying not to dwell on regrets and misgivings.

Lee, Gatlinburg, TN

Sara, her husband, and daughter did not know what questions to ask. Was the "small lesion" necrosis or tumor? There was no single best choice in this situation. The boost can improve chances for longer survival. What was a "choice," however, was to be informed in advance about the upside and downside consequences of the choices. Why didn't Sara and her husband ask the questions? Did they not want to challenge the doctor, particularly in light of his previous success? Were they afraid to hear the downside? Again, to me this sounds much like the lesson from *The Garden of Eden* and fear of challenging a higher authority (see Chapter 2).

Regardless of the reasons, Sara's daughter now has to rely on the Internet to get this information, after-the-fact.

WHOLE BRAIN OR STEREOTACTIC RADIATION TO INDIVIDUAL METASTATIC TUMORS: THE CHOICE THAT COULD AFFECT YOUR QUALITY OF LIFE?

The recommendation of whole (total) brain radiation therapy for multiple metastases or diffuse tumor has been a reflexive one in many practices (see Chapter 15: Brain Metastases[1]), with not much attention paid to side effects of importance to patients. Most studies just report survival,[16] not quality of survival.

What are these questions about quality of survival? They are simple but important:
1. Will my memory be intact?
2. Will I recognize my spouse or friends?
3. Will I still be able to care for my daily needs like getting dressed, fixing a cup of coffee, and going unassisted to the toilet?

The issues of quality of life and brain function are important and open to different meanings. A major debate among physicians exists as to whether people with less than six metastases should receive whole brain or individual tumor (stereotactic) radiotherapy (SRT). Your age, tumor type and location are all variables. After hearing the information, you and your family should make an informed decision about which treatment to choose, rather than having someone else

> For your specific radiation therapy, understand both the risk and benefits.

makes this decision for you. While no one would want to prescribe a potentially toxic therapy that is not needed, there are differences between older and modern approaches, with much at stake. Only you will have to deal with the consequences, both good and bad. This is why you *must* be informed.

For untreated multiple brain metastases, average survival is less than three months. But for treated metastases, survivals of six to 18 months are increasingly common for people under 60 years of age with high functional scores.[17]

> **Example 3:** Barry is a 71-year-old certified public accountant (CPA) and professor at the local college who was diagnosed with prostate cancer in 1993 and colon cancer in 1998. Both were successfully treated. In December

2000, he found it increasingly difficult to use his adding machine and recall words of federal accounting law. His family noticed new irrational behaviors. An enhanced brain MRI demonstrated three deep metastases with small amounts of bleeding around each tumor -- two in the left parietal lobe (front-middle) and one in the left temporal lobe (side). There was no evidence of active prostate or colon cancer. His local radiation oncologist recommended whole brain radiation. This case was presented to our Tumor Board.

While neither of Barry's original tumor types is usually responsive to chemotherapy, both (prostate and colon carcinoma) are sensitive to radiation. Given the deep location of his tumors, there would be no advantage in having a surgical resection or biopsy prior to radiation treatment, since radiation would have been given in either case. (The only exception would be if he had a *large* brain hemorrhage around the tumor, which would need to be removed by surgery before radiation treatment.) Usually, biopsy and surgical removal are warranted, because removal of brain metastases near the surface gives more immediate relief from pressure-related problems.

Barry opted for localized stereotactic radiation to each of the three tumors, after the complex considerations of his case were explained to him.

You need to ask the radiation oncologist about the *likelihood* that the therapy will cause you or your loved one to be unable to perform tasks #1-3 above, affecting quality of life. This is tough stuff... but it is critical to have this information when making difficult decisions about how you want to live or how you may not want to die.

What Do I Need to Know about Radiosurgery Before I Receive It?

What benefits will it provide and what harm may result from its use? What are its advantages? There is no question that Radiosurgery can be beneficial for selected patients; however, studies have not yet established the benefits versus side effects for many types of cancer. Possible side effects of necrosis or later dementia are anything but easy. Unfortunately, Radiosurgery has been used for some tumors that really require different approaches, like lymphomas (see Chapter 20: Early & Later Side Effects of Treatment or the Brain Tumor).

◻ **Bottom Line** I do not suggest that you blankly avoid all or one type of radiation therapy, because of the potential for longer-term side effects.

Be cautious of associations dedicated to providing information about Radiosurgery and its relative merits.[18] For example, the International Radiosurgery Support Association has the following advice under "Brain Tumors-Biopsies" on their web site information page www.irsa.org:

> *Surgical biopsies of brain tumors are no longer considered absolutely necessary because of the development of new imaging techniques. Current scanning ability with contrast dyes, CT and MRI scans, enables the diagnosis of a brain tumor as malignant or benign, without opening the skull for a biopsy. There has always been controversy over whether the act of obtaining a biopsy may allow the spread of cancerous cells to other brain areas.[18]*

These statements could inspire controversy, and outright denial, among many oncologists. Yet the public, for whom this is intended, would likely accept this as fact. The question one has to ask is, "How unbiased is this information?" All the medical advisors listed on the International Radiosurgery Support Association web site appear to run Radiosurgery centers. Contrast the above web site information with that from the Brain Tumor Foundation (a group at NYU, that has a Team approach) that I believe is more straightforward and informative about the actual risks (go to http://www.braintumorfoundation.org/tumors/gamma.htm).

Unfortunately, it has become profitable to set up high-tech, outpatient radiation therapy units (e.g., X-Knife, or GammaKnife Radiosurgery Centers) that advertise phenomenal results, and carefree treatment in less than an hour without bother to the patient. Beware of anything that sounds too good to be true! (See also Chapter 5: The Team, for questions to ask.[1])

Let me provide examples, from my practice, of how well-intentioned patients can do themselves a disservice by blindly following Internet advertisements and recommendations:

> Hernando is a 45-year-old CEO of a telecommunications company who came to see me in Winter 1998 with an unbiopsied brain tumor. He was scheduled to receive Radiosurgery from a local GammaKnife Center the next day. Due to the confusing MRI scan appearance of the tumor, we recommended an open biopsy before any treatment decision. As we suspected, he had a lymphoma, not a primary brain tumor. He should have chemotherapy and immunotherapy first, since radiation sensitizes the brain to future damage from one very effective chemotherapy drug called methotrexate. Hernando subsequently received chemotherapy and then became one of

the first patients to receive a lymphoma-specific antibody therapy for a brain lymphoma. He also received conventional radiation, but only after the other therapies had been completed. Hernando is still working and remains tumor-free five and a half years later.

"Simple," "fast," and "painless" outpatient Radiosurgery would have been the *wrong* treatment for Hernando and would have precluded more effective treatment options. Although GammaKnife therapy would have made the "tumor" disappear, the lymphoma would have returned elsewhere. If he later received the appropriate chemotherapy, he could have suffered intolerable brain damage because of previous exposure to radiation.

Here is another example of why one must guard against quick and easy solutions for unbiopsied "tumors":

My husband is in week seven, post GammaKnife, and he has really gone downhill fast. He only has stamina for going to the table to eat and to the bathroom for a quick shower. We are returning to the doctor to see if we can decrease the Decadron, the necessary evil for now.

Our diagnosis was a BB-size lesion on the brain stem. It was "inoperable," so we can't have a biopsy done. We are hoping for some answers from the doctor tomorrow. I have a feeling that people like you are going to be our best source.

Lucille M., San Diego, CA

The brainstem cannot tolerate high intensity dose treatment; and this may not even have been cancer. This highlights the importance of having a biopsy-proven diagnosis from an experienced, unbiased *team*. One potential problem in dealing with commercial Radiosurgery centers is that they are not a "team" (my definition, Chapter 5).[1]

Radiation and chemotherapy represent a balancing act between increased life span versus brain damage that can affect one's quality of life, performance of daily activities, and the general "essence" of the person.

The bottom line before receiving radiation or any therapy:
- Be informed.
- Ask questions.
- Do your own research.

- Obtain second opinions
- Ask more questions.
- Do not be afraid!

CHEMOTHERAPY

Detailed information about individual drugs and their side effects can be found in Chapter 19: Cancer-fighting drugs: Chemotherapy, Antibiotics, Marrow Stimulants and Their Side Effects.

Most often, the choice and administration of chemotherapy is in the hands of your oncologist. An exception is the neurosurgeon who implants Gliadel wafers (see below) or places a reservoir for chemotherapy into the brain or spinal fluid.

The belief that chemotherapy can be effective in the treatment of brain tumors is a relatively recent one, beginning in the late 1960s. Drugs found useful for other cancers were evaluated much later in patients with brain tumors. The concept, that only drugs that cross the intact "blood-brain barrier" would be effective, contributed to doubts about their effectiveness since they cannot reach the tumor. It was later shown that the tumor blood vessels are leaky and allow the drugs into the tumor. Finally, in 1980 Dr. Michael Walker reported that BCNU plus radiation improved survival compared with radiation alone for adults with *glioblastoma multiforme* (grade 4 astrocytoma).[19] That survival difference was a modest but real *average* of eight to 10 weeks of life extension.

> The "blood-brain-barrier" is not the major problem. It has been lack of effective chemotherapy.

The Food and Drug Administration (FDA) approved intravenous Carmustine (BCNU) (and its oral counterpart, CCNU, called Lomustine) in 1979 for treatment of brain tumors. These remained the only approved drugs until 1998, when a new oral (pill form) drug called temozolomide (Temodar in the USA; Temodal elsewhere) was developed and approved for recurrent grade 3 astrocytomas, including oligodendrogliomas.[20] The FDA did not approve its use for *glioblastoma multiforme* and required additional studies until 2005. Temodar is close to being an ideal agent. There are now clinical trials testing Temodar with other drugs, such as Vitamin A (Accutane), thalidomide and others for a wide variety of tumors, including childhood cancers, melanoma, and brain metastases (See Table 17-8).

Table 17-8 Major Chemotherapy Approaches & Treatment Options

Chemotherapy (FDA-approved or useful)

1. Temodar
2. BCNU / CCNU
3. P-C-V (procarbazine, lomustine, vincristine)
4. Gliadel
5. Decadron
6. Intrathecal therapies

Chemotherapy in active trials (Chapters 19, 21)

1. CPT-11
2. Tamoxifen
3. Accutane
4. Thalidomide
5. Gleevec

WHAT ARE THE DIFFERENT TYPES OF CHEMOTHERAPY?

Systemic Chemotherapy

This is the most common form, whether by pill or injection. It is absorbed and travels by the blood (system) to the tumor. Temodar and BCNU/CCNU remain the only FDA-approved medications for brain tumors. Other drugs have been used to treat brain tumors, because the FDA approved their use for other cancers. This is called "off label" use and is permitted by the FDA, but sometimes refused by insurance companies One effective combination is called "P-C-V" (procarbazine, CCNU, and vincristine) which originally contributed to the cure of Hodgkin's disease. This PCV combination provides a significant survival advantage for patients with anaplastic astrocytomas (grade 3)[21,22,23] and oligodendrogliomas[24,25,26] but not for those with *glioblastoma multiforme*. Commonly-used, but not FDA-approved chemotherapies are also discussed in Chapter 19: Cancer-fighting drugs: Chemotherapy, Antibiotics, Marrow Stimulants and Their Side Effects.

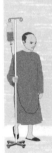

Regional or Local Chemotherapy

One example is the Gliadel wafer, placed inside or around the tumor. Gliadel is a BCNU-impregnated biodegradable wafer, up to eight of which are placed in the tumor cavity at the time of surgical removal of newly diagnosed and recurrent malignant gliomas. The BCNU leeches out of the wafer into the tumor area over a period of 2 to 14 days, and the wafers are later absorbed.

Gliadel wafers avoid systemic toxicities of low blood counts and lung or liver damage found with intravenous BCNU or CCNU. The major disadvantage of Gliadel wafers is that it is a one-time therapy. In addition, delayed healing, spinal fluid leaks, post-operative brain swelling, and infections can occur. In spite of these side effects, a major clinical trial demonstrated an average survival increase of eight weeks compared with patients who did not receive it.[27] Unfortunately, government and private health insurance companies have not been reimbursing physicians or hospitals for this medication.

Intrathecal Chemotherapy

This is a form of regional therapy that is injected through the spine via a thin needle or into a small reservoir under the scalp that is connected to the ventricles (fluid cavities in the brain) with a thin tube. It is used to treat "leptomeningeal spread," also called "neoplastic meningitis." This thin layer spread occurs when cells from brain tumors or metastases travel by the cerebrospinal fluid and grow throughout the nervous system. Drugs that can be safely given by the intrathecal approach include: methotrexate (Trexall), thiotepa (Thioplex), cytosine arabinoside (Ara-C, Cytosar-U) and Depocyte. The latter is a long acting form of Ara-C that received FDA approval for the treatment of leukemia and lymphoma of the nervous system (see Fig 17-3 showing pathways of the ventricular system).

UNANSWERED QUESTIONS ABOUT TREATMENT

How Long Can You Take Chemotherapy?

There is no consensus among doctors for how long a patient should be on Temodar, for example. Patty's observations as a patient (below) ring true as doctors are finding out how to best use this new drug.

George on the Jersey shore was also told 12 months and no more. The doctor finally gave in so he could do 3 more for a total of 15 cycles. Another woman from New Jersey has completed 36 rounds. Bob was told he "had to stop" the Temodar since it was 24 months and he could risk getting leukemia and it couldn't go past this. Another woman from Alabama has a daughter who was told that she had to stop Temodar after 24 months, as you are "not allowed" to remain on it any longer. They were not even given other options. Her tumor came back at her 6th month MRI. She is now so furious.

It is sad that a one-minute decision by a doctor could change somebody's entire life. This is where the second, third and even fourth opinions are definitely necessary. They need to realize that the 24-month Temodar thing is not etched in stone. Nor is any other treatment for that matter.

Patty, an oligo survivor. Woodbridge, NJ

Should You Take Procarbazine, CCNU and Vincristine (PCV) or Temodar?

A question raised by a "successfully" treated patient brings up issues of informed consent and knowledge of pros and cons of different therapies. Here, current practice is ahead of the results from clinical trials. Temodar is being used extensively because of its low side effect profile and oral use. The historic gold standard is still PCV therapy for anaplastic astrocytoma and oligodendrogliomas.

I was diagnosed in 1992 after suffering a Grand Mal seizure. An 8 cm. lesion was resected from my right temporal lobe, a mixed glioma Grade-II (mostly oligo). This was followed up with six weeks of fractionated radiation (5760 rads). The tumor site remained inactive until 1998 with a recurrence in adjacent tissue showed up in a contrast-enhancing MRI. A second surgery successfully removed all visible enhancing areas and I have almost no neurological deficit (upper left visual quadrant). Recurrence appeared the following year and I began Temodar and completed 30 cycles with exceptional results. All visible tumor disappeared. However, within the last four months a recurrence has grown to 1 cm. Next week, I will undergo a GammaKnife treatment, but I have ambivalence about starting the recommended PCV treatment.

I know that it has been proven that PCV is probably the most effective treatment. It is also widely accepted that no chemotherapy will "cure" the condition. Thus, if PCV is truly a one-time shot (i.e. Silver Bullet), then should I save this treatment for the time when the tumor becomes inoperable or changes its histology? Should I use Temodar or a watch and wait approach regarding the PCV?

George, Los Angeles, CA

Comment: This is complex. This reader does not realize that PCV has cured many people with this tumor. Yes, it is not perfect. But with two recurrences without any data to say intensive treatment should be saved, I would throw everything at the tumor. Rely on new drugs… if it should return.

Table 17-9 Experimental Options for Treatment

1. Newer approaches (see Chapter 21)
2. Vaccine therapies
3. Gene therapies
4. Receptor based therapy
   Anti-receptor antibodies(VEGF, EGFR)
   Transferrin-Diphtheria Toxin (TransMid)
   IL13 (interleukin-13) & PE38QQR (bacteria toxin) (NeoPharm)
5. Signal transduction inhibitors
6. Anti-angiogenesis agents
7. Viral therapies

You Do Not Like the Choices that Are Given to You?

There are at least seven things a person can do to expand his/her options:

1. See Chapter 5 and review the questions to ask your Team.[1]
   - What questions do I ask each specialist?
   - Which physician is responsible for what part of my care?
2. See Chapter 6 for Getting to an Expert for a second opinion.[1]
   - Get organized to go for a second opinion.
   - Find out more about newer therapies from an expert. (See Table 17-9).
3. See Chapter 7: The Referral Hospital[1]
   - They may have different conventional and experimental options.
4. See Chapter 4: Searching the Web/Internet and Other Resources
   - The tumor has recurred? And there are no "standard" therapies left for me?
   - Find out how to surf the Internet to find major brain tumor centers that offer newer, more experimental approaches.[1]
5. See Chapter 21: Clinical Trials
   - This will provide totally new and different approaches for you to consider.
   - An example of possible benefit from a clinical trial: Patients with recurrent grade 4 astrocytoma (*glioblastoma multiforme*) found leading centers in Europe and participated on a Phase 2 trial of Temozolomide and radiation. They had better survival than historical controls.[28] (See also Table 17-9.)

> Part of fighting a brain tumor is the realization that you DO have choices.

6. See Chapters 10 to 15 and read more about your specific tumor.[1]
7. See Chapter 18: Complementary and Alternative Medicine (CAM) for Brain Tumors. Review this information about treatments, if this is of interest to you.

Table 17-10 Internet Resources for Treatment

Subject	Web Site or Information Source
Brain Mapping Function Loss	http://www.radiology.wisc.edu/Med_Students/neuroradiology/fmri http://seizure.health.ufl.edu/clinical/mapping.htm.
Brain Mapping-Word/speech recognition	http://www.radiologyinfo.com/content/functional_mr.htm http://en2.wikipedia.org/wiki/Magnetic_resonance_imaging (MRI) http://www.radiologyinfo.com/content/functional_mr.htm (Functional MRI)
Cancer Information Service	Toll-free call 1-800-4-CANCER (1-800-422-6237) ; Monday through Friday 9:00 a.m. to 4:30 p.m. Deaf, hard-of-hearing callers with TTY equipment, 1-800-332-8615. A trained Cancer Information Specialist can answer your questions. The National Cancer Institute (NCI) has booklets and other materials. They can be ordered by telephone from the Cancer Information Service at 1-800-4-CANCER (1-800-422-6237), TTY at 1-800-332-8615.
The NCI's LiveHelp	http://cancer.gov/livehelp/vp/vp_sq.html service, a program available on several of the Institute's Web sites. Service available from 9:00 a.m. - 5:00 p.m. Eastern time, Mo - Fri. Information Specialists help Internet users find information on NCI Web sites and answer questions about cancer.
Chemotherapy-BCNU	http://www.virtualtrials.com/bcnu2.cfm.
Chemotherapy-Temodar	http://www.virtualtrials.com/temodar
General Sites	www.virtualtrials.com http://www.cancer.gov/templates/doc_wyntk.aspx?viewid=b5500bd0-3da6-496a-8080-3052a630ba57
Hydrocephalus	http://www.nhfonline.org/page7.html http://www.patientcenters.com/hydrocephalus/news/differences.html http://www.nyneurosurgery.org/hydro_shunt.htm http://www.hydroassoc.org
Image Guided Surgery	http://www.virtualtrials.com/Schulder.cfm

Radiation -Cyberknife	http://www.cksociety.org/
Radiation -GliaSite	http://www.docguide.com/dg.nsf/PrintPrint/FC3432F083893ED985256D7B004E2E65 http://www.proximatherapeutics.com/index_glia.asp
Radiation- Proton	http://www.llu.edu/proton/ http://neurosurgery.mgh.harvard.edu/ProtonBeam/Default.htm
Radiation Therapy	http://my.webmd.com/content/article/4/1680_50263?src=Inktomi&condition=Health_Topics_A-Z
Radiosurgery	http://www.irsa.org/radiation_injury.html http://www.braintumorfoundation.org/tumors/gamma.htm
Surgery	http://www.braintumorfoundation.org/neurosurgery/ss3_1.htm http://www.yoursurgery.com/ProcedureDetails.cfm?BR=4&Proc=19 (Skull anatomy)
Surgery-awake	http://www.unsaonline.com/understanding/awakecraniotomy.html
Surgery-shunts Hydrocephalus	http://www.yoursurgery.com/proceduredetails.cfm?br=4&proc=44

CHAPTER 18

Complementary and Alternative Medicine (CAM) for Brain Tumors

I've never thought of myself as a cancer victim. I live on a journey with cancer. Death comes to all of us, but until that time, I intend to focus on the quality of life, not the end of it. Some of my doctors told me that I was living with false hope. I said, "Well that's fine, let me hang on to it."

In October 2004, Cheryl will reach her seven-year benchmark since her diagnosis. When asked from where her wellspring of hope stems, she replies, It's a choice. I've been depressed…it's the pits. Fear and doubt create misery, and so can negativity. Since my diagnosis, I live with more hope and faith than ever.

Cheryl. Glioblastoma survivor.

- Echinacea
- Natural immune stimulants
- Yunnan Paiyao; blood platelet stimulants

Other Popular alternative therapies
- Antineoplaston therapy
- Cancell/ Entelev/ Protocel
- Coral calcium

ALTERNATIVE MEDICAL SYSTEMS
Acupuncture and traditional Chinese medicine
Ayurvedic medicine

MANIPULATIVE AND BODY-BASED THERAPIES
Yoga
Massage
Therapeutic touch
Reiki

MIND-BODY THERAPIES
Meditation
Prayer and spiritual healing
Hypnotherapy
Education therapy
Support groups
Psychotherapy
Relaxation training
Aromatherapy
Music therapy

Key search words

- CAM
- holistic
- oriental medicine
- Burzynski
- copper
- nutrition
- acupuncture
- meditation

- complementary
- ayurvedic
- herb
- mushroom extract
- chelation
- aromatherapy
- yoga
- mind body

- alternative
- TCM
- melatonin
- protocel
- laetrile
- massage
- psychotherapy

CAM is a general term for many types of therapy that are not part of the history and style of disease-based, Western medicine as practiced in North America for most of the last century. The major divisions of CAM, as expressed by the National Center for CAM (NCCAM), are illustrated in Table 18-1[1]; there is often overlap among them. People with brain tumors often turn to these therapies when either *conventional* medication is no longer working or side effects have become unacceptable. Many of my patients who have had severe side effects from drugs have said, "There must be a better way to help me!" Yes, I agree.

FREQUENTLY ASKED QUESTIONS

WHAT IS COMPLEMENTARY AND ALTERNATIVE MEDICINE (CAM)?

More than sixty percent of people with brain tumors and other cancers use non-traditional medications and approaches to help them feel better or fight their cancer.[2] Many credit CAM with saving their lives. However, there is a dark side. Although they are *natural* or *organic*, some CAM medications can be harmful. Knowing what they do and how they work will help you decide if a specific CAM is for you.

There is scant scientific evidence that CAM can *cure* brain tumors. However, it can definitely improve quality of life, reduce side effects, and possibly improve treatment efficacy. The effects of CAM are often subtle, however, and they may take weeks to show. Thus, waiting until symptoms are intolerable or advanced may not be the best approach. I have chosen to highlight selected therapies that are regularly discussed on the Internet and in support groups. Some Internet discussions are filled with misinformation; I will attempt to clarify this with facts.

Complementary and alternative care in the United States and elsewhere else is huge. Forty percent of Americans used CAM in 1997. They made more visits to providers of *unconventional* therapy than to their primary care physicians (629 million vs. 386 million visits).[3] Its power can be estimated by its effect on our economy. Estimated expenditures in 1997 amounted to approximately $21.2 billion, two thirds of which ($12.2 billion) was paid out of pocket. These figures compare with $9.1 billion spent out of pocket annually for all hospitalizations in the United States and $29.3 billion spent annually on all US physician visits in the country.

> Complementary treatments intend to make you feel better and lessen uncomfortable symptoms.

What Is the Difference Between Complementary and Alternative Therapy?

Complementary treatments intend to make you feel better and lessen uncomfortable symptoms like nausea (lemon or ginger, acupuncture); pain (capsaicin pepper extract or sugar); diarrhea (spearmint tea or rice water); or headaches (acupuncture). Some CAM therapies claim to boost the immune system, treat high blood pressure, or fight cancer. They are used along with more traditional therapies like surgery, radiation, or chemotherapy. People often take these treatments with or without their physician's knowledge.

Alternative therapy used to mean cancer treatment, *instead* of conventional therapy. Such treatments include herbs like the maitake mushroom or boswellia; trace metals like selenium or chelated copper; raw or purified extracts from plants (laetrile-krebiozen), fish (shark cartilage), or urine (antineoplastons). Many people actually use these alternative treatments along *with* conventional therapies. Perhaps antineoplastons (see below) might qualify as a major *alternative* therapy for brain tumors.

> Alternative therapies used to mean treatment in place of conventional therapies.

Table 18-1 Major Areas of CAM Therapy

Domain	Therapies and applications		Functions
Alternative Medical Systems	1. Homeopathic medicine (HM)	Minute doses of plant extracts, minerals, nutrition (1)	Stimulates the body's defense mechanisms against cancer
	2. Naturopathic medicine (NM)	Counseling (1) Pharmacology (2) Hydrotherapy, physical therapies (2)	
	3. Ayurvedic medicine (AM)	Herbal medicine (2,3,4) Massage (3,4)	Helps chronic pain, nausea, appetite
	4. Traditional Chinese medicine-(TCM)	Acupuncture (4) Movement (3,4)	

Biologically-Based Therapies	Same as above plus Herbs Nutritional supplements Special diets Natural compounds	Herbal remedies, plant preparations, (1) Vitamins, dietary supplements [shark cartilage, mushroom extract] (2) Macrobiotics (3) antineoplastons (4)	Alleviate symptoms or control cancer
Manipulative & Body-Based Methods	Chiropractic Osteopathic manipulations Massage Physical therapy Yoga	Touch, pressure (1,2,3,4) Movement (4,5)	Symptom relief
Energy Therapies	Reiki Therapeutic Touch Electrical devices	Manipulate energy biofields within/ around body without direct contact (1,2) Bio-electromagnetic therapies [electromagnetic fields of pulsed, alternating or direct current] (3).	Symptom relief
Mind-Body Interventions	Art therapies Biofeedback Hypnotherapy Meditation Psychotherapy Spiritual counseling Others practiced by healers	Enhance the mind's capacity to affect bodily function and symptoms	Symptom relief, coping

(n) number refers to therapy types 1-4.

WHAT IS THE DIFFERENCE BETWEEN CAM FOR CANCER PREVENTION VS. CANCER THERAPY?

There is often confusion between the uses of herbs, special diets, or *hands-on* approaches for treatment, as opposed to prevention. Symptom management, cancer prevention, and cancer treatment are often confused as a combined, single concept. However, just because something *causes* cancer does not mean that its removal or a process will necessarily *cure* it. For example, cancer is highly related to lifestyle choices and can take years to develop. Once smoking damages cell function to the point of causing lung cancer, it is not nearly as easy to stop the tumor, in contrast to having prevented the problem by not smoking in the first place. There is evidence that people who eat macrobiotic diets (increased dietary intake of soybean and avoidance of meat and certain vegetables) have a *decreased* chance of getting *some* cancers. That is different from saying that macrobiotic diets can *cure* cancer, once it is present. For the rare five percent of all brain tumors that are *genetic* (see Chapter 24: Heredity and Other Causes of Brain Tumors), there are no known CAM therapies that prevent their development.

Unfortunately, few studies of alternative therapies have shown effective shrinking of tumors. This is not to say they do not promote general health. Indeed, there is strong evidence that complementary treatments *relieve* symptoms. They just have not been well investigated for their curative effects. Thus, anyone wishing to use these as treatments is an individual experiment, choosing to take the word of others. I will provide examples of purported cures for cancer that do not have scientific evidence to support them and point out treatments for which there are studies to support their use.

> Complementary approaches: can make you feel better and improve quality of life.

One web site, http://www.hopeforcancer.com/protocol.html, offers the following:

> *"cancer killing products" that provide maximum RESULTS in combination… and [are] based on the combined experience of many folks sharing these products, producing 'phenomenal results'. Their promise: This IS what we have done successfully for our families and loved ones and hundreds of others just like you!*

> Few studies of alternative therapies demonstrate shrinking of brain tumors.

The following is their "three-pronged assault on cancer":

1. Kill cancer. Kill cancer cells via apoptosis, or natural cell death. Ellagic acid literally reactivates cancer cells' self-destruct mechanism causing them to die — gently & safely.
   Ellagic Insurance Formula (List price $79.00)
   http://www.hopeforcancer.com/ellagic.html
2. Make your body an anti-cancer environment. Surround your cells with a calcium bath and raise the body pH above 7.3. Cancer cannot grow and survive in that environment. Coral Calcium Daily (List price $24.95)

▸ **Bottom Line** People who eat macrobiotic diets have a decreased risk of getting some cancers. That differs from macrobiotic diet's ability to cure cancer once it is present.

3. Strengthen your body. Provide essential nutrition to feed and nourish the body during this cancer "war." Receive optimum nutrition from your food with the help of potent enzymes and fulfill all your body's vitamin / mineral requirements with the full-spectrum vitamin / mineral supplement.

I do not mean to deny hope to anyone, but the web site listed above is just one of hundreds that provides misleading and unverified information. Their 33 downloadable pages contain *nothing* about patient cancer treatment; all is prevention. Yet their web site says:

> *Pure, natural form of Ellagic Acid with Graviola. The most potent source of Ellagic on the market! Allows cancer cells to self-destruct like normal cells and then be removed by the body. Helps, literally eliminates cancer from the system. Clinically impacts many forms of cancer.*

In Chapter 4: Searching the Web,[4] I provide some guidelines for evaluating sites like these.

How Might CAM Benefit a Person with a Brain Tumor?

You may have discomfort and pain that is directly or indirectly related to the tumor or treatment for it, such as muscle wasting from steroids; injuries; strains; muscle spasms; steroid-induced pain in muscles, tendons, or bone; headache; difficulty sleeping; or nausea. The good news is that there are complementary approaches that can make you feel better and improve your quality of life. These include acupuncture; a massage from a trained massage therapist; herbs that have

Tell your doctors about all supplements and medications & other treatments you take.

a relaxing effect on the body without causing severe side effects; and herbs that reduce inflammation. For example, nausea during or after chemotherapy might be alleviated with raw ginger, ginger extract, or acupuncture. Many traditional doctors may not know about these remedies, but they can refer you to a CAM expert. Your local brain tumor or cancer society also can suggest CAM consultants.

Beware. Seemingly healthy, *organic* drugs can harm you. A recent study combining high-dose beta-carotene, the form of vitamin A present in

Organic means it is not a mineral, like iron or zinc.

carrots, with chemotherapy for lung cancer was associated with *earlier* recurrence of the cancer! The study was stopped.[5] This is another reason to tell your doctors about all the *supplements* and *medications* you are taking and any other treatments that you are undergoing (see Chapter 3: Getting Organized).

Will adopting a more "healthy" lifestyle with exercise or diet cure a brain tumor? Probably not by itself, but it will help unburden your body, facilitate your recovery, fortify your body's healing ability, and enhance your quality of life. It probably wouldn't hurt for you to lose a few pounds if you are overweight, but do not go crazy trying to do it.

WHY IS THERE SO MUCH DISCUSSION ABOUT CAM IN THE MEDIA?

Discussions about CAM that now take place regularly among people with brain tumors and other illnesses never took place 20 years ago. Why? A few reasons follow:

- Patients want to become more knowledgeable about how CAM might be helpful to them.
- Patient-driven organizations (ABTA, NBTF, BTS) provide seminars and meetings to teach about these treatments (see Chapter 3: Table 3-1).
- Books, magazines, and the Internet disseminate CAM information.
- Most physicians know little about CAM-based therapies and how they work. Patients have taken a more active role.
- The private sector sees CAM as a money-making enterprise and has created a billion-dollar industry through savvy marketing campaigns.
- The United States Government established the National Center for Complementary and Alternative Medicine (NCCAM), which is devoted to testing natural compounds, funding research, and providing helpful information (see Table 18-6).

WHY DOESN'T YOUR REGULAR DOCTOR OFFER CAM TO YOU?

The answer requires a little history. Western medicine since 1900 has advanced the public's health in large part due to the conquest of infectious diseases, which used to kill or maim (examples: yellow fever, typhus, tuberculosis, polio, smallpox, syphilis, "strep" throat). Medicine's success was propelled by changes in public health preventive measures: adequate food and shelter, clean water and sewage treatment, as well as antibiotics and immunizations. The current medical model still focuses on the treatment of life-threatening disease after diagnosis. Patients, and

□ **Bottom Line** ➤ Natural means it occurs in nature, not necessarily pure or effective.

later insurance companies, paid for these services, based on physician expertise and sophisticated equipment, regardless of whether the disease was an ulcer, kidney failure or pneumonia.

While cancers are similarly diagnosed and treated, the therapy is not as curative as antibiotics have been for infections. This has led patients to desire two distinctly different types of attention from their physicians: Advice and treatment directed toward prevention of fatal illnesses; and alleviation of suffering, when the disease cannot be reversed.

Table 18-2 Reasons Why CAM Is Not Offered By Physicians
1. Herbs, techniques of CAM are outside the realm of expertise of most physicians.
2. Less training and fewer rewards for attending to issues of comfort.
3. Doctors see their role as "disease-fixers." If they cannot fix the problem and get reimbursed, then the health care system promotes moving on to the next patient.
4. Requests for a different tradition (CAM) appear as a rejection of the physician's efforts.
5. Positive financial reward is given for prescribing procedures: x-ray, operation, injection, documented special exams.
6. Little compensation is given for time spent discussing illness prevention, lifestyle, or foods contributing to long-term health; staying through a crisis; and listening to discomforts facing a dying patient.
7. Detailed documentation of advice is required for billing; reimbursement levels are low.

The satisfaction of these needs could not have come at a worse time in the social and economic development of American medicine. Doctors have been moved from the top to a much lower level in the food chain of value and financial reward. Your questions about yoga, herbs, diets, and Ayurvedic (Eastern) medicine (described later in this chapter) are dismissed or not supported. So if a physician suggests acupuncture or yoga, he or she cannot directly bill for that suggestion. There is no incentive for a doctor to think about CAM—despite his best efforts or intentions. You, the patient, may find yourself "jumping ship" and going to the other side... and no one is satisfied (see Table 18-2).

> The American medical model focuses on treatment of life-threatening disease after diagnosis, rather than prevention.

If Western medicine had answers (read: cure), there would not be a problem. We physicians continue our successful habit with the older model of cure (antibiotics for pneumonia or bypass surgery for blocked arteries) or quarantine (as in SARS, TB or Mad Cow disease), while we await solid proof of the effectiveness of alternative remedies. Meanwhile, the public hears almost daily news flashes of a new wonder drug or "stem cells" that may lead to the cure of brain or breast cancer.

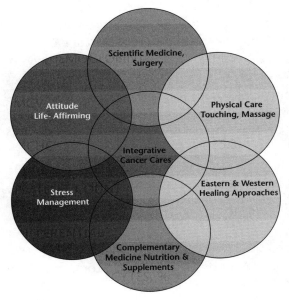

Figure 18-1 Ideal Integrative Cancer Care Model

Furthermore, physicians have left a "caring" gap in the process. Many patients find the care they seek in CAM practitioners, who typically acknowledge both the physical and emotional well-being. Those who are dying of cancer and suffering without relief are particularly inclined toward receiving care from someone who promises a steadying hand and a cure for their ills. Enter knowledgeable CAM practitioners who may have something valuable to offer. Unfortunately, enter, too, those who exploit patients with their promise of cure or even have you pay for information that is actually available free on many Internet sites.

(http://www.holisticcancersolutions.com/braintumorsarticle.htm).

Some physicians have attempted to bridge the knowledge gap with an "Integrative Cancer Care Model."[6] This approach is what most people would want, if given the choice (Figure 18-1). However, with increasing specialization, it is doubtful that one provider, HMO, or center will provide all of these, or that insurance will cover their charges. You can use this checklist as a model for the care that you are seeking. (See also table 18-3.)

> Many alternative practitioners exploit patients with promise of cure or have you pay for information available free on the Internet.

What Training Do CAM Practitioners Have?

Only a select few CAM practitioners have completed training that leads to becoming a medical doctor (an M.D. degree). Most CAM practitioners are trained in Traditional Chinese or oriental medicine (TCM) and are Board certified in most states. Others who have training in specialties, such as psychology or massage, may

| CAM practitioners come with varied backgrounds and different training. |

or may not be licensed. Still, others are experts in folk medicine, for which formal training is not available in the United States. The Curandero of the Latin-American community or Conjur women in African-American communities, for example, may be respected, knowledgeable community members who advise and treat conditions as varied as stress management, childbirth, abdominal pain, and diarrhea.[7] Strangely enough, the financial reward can be better for the CAM practitioner than for physicians treating a *conventional* diagnosis, because insurance plans rarely reimburse for this therapy.

What Are the Major CAM Approaches For Cancer Treatment and Symptom Reduction?

I address traditional, Western medical treatment of pain and nausea in Chapters 9 and 19. In this section, I show how pain and other bothersome symptoms might be effectively treated using a combination of Western and complementary therapies (see Table 18-3). Remember, people are individuals, and what is effective for others may not work well for you. Keep in mind also that there may be clinical trials offering CAM therapies for which you may be eligible to enroll (see Table 18-6).

Table 18-3 Integrative Approaches to Symptom Relief

Symptom	CAM	Western Medical

Pain:
• Neuropathic
  –sensitivity to touch,
  burning, pins-needles
• Muscle-tenderness
• Central
	Acupuncture, moxibustion,
	  capsaicin cream [8]
	Heat, massage
	Hypnosis
		Elavil, Ibuprofen (Advil)
		Opioid (codeine, morphine),
		Physical Therapy

Fatigue	Bach Flower Remedy - Olive "Green Drinks," Chinese herbs, Rest	Ritalin Provigil, Prozac-SSRIs
Nausea	Acupuncture Hypnosis, distraction Ginger root/ tea/ lemon, Iberogast	Kytril Zofran Compazine Marinol [9]
Swelling	Boswellia, Bromelain	dexamethasone
Appetite	Iberogast, "Sweetish Bitters"	Megace
Depression	Bach Flower Remedy - Gorse Rhodiola - Arctic Root Avoid St. John's Wort (see Interactions-below)	Prozac, Zoloft, SSRIs
Poor Nutrition	Diet Appetite stimulant Culturally sensitive foods	Megace Commercial supplements (Ensure)

A Word about Nutrition

What we eat plays an important role in our health. Scientists know more about how diet can cause or prevent cancer than how nutrition can cure it. Earlier, I cited the example of how a macrobiotic diet is linked to *reduced* breast and colon cancer risk,[10] yet it will not necessarily fight or cure a brain tumor (see Table 18-6).

However, it is encouraging that one nutritionist has submitted evidence to the National Center for Complementary & Alternative Medicine (NCCAM) regarding the effectiveness of a nutritional approach in 101 cases of *glioblastoma multiforme*. A preliminary review suggested a possible survival benefit from a particular nutritional program. The submission is under further review.[11]

The Histidine- and Methionine-Free Diet

About 25 years ago, grade 3-4 astrocytomas were treated with dietary restriction of a single amino acid (most often histidine) that the tumor used for its metabolism. This diet restriction protocol proved to be more effective on its own, than when coupled with BCNU chemotherapy.[12] No further studies have been reported.

CAN DIETARY SUPPLEMENTS MEAN THE DIFFERENCE BETWEEN LIFE AND DEATH?

There is confusing and conflicting information about supplements. Do they help tumor cells grow... or do they kill them? An e-mail below summarizes one caregiver's dilemma:

> *I started and stopped Mack on CoQ$_{10}$ several times. I will read something very good and start him on it, and then read something not so good and stop... back and forth. The bad part is a theory that it may interfere with... chemotherapy by protecting the cells. This confuses me especially when I read that many drugs and supplements "inhibit cancer cells while not interfering with... healthy cells." I do not have a CAM doctor and am trying to find one. I do not have the money to consult with a well-known nutritionist for patients with brain tumors.*

> Martha L. Chicago, IL

| There are excellent web sites to check out info about herbs and other supplements. |

Unfortunately, there are many scam artists in this $17 billion a year industry that capitalizes on the vulnerability of cancer patients who are desperate to seek treatment and relief. Read the passage below that appeared on a brain tumor e-mail list:

> *We have investigated a treatment called MYGA III that stops any cancerous growth and often reduces the tumor size by 30 percent within 24 hours! This therapy, very recently developed by a U.S. scientist, is... well documented, and it is being used in a number of clinics and hospitals in foreign countries. We were given information on a device that targets internal tumors with complete success (Pulse Modulated Microwave), and several oral medications that control prostate cancer. McGill University scientists have developed an over-the-counter oral medication that*

| If a promotional statement sounds too good to be true, it probably is! |

▯**Bottom Line** Presentation or advertisement of alternative therapies on web sites does not mean endorsement or even that that are effective.

is patented in Australia, U.S.A., and Canada as an anti-cancer medication. Despite the huge number of impressive and successful in vitro and in vivo studies carried out with the product, only a handful of doctors in North America ever heard of it. These are but a few examples of the many alternative cancer therapies you will find in our reports. See http://www.holisticcancersolutions.com/CancerTextPage.htm for more information.

The problem? At least two desperate people with cancer died from receiving contaminated MYGA III, so the FDA ordered the product removed from the United States' market. (http://seattlepi.nwsource.com/local/22927_cancer14.shtml).

The supplement industry is loosely regulated, so products can be marketed without proof of safety and efficacy that is required of substances classified as official drugs by the FDA. As long as manufacturers do not claim that their products should treat or cure disease, they are not *drugs* as defined by the FDA. The government cannot take a supplement off the market, unless there is proof that consumers have been harmed. For more information on frauds, see Table 18-6.

WHAT DO HERBS AND OTHER SUPPLEMENTS COST?

The e-mail excerpt below gives an example of the challenge that patients and families face regarding herbs and other forms of dietary supplements:

Twenty year-old Michael has been looking into alternative treatments for his low-grade astrocytoma. He takes Chinese herbs ($110 for 14 days) prescribed by Dr. Zoltan Xhu from the Chinese medical practice in Sydney and made up in Canberra by a Chinese herbalist. There are 10 ingredients, including scorpion and fungi which he boils for 45 minutes in a clay pot and then drinks the fluid. He alternates these herbs with some natural herbal tinctures ($62 a month) prescribed by the Robina naturopath, Dr. Tony Kovaks, and made up in Canberra from Griffith shops. I am sure both treatments are helping his general health and attitude.

Someone has now told him about food supplements to cure or aid other conventional treatments that would be $1,015 per month. The food supplements are from a U.S. company, Mannatech, and are distributed by network marketing. They have a range of products including ones supposed to be good for cancer and… other illnesses. They include "Ambrotose," Catalyst, Phytaloe, and Sport. Michael was initially excited by the science behind the *products. But a rather high pressure sales person, the high cost, and other info made him rather suspicious despite the testimonials on various sites.*

Anonymous, Austin, TX

Costs can range from a few dollars to thousands per month. It is also good to know that some herbalists and nutritional consultants have financial aid programs and will take low-income clients at reduced cost.[13]

WHAT SHOULD A PATIENT DO WITH CONFLICTING OR NO INFORMATION ABOUT HERBS AND OTHER SUPPLEMENTS?

Follow these eight guidelines:
1. Ask your CAM doctor for evidence of effectiveness for your symptom or type of tumor.
2. Ask about potential interference with any medications that you are taking.
3. Seek information from Office of Cancer Complementary and Alternative Medicine. This is a web site for the National Cancer Institute, which has good information on dietary supplements and drug interactions: http://www3.cancer.gov/occam.
4. The Longwood Herbal Task Force (originated in Boston by the Children's Hospital, and College of Pharmacy and Dana Farber Cancer Institute) has a user-friendly web site that offers a comprehensive, balanced description of many herbs, their clinical uses, and evidence for effectiveness (http://www.mcp.edu/herbal).
5. A review of common herbs can be found at the American Academy of Family Physicians' web site: http://www.aafp.org/afp/981001ap/zink.html.
6. The web sites for the United States Department of Agriculture, Mayo Clinic, Memorial-Sloan Kettering Cancer Center, and M.D. Anderson Medical Centers also offer information on dietary supplements (see Table 18-6).
7. Heed warnings about the adverse effects of herbal products.
   The following was posted on the government's Office of Cancer Complementary and Alternative Medicine web site:
   "Potential Risk of Kava-Containing Dietary Supplements" "The FDA Center for Food Safety and Applied Nutrition (CFSAN) notified healthcare professionals and consumers of the potential risk of severe liver injury associated with kava-containing dietary supplements. Supplements containing the herbal ingredient kava are promoted for relaxation (e.g., to relieve stress, anxiety, and tension), sleeplessness, menopausal symptoms and

other uses. Kava-containing products have been associated with liver-related injuries, including hepatitis, cirrhosis, and liver failure. Given these reports, persons who have liver disease or liver problems, or persons who are taking drug products that can affect the liver, should consult a physician before using kava-containing supplements." See also MedWatch 2002 Safety Information entry for the types of information available on the web:
http://www.fda.gov/medwatch/SAFETY/2002/safety02.htm#kava

8. Try to enroll in a clinical CAM trial. If you do receive these compounds, it will be under controlled conditions and side effects will be carefully monitored.

CAM THERAPIES WIDELY ENCOUNTERED AND USED BY CANCER PATIENTS

CAN DIETARY SUPPLEMENTS INTERFERE WITH YOUR CHEMOTHERAPY?

The quick answer is yes! Unexpected or severe side effects and death have occurred with *natural* products. Innocuous herbs also can affect your chemotherapy program. See Table 18-4 and the three examples below:

Turmeric (Curcumin)

Irinotecan (CPT-11 or Camptosar) chemotherapy is under active investigation for brain tumors. It is *neutralized* (made ineffective) by curcumin, a component of the common spice turmeric. Test tube studies showed that curcumin inhibited the anti-cancer effects of several chemotherapy drugs: CPT-11, mechlorethamine (nitrogen mustard), and doxorubicin.[14] Does it have the same effect on brain tumor cells? We do not know. Should you avoid (Indian) food containing turmeric while receiving CPT-11? The answer is probably yes.

St. John's Wort

Concurrent administration of St. John's wort (300 mg. three times per day) with the chemotherapy drug Irinotecan can decrease its blood levels by 42 percent! Moreover, these decreased levels

> Taking St. John's Wort can reduce chemotherapy effectiveness to the point of treatment failure.

may last up to three weeks after discontinuation of the herb.[15] St. John's Wort increases the enzymes in your liver that metabolize many drugs, and thus lowers the drug level in the bloodstream. The same enzymes affected by St. John's wort also metabolize more than 50 percent of all anti-cancer drugs. This list includes

□ **Bottom Line** ➤ Natural products and herbs can inactivate your chemotherapy.

tamoxifen, Cytoxan, etoposide, vincristine, and taxol and taxotere. Thus, taking St. John's Wort before or during chemotherapy can reduce the effectiveness to the point of treatment failure.

Table 18-4 Information & Precautions for Popular Complementary & Alternative Therapies	
Dietary supplements that affect your chemotherapy • Turmeric (curcumin) • St. John's Wort • Beta-carotene Plant products (botanicals), minerals for alternative tumor therapy • Coenzyme Q10 • Copper chelating drugs • Evening primrose (starflower or borage) • Laetrile • Melatonin • Mistletoe (iscador) • Mushrooms • Red ginseng A and B • Essiac tea Natural Compounds-symptom relief • Boswellia • Bromelain • Echinacea • Natural immune stimulants • Yunnan Paiyao; blood platelet stimulants	Other Therapies • Antineoplaston therapy • Cancell/ (Entelev, Protocel) • Coral calcium Alternative Medical Systems • Acupuncture and traditional Chinese medicine • Ayurvedic medicine • Homeopathy Physical and Touch • Yoga • Massage • Therapeutic touch Mind-Body • Meditation • Prayer and spiritual healing • Hypnotherapy • Education therapy • Support groups • Psychotherapy • Relaxation training • Music therapy • Aromatherapy

Beta Carotene

Clinical trials have shown that supplementation with beta-carotene (the precursor form of Vitamin A that is found in raw foods like carrots) can decrease the risk of *developing* some cancers.[16,17] Beta-carotene is a strong anti-oxidant; therefore, it may appear logical that beta-carotene supplementation is a potentially effective anti-cancer accompaniment to chemotherapy. Many people with brain tumors take Vitamin A or beta-carotene to help fight their tumor. Unfortunately, a recent clinical trial testing chemotherapy with beta-carotene for lung cancer therapy found that cancer grew *faster* in patients who received *both* medications. Can beta-carotene make brain tumors grow faster? We do not know. "Logical, common sense" therapy can sometimes be harmful and routine recommendation of supplements is difficult, if not impossible, to make.

WHAT PLANT PRODUCTS (BOTANICALS) AND NATURAL PRODUCTS HAVE BEEN USED IN ALTERNATIVE THERAPIES?

Herbs have an historic role as cancer therapies. For example, the drug vincristine comes from the common vinca plant, and taxol originally was purified from the bark of the Pacific Yew tree. Both are effective against primary and metastatic brain tumors. However, the effectiveness of herb *supplements* as anti-cancer agents is unproven, scientifically. This has not slowed their popularity. Over 65 percent of brain tumor patients use herbal therapy or vegetable-derived supplements.[18] Medicinal mushrooms, echinacea, and Essiac appear to be the most popular. Bromelain, boswellia, coenzyme Q_{10}, evening primrose (starflower) with omega-3 fats also are part of an anti-tumor cocktail. Most reports of their effectiveness are "test tube" studies.[19,20,21] Do they help? Are they harmful? Unfortunately, scientific information is limited. (See Table 18-4.)

Coenzyme Q_{10}

Coenzyme Q_{10} circulates in our blood and is a component of dietary phytoestrogens that display anti-oxidant and anti-cancer activity against breast and prostate cancer in the test tube.[22] Vegetables, particularly soybeans, are a primary source. Most clinical studies of coenzyme Q_{10} have focused on its prevention of oxidant-injury damage to the heart from chemotherapy drugs like adriamycin.[23] Many Internet sources promote it as a supplement for treating cancer. It has no proven role in brain tumor therapy (see Table 18-6).

Copper Chelating Drugs

Copper may be important in cancer cell metabolism and the formation of blood vessels that feed tumors. The metal-binding drug penicillamine attaches to copper which then is excreted into the urine through the kidneys. Drugs containing molybdenum also bind copper. There are several web sites with information about copper, anti-angiogenesis, and cancer (see Table 18-6). One web site details a clinical trial led by Dr. Steven Brem at Moffitt Cancer Research Center in Florida that uses copper chelation (binding) to treat *glioblastoma multiforme* and other brain tumors. There, an explanation of anti-angiogenesis (blood vessel formation) and pharmacies that dispense copper chelators are cited. I do not recommend use of these products outside of a clinical trial.

Evening Primrose (Starflower or Borage)

The evening primrose or starflower, also called borage, contains gamma linolenic acid (GLA), an omega-3 fatty acid, which kills brain and prostate cancer cells in the test tube. It also arrests the spread of malignant tumors by limiting blood vessel growth. The combination of GLA and tamoxifen improved chemotherapy response in 38 breast cancer patients, compared with a control group of women who took tamoxifen only.[24] Starflower oil containing 24 percent GLA also is present in evening primrose oil used to treat premenstrual problems. One uncontrolled study showed that it caused an astrocytoma to shrink when directly applied to the tumor.[25] Despite the generally encouraging information, there is controversy about whether or not it may cause tumors to grow, depending on dosage.

Laetrile

Laetrile was used worldwide as an anti-cancer treatment up until the 1970s. The FDA in the United States never approved it. *Laetrile* is another name for the chemical amygdalin, a plant compound that contains sugar and produces cyanide. Amygdalin is found in the pits of many fruits and raw nuts as well as in lima beans, clover, and sorghum. For those who believe that laetrile kills cancer, cyanide is assumed to be the active component.

Though the names laetrile, Laetrile, and amygdalin are treated interchangeably, they are not the same compound. The chemical make-up of Laetrile patented in the United States is different from the laetrile (amygdalin) produced in Mexico. The patented Laetrile is a semi-synthetic form of amygdalin, while the laetrile manufactured in Mexico is amygdalin from crushed apricot pits. Two United States' studies in the 1970s found no significant anti-cancer activity from Laetrile, though brain tumors were not studied (see Table 18-6).

Melatonin

Melatonin is a hormone secreted by the pineal gland in the brain that responds to and regulates our day-night rhythms. One study of 30 brain tumor patients showed a survival benefit for patients receiving melatonin while undergoing radiation for *glioblastoma multiforme*.[26]

Mistletoe (Iscador)

Extracts of mistletoe can either stimulate or inhibit brain tumors. One German study found an increase in overall survival among patients receiving surgery and radiation plus mistletoe extract.[27] This same compound stimulated tumor growth in an experimental study.[28] These mixed results make it difficult to recommend mistletoe as therapy.

Mushrooms

Credited with medicinal properties for hundreds of years in China, mushrooms are widely advertised as having anti-cancer effects. Extracts from the shiitake mushroom (*lentinus edodes*), maitake mushroom (*grifola frondosa*), *coriolus vesicolor*, Cordyceps (*cordyceps sinesis*), and *ganoderma lucidum* have been investigated with positive results in mice.[29,30,31,32,33] In a randomized, controlled clinical trial (the gold standard for research), 111 patients received either *coriolus vesicolor* extract or a placebo after surgery for colorectal cancer. Survival was significantly higher in patients who received the extract. The extracts have not been tested in brain tumor patients.

Cordyceps sinesis, an ancient Chinese herb, may improve immunity and free-radical scavenging and thus protect DNA. Direct exposure of tumor cells to Cordyceps sinesis in a test tube inhibits tumor growth. In a clinical trial, water extracts of natural Cordyceps (10 g/kg, p.o.) or its fermentation products (5 g/kg, p.o.) *enhanced* the anti-cancer effects of vincristine. In other words, significantly more patients tolerated their chemotherapy and radiation better in combination with the herb. In contrast to the control group, blood counts were within normal range after chemotherapy and radiation therapy. Fifty patients in two studies showed more than 70 percent improvement of all symptoms. Tumor size shrank 25 to 50 percent in about half of patients who received the combination. In two patients, the tumor disappeared completely; one patient had tumor enlargement. This herb also has anti-inflammatory effects.[34]

Red Ginseng A and B

Red ginseng A and B have RH2 factor, a strong anti-oxidant and immune stimulant with cancer preventive and protective effects in mice. Solutions of ginseng A (at 0.5 mg/ml) and ginseng B (at 0.1-0.25 mg/ml) stimulated T-lymphocytes and stopped tumor cell growth in the animals. Red ginseng B was found to be more potent than red ginseng A.[35] No scientific clinical trials in humans have been reported.

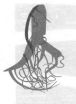

Essiac Tea

Essiac is an urban legend that deserves background information. It was popularized in Canada during the 1920s, when Rene Caisse (essiaC spelled backwards), a Canadian nurse, advocated it as a cancer treatment. Essiac is an herbal tea formula (derived by an Ojibwa Native American medicine man) that Caisse obtained from a breast cancer patient who claimed to have been cured by it. Caisse modified the formula and produced both injectable and oral forms. In 1938, members of the Royal Cancer Commission of Canada concluded that there was limited evidence for effectiveness. From 1959 until the late 1970s, Caisse worked with an American physician to conduct clinical studies and promote its use. This collaboration led to the development of the eight-herb formula now marketed as Flor-Essence. There are no results of clinical studies in peer-reviewed, scientific journals (see Table 18-6).

Essiac and Flor-Essence are proprietary herbal tea mixtures produced by different manufacturers. Essiac contains four herbs: burdock root (*arctium lappa*), Indian rhubarb root (*rheum palmatum,* or Turkish rhubarb), sheep sorrel (*rumex acetosella*), and inner bark of slippery elm (*ulmus fulva* or *ulmus rubra*). Flor-Essence contains the same four herbs as Essiac, plus four *potentiating* (increasing effectiveness of other) herbs: watercress (*nasturtium officinale*), blessed thistle (*cnicus benedictus*), red clover (*trifolium pratense*), and kelp (*laminaria digitata*). [The manufacturers of Essiac and Flor-Essence both claim that they market the original herbal mixture.] One company manufactures Flor Essence, but several companies produce and market Essiac-like products.

Essiac and Flor-Essence are said to "detoxify" the body and strengthen the immune system. Proponents of Essiac further claim that it relieves pain, improves overall quality of life, may reduce tumor size, and may prolong the survival of patients with various types of cancer. There are no well-documented studies of Essiac tea in patients with brain tumors.

As a physician, I have no direct knowledge of any of the components in this tea. My concern about the use of such a mixture, which to me sounds like a potion from Shakespeare's *Macbeth*, is illustrated by the following e-mail to a support group from a well-meaning caregiver. How can anyone answer her questions with information about side effects or drug interactions? There is no scientific data available with which to guide her. This highlights the vulnerability of patients and the need for research. Note that she was not aware of the curcumin interaction discussed earlier:

Now that all of William's treatments are almost done, we feel like we're doing nothing...if he starts drinking Essiac tea, it will help him. I remember someone mentioning that they actually had tumor shrinkage after drinking this stuff. Sounds like a great thing to try. I am going to list a few questions. Can you Essiac users give me some info?

The store...carried...Flor-Essence...it's more expensive. We are going to try the liquid concentrate stuff...instead of the brew-your-own. The lady at the store said to take an ounce a day. The Flor-Essence pamphlet says to take 2 ounces twice daily...for "detoxification," and... 2 ounces twice daily for one month in the spring and fall of each year "for maintenance." Is this as effective as the Essiac brand?

Do any of you find a difference with liquid concentrate vs. the brew-your-own? How much...do you drink each day? Any side effects? How many...saw shrinkage in your tumor? How long did it take? We are also taking red clover & burdock root, mistletoe, shark liver, curcumin, and CPT-11.

What Plant Products (Botanicals) Are Useful for Symptom Relief?

The information is summarized in Table 18-4.

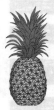

Boswellia

Boswellia (boswellic acid) may have useful anti-water retention effects (like steroids) and is prescribed by many practitioners. Test tube studies of boswellia have been conducted, but only one clinical Phase 2 palliative therapy trial in children was been reported. No tumor responses were noted in 19 patients.[36]

Bromelain

Bromelain is a digestive enzyme from the pineapple that can alleviate swelling.[37] It also prevents or breaks down blood clots; in large doses, it may cause bleeding. Although not tested for anti-cancer activity, it may have some cancer-fighting properties, since it is able to lower levels of TGF-beta, a cytokine that stimulates tumor growth.

Echinacea

Echinacea leads the list of herbs publicized for the treatment of colds. Many brain tumor patients use echinacea as an immune-stimulant during chemotherapy, with the hope of decreasing risk of infection.[38] No data exists on this use for brain tumor patients. This herb possesses immune-stimulating properties that include increased phagocytosis, stimulation of interleukins IL-1, IL-6, and tumor necrosis factor (TNF). Research on echinacea in the prevention and treatment of colds has yielded mixed results.[39,40] Many herbal experts also caution against the use of echinacea for more than 10 days, citing that it may decrease immunity after that.[41]

Natural Immune Stimulants

Many products and companies use immunology "buzz words" like *natural killer cells* and link these with cancer. This proves nothing. For example, ImmPower is advertised and distributed over the Internet by Beachwood Canyon, Naturally, Ltd., Advanced Dietary Supplements. The company states:

> *Working With Nature and Developed over 15 years ago in Japan, ImmPower has been well researched for effectiveness and safety. Today it is the best-selling supplement in Japan, used to support a strong immune system by activating the body's Natural Killer Cells, T-Cells and Macrophage activity. 10 published articles in peer-reviewed journals show that taking ImmPower, AHCC: Maintains Peak Natural Killer Cell Function, Supports Enhanced Cytokine Production, Promotes Optimal T-Cell and Macrophage Activity.*

The main ingredients in ImmPower are reported as mushroom mycelia extract, candelilla wax, and cyclodextrin microcrystalline cellulose. There are many claims for its effectiveness in decreasing metastases, but most are misleading or not based on solid criteria. What does it do for cancer? Can it be toxic or contain dangerous contaminants? Your guess is as good as mine.

There are several clinical trials using brain tumor cells and the body's own white cells (called dendritic cells) to fight brain cancers. See www.virtualtrials.com for a list of these. The principle is either to eradicate the tumors with infusions of the patient's own engineered, expanded cytotoxic T cells or to promote a longer lasting immunity by actively immunizing the patient against the tumor, after it has been partially or completely resected.

Yunnan Paiyao and Blood Platelet Stimulants

Platelets in our blood plug minute holes to prevent bleeding. Message boards and e-mails perpetuate the myth that the Chinese herb formula *Yunnan Paiyao* increases platelet count and helps the body recover from the effects of chemotherapy. During the Vietnam War, Viet Cong reportedly carried it in their first aid kits for gunshot wounds.

The myth is not in accord with the facts! *Yunnan Paiyao* causes platelets to clump and its effect lasts for three to four hours. Yes, it can stop traumatic bleeding; but this comes at a price, since it consumes and depletes platelets and does not regenerate them! Continued use could lower your platelet count (Table 18-6). Below is an example of a recent e-mail that perpetuates the misinformation:

> *We have come across a wonderful herbal approach to increasing platelet counts. It is a Chinese patent medicine called <u>Yunnan Paiyao</u>...prescribed to us by our TCM/ Naturopathic Doctor. My wife's platelets were just slightly above 100 and after 3 days of treatment, they rebounded to 168. However, her WBC still remains low for which we are still working on improving this. The medicine is inexpensive.*

There are other recipes for blood stimulants: alkyglycerols (100 mg. alkyglycerols 3x/day with meals, for platelets); red root (1-2 tsp. 4x/day), a tea developed by Native Americans known as New Jersey tea; and tahini (1-2 tbsp/day). To the best of my knowledge, none of these is accompanied by studies showing their value. Are they beneficial or harmful? I do not know.

WHAT ARE OTHER POPULAR ALTERNATIVE THERAPIES?

Antineoplaston Therapy

Dr. Stanislaw Burzynski developed antineoplaston treatment for many cancers including brain tumors. It is often mentioned by the lay public in North America as the first choice of alternative therapy for people with brain tumors. The treatment and its founder have had a rocky history over the past 25 years. One scientist questioned his background and methods but did not assess the clinical success issues. An objective review of antineoplastons appears in <u>http://www.mcphs.edu/herbal</u> or <u>http://www.mcphs.edu/herbal/antineoplastons/antineoplastons.cis.pdf</u> (see Tables 18-4, 18-6).

> Antineoplastons may be available on a clinical trial basis as an alternative therapy.

Antineoplastons are a mixture of synthetically produced peptides, amino acid derivatives, and organic acids, originally purified from human urine. Dr. Burzynski postulates that antineoplastons are part of a natural defense system against cancer that does not depend upon the immune system.

There have been substantial claims and case reports of successful treatment of brain tumors in both children and adults from the Burzynski Institute in Texas.[42] Many reports are in the institute's own journal, not subject to outside physician review. The National Cancer Institute evaluated seven patients who had reportedly responded to treatment in 1991. They concluded that those patients seemed to have benefited from the therapy.[43] A phase II trial was then endorsed by the National Cancer Institute and several major centers. Only nine patients were enrolled on the study by Dr. Burzynski by 1995, although hundreds had been treated off protocol. Results of the study were inconclusive due to the small sample size.[44] Currently, the Burzynski Research Institute is recruiting patients for a phase II trial of antineoplastons for different types of brain tumors. These results are not available to the public over the institute's web site.

One major problem and source of controversy has been Burzynski's reporting methods and comparisons about his treatment. For example, the following press release describes Dr. Burzynski's results:

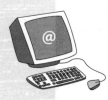

> *Antineoplaston's astonishing success rate vs. standard treatments is starkest with brain tumors. Burzynski has about a 65 percent response rate for all types of brain cancers, whereas chemo and radiation achieve five-year cures in less than 1 percent of all cases. Chemotherapeutic agents rarely reach the brain (because of the "blood-brain barrier") whereas antineoplastons do!*
> http://www.weeklyuniverse.com/2003/burzynski.htm

The news release above implies that an astonishing 65 percent of Burzynski's patients respond *and are cured* while "standard therapy" has a 1 percent success rate. The latter conclusion is just not true. With all brain tumors considered, about 30-50 percent of patients are alive five years after standard therapy. Even in *glioblastoma multiforme* patients, who have the worst prognosis, two to five percent of patients are alive at five years. In interpreting the above claim, it is important to note that some Burzynski *successes* were achieved in people with low-grade tumors that have longer survivals. Finally, while the blood-brain-barrier does exist in normal brain, most malignant tumors lack this barrier, as evidenced by their permeability to contrast dye used with CT or MRI scans. Therefore, drugs reach the tumor; they are just not effective. For a National Cancer Institute report on antineoplastons, see (http://www.heall.com/body/altmed/treatment/antineoplastons.html).

The Burzynski Institute revamped its web site (http://www.cancermed.com/). Their previous version contained detailed information on antineoplastons, including an extensive bibliography, copies of all open research protocols, and reprints of some independent inspections. The current webpage [as of March 2005], is much slicker than the old one, but does not contain the word *antineoplaston*.[45]

Does Dr. Burzynski's therapy offer a reasonably priced, realistic alternative? I am not sure. Traditional medical oncologists clearly do not have a reliable, successful treatment for *glioblastoma multiforme*, brain stem gliomas, or many recurrent gliomas. I suggest that anyone wanting this experimental therapy receive it on a clinical trial basis (see Chapter 21: Clinical Trials). The major disadvantages of the treatment are that it costs more than $10,000 every four to six months (no insurance coverage is available) and patients have to travel to Dr. Burzynski's clinic in Houston, Texas to receive the treatment. Additional information on antineoplaston therapy is available at www.virtualtrials.com and the NCI site http://cis.nci.nih.gov/fact/7_43.htm.

Cancell/ Entelev/ Protocel

Cancell (called Entelev and Protocel, also known as Sheridan's Formula, Jim's Juice, Crocinic Acid, JS–114, JS–101, 126–F, and Cantron) is promoted as a treatment for cancer and other diseases. Cancell has been produced in several forms by two manufacturers since the late 1930s. The FDA has not approved the formula but has attempted to investigate its components, reported as inositol, nitric acid, sodium sulfite, potassium hydroxide, sulfuric acid, and catechol. However, the exact composition of Cancell/ Entelev/ Protocel is unknown.

According to the original manufacturer, Cancell/ Entelev/ Protocel changes cancer cells so that they are identified as *foreign* and then destroyed. The second manufacturer states that Cancell/ Entelev/ Protocel

> Neither coral calcium nor Cancell have any proven role in controlling or shrinking a brain tumor.

changes cancer cells so that they *self-digest* and are replaced by normal cells. The waste materials produced by self-digestion supposedly are eliminated through urine, perspiration, and other body fluids. Independent tests on one form of Cancell/ Entelev/ Protocel found 12 different compounds, none of which is known to be effective in treating any form of cancer (see Table 18-6).

Coral Calcium

Coral calcium appears in many advertisements as a cure for all types of cancer. Excess calcium, however, can increase the risk of constipation, kidney stones, and blood clots. There is no evidence to support its efficacy in treating cancer. Recently the government initiated proceedings against a supplier of coral calcium who had a large Internet following:

> The Federal Trade Commission (FTC) filed a case (May, 2002) against marketers of a dietary supplement called Coral Calcium Supreme with making false and unsubstantiated claims about their product's health benefits. The FTC has charged that Kevin Trudeau, Robert Barefoot, Shop America LLC and Deonna Enterprises claim that their product can treat or cure all forms of cancer, multiple sclerosis, lupus, chronic high blood pressure and heart disease. The statements made in a nationally televised 30-minute infomercial and through statements in brochures accompanying the product are unfounded and unsupported... The FTC is looking for permanent injunction and financial restitution to consumers who purchased Coral Calcium Supreme. ...the FTC and... FDA have issued warning letters to dozens of web site operators making similar claims for coral calcium products...

ALTERNATIVE MEDICAL SYSTEMS

ACUPUNCTURE AND TRADITIONAL CHINESE MEDICINE

The aim of traditional Chinese medicine (TCM) is to correct imbalances in yin (-) and yang (+) (the two opposing aspects of life energy, called *qi* or *chi*) and the five elements (wood, earth, fire, water and metal). (See Figure 18-2.) In TCM theory, there are pathways or meridians, throughout which *qi* flows in the body. TCM views diseases as an *imbalance* of energy and elements. It facilitates healing by restoring balance and harmony. Acupuncture is the most familiar of several therapies that make up traditional Chinese medicine (TCM); it is effective for relief of headache, tension, and nausea and vomiting from chemotherapy. Acupuncture is part of a comprehensive program that includes herbs, special diets, movement, massage, and meditation. It is almost never a sole treatment. For methods and functions, see Table 18-1.

Acupuncture is an ancient practice of inserting needles into specific points along meridians in order to unblock energy and restore balance. Modern acupuncture has

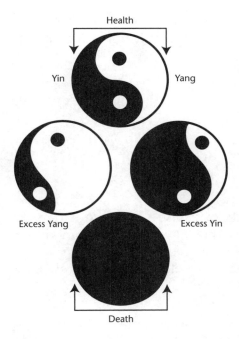

Figure 18-2. Balance of Ying and Yang in health and Disease

adopted novel point-stimulation technologies such as magnets and lasers, in addition to fine needles. Recently, electric stimulation of the needles achieved more profound effects. Using functional MRI scans, investigations have confirmed that acupuncture points for certain organs, often far removed from the actual organ, stimulate the same location in the brain as physical stimulation of the organ itself.[46,47]

Pain researchers note that stimulation of acupuncture points activates nerve fibers that allow release of the body's own endorphin and enkephalins (natural morphine-like chemicals) inside the central nervous system. These effects are blocked or reversed by morphine-inhibiting agents. Release of other neuropeptides and hormones (for example, adrenocorticotropic hormone [ACTH], thyroid-stimulating hormone [TSH], gastrin, substance P) also occur. This release affects pain perception as well as heart, respiratory, immune, and gastrointestinal functions. [48,49,50]

There is clear evidence for acupuncture's effectiveness in treating chemotherapy-induced nausea and vomiting. In 130 cancer patients who had a history of chemotherapy-induced nausea and vomiting, P6 type electro-acupuncture for 5 minutes (at 10 Hz.) either completely alleviated or reduced vomiting in 97 percent of the patients.[51] Acupuncture can relieve headache [52] and back pain.[53] Twenty-four out of 41 patients reported reduced migraine or muscle pain levels after acupuncture therapy; in contrast, only three of 36 patients with medical treatment alone reported reduced pain.[54] (See Table 18-6 for TCM web sites.)

> Acupuncture and TCM are helpful for symptom relief of headache, pain and nausea.

AYURVEDIC MEDICINE

Ayurvedic medicine, or Ayurveda, is a system of healing that originated in ancient India and is practiced by 80 percent of the Indian population. In Sanskrit, *ayurveda* means "knowledge of living" or "science of longevity." Ayurvedic medicine emphasizes seven approaches to improved health and shares features in common with traditional Chinese medicine:

1. Diet;
2. Detoxification and purification;
3. Herbal and mineral remedies;
4. Yoga;
5. Massage therapy;
6. Breathing exercises; and
7. Meditation.

Ayurvedic physicians seek to discover the roots of a disease, before it gets so advanced that radical treatment is necessary. Thus, Ayurveda has limitations for treating advanced medical conditions or injuries requiring invasive surgery. Ayurvedic techniques are used in a complementary way along with chemotherapy and surgery to assist in recovery and healing.[55]

Aided by the efforts of Deepak Chopra, Ayurveda has become an increasingly accepted complementary medical approach. In North America, there is no standardized program for the certification of Ayurvedic practitioners. Many have primary degrees as M.D., homeopaths, or naturopathic physicians, with additional training in Ayurveda.

Diagnosis and treatment in Ayurveda differs from that of western medicine and first uses *dosha* to classify people into one of the three characteristic body types: *vata* (air), *pitta* (fire), or *kapha* (water). Ayurveda analyzes the individual's unique *dosha* pattern or *prakriti. Panchakarma,* an intensive Ayurvedic cleansing and detoxification program, is employed, along with *meditation* (a technique of calming the mind) to hasten healing. Ayurveda assumes belief in *prana,* the basic life energy, and employs *yoga* to exercise the breath. Many people may be a combination of dosha types, not just one. (See Table 18-5.)

Table 18-5 Ayurvedic Medicine: Three Major Dosha Patterns in People

Character-istics	Vata	Pitta	Kapha
Physical	Thin, prominent features; cool, dry skin; constipation; cramps	Average build; fair; thin hair; warm, moist skin; ulcers; heartburn; hemorrhoids; acne	Large build; wavy, thick hair; pale; cool, oily skin; obesity; allergies; sinus problems; high cholesterol
Emotional	Moody; vivacious; imaginative; enthusiastic; intuitive	Intense; quick tempered; intelligent; loving; articulate	Relaxed; not easily angered; affectionate; tolerant; compassionate
Behavioral	Unscheduled sleep and meal times; nervous disorders; anxiety	Orderly structured sleep and meal times; perfectionist	Slow; graceful; long sleeper and slow eater; procrastination

Detoxification theoretically rids the body of toxins from environmental poisoning, such as smog, mercury, or microwaves. It uses herbal laxatives and high fiber foods, like psyllium seeds, to cleanse the digestive tract and promote elimination. Colonics cleanse the lower intestines. Digestive enzymes are prescribed to improve digestion, and acidophilus and other friendly bacteria are reintroduced into the system with nutritional supplements. Fasting is another method in detoxification.

A COMMENT ON DETOXIFICATION

Environmental medicine with attention to pollutants is gaining more respect, but detoxification in cancer treatment has little recognition within the medical establishment. Research on it is largely testimonial, consisting of personal accounts of healing, without statistics or controlled scientific experiments. In the alternative medical community, detoxification is an

> Detoxification is recommended often but has little scientific proof for fighting a brain tumor.

essential and widely accepted treatment for many illnesses and chronic conditions. Many Ayurvedic institutes can advise you on the appropriateness of detoxification. (See Table 18-6 for web sites and the Gale Encyclopedia of Alternative Medicine web site for more information on detoxification.)

MANIPULATIVE AND BODY-BASED THERAPIES

Physical manipulation and therapies involving touch are part of an Ayurvedic, naturopathic, traditional Chinese medicine, or other CAM approaches. Many people report that they feel better after a massage or therapeutic touch. There have been few clinical trials in people with cancer to document positive results using these techniques. I have found no studies that address their effectiveness specifically for people with brain tumors. Nevertheless, they offer a drug-free, painless, easy and probably effective way to gain relief from discomfort. This makes them reasonable to consider as a part of overall therapy, if appropriate cautions are observed (see under Yoga below).

YOGA

Yoga teaches self-control through a series of postures, breathing exercises, relaxation, and meditation techniques. The ultimate goal of yoga is *self-realization* – attainment of complete physical, emotional, mental, and spiritual potential. A more limited goal of yoga is to restore the whole person to balance, thus optimizing health. A study involving 50 cancer patients who received yoga therapy found that 11 of 50 experienced improved appetite, sleep, and digestion; 10 reported elevated feelings of peace and tranquility.[56]

Precautions: Most yoga exercises employ postures that emphasize relaxation and avoidance of muscle stress or pain. However, some yoga poses are quite strenuous and can lead to injury that may limit activity. Understand the kind of yoga you will be practicing *before* you start, as there are different kinds and levels taught. Always know what to expect before joining a class. As with any exercise program, those who have not been physically active, are overweight, are on steroids, have high blood pressure, have lost muscle or bone density, have arthritis, or have spinal disk injuries should consult their physician before engaging in yoga.

In order to prevent injury, it is important to learn the yoga postures correctly, to be aware of the physical sensations that might occur during practice, and to refrain from movements that are painful – particularly when unsupervised. Some practioners recommend avoidance of inverted (upside down) postures. Some postures may release cytokines or adrenaline, which can cause you to feel faint or anxious. Qualified instructors will prepare and teach you not to panic because of these sensations. For all these reasons, I recommend a well-trained Ayurvedic yoga teacher.

> Yoga, massage, and Therapeutic Touch can be effective in making you feel better.

MASSAGE

Massage therapy can alleviate pain or physical discomfort. Four studies attest to the benefits of massage in cancer patients. Two types, Swedish and Shiatsu, increase relaxation, stimulate blood and lymph flow, decrease heart rate, and induce "purification of the immune system."[57] All 48 cancer patients who received a massage treatment enjoyed the massage and felt more relaxed. Fourteen experienced long-term relaxation that continued after treatment. Sixteen patients experienced a reduction in pain; but eight reported a negative experience during the massage treatment.[58] A second study compared massage with more personal attention in 41 hospitalized adult cancer patients. In those who received therapeutic massage, there was improvement in scores for pain, sleep quality, symptom distress, and anxiety, while participants in the control group only reported less anxiety.[59] In another study of nine cancer patients, pain decreased 60 percent, anxiety decreased 24 percent, and relaxation increased 58 percent overall.[60]

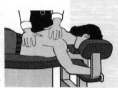

There has been a school of thought that advised against massage for people with cancer due to concerns that massage may spread disease. Current thinking has moved away from this viewpoint to accept massage as a mild physiological stimulus similar to exercise, when proper precautions are used. Such precautions are taught to massage therapists at places such as Memorial Sloan-Kettering Cancer Center (see Table 18-6).

THERAPEUTIC TOUCH

Therapeutic touch attempts to affect an energy field surrounding the patient. It has three basic steps:
- Centering: the practitioner begins therapy by assuming a meditative form of awareness.
- Assessing: the medical practitioner holds his or her hands above the patient's body, and then moves them from head to toe to "assess" the energy field of the patient.
- Directing energy: the practitioner "redirects" areas of accumulated tension, restores balance, and re-establishes energy flow to depleted areas.

The reported effects of therapeutic touch include decreased pain, anxiety, and diastolic blood pressure. These effects have a low standard of documented "proof."[61,62]

REIKI

Reiki is another energy therapy that may or may not involve hands-on contact by the therapist. It attempts to reestablish energy balance in areas of the body that are experiencing disease and discomfort, thus promoting healing, pain reduction, and increased quality of life. Reiki therapists direct this therapy toward 18 specific areas of the body; 18 of 20 patients reported lower pain scores after one Reiki treatment.[63] More than 26 percent of cancer patients have used some form of "energy healing" in the previous year.

THERAPIES USING MIND-BODY CONNECTION & MEDITATION

We understand now how meditation might work to help the body function better at times of stress. Early studies reported subjective, "touchy-feely" results, which did not meet scientific standards for proof. For example, one study from the 1980's stated that "all" cancer patients who used meditation therapy showed less anxiety and depression and experienced less discomfort and pain as a result. Actual increase in quality or length of life was uncertain.[64] In a subsequent study, meditation contributed to a 92 percent improvement in well-being (feeling more peaceful). Sixty percent of the patients felt more energetic and 52 percent demonstrated increased tolerance for radiation therapy (fewer adverse effects).[65]

MEDITATION

How does meditation affect the brain? Many people think that meditation quiets the mind and gives the brain a vacation. Just the opposite is true! Deep meditation in Buddhist monks is associated with increase activity in many regions of the brain.[66] Scientists have mapped out how the brain responds in a (Zen) state of meditation. Here's what researchers know so far:

> Meditation can contribute to fighting your brain tumor more effectively.

1. Concentrating fully on an object promotes activity in your frontal lobe, which controls motivation.
2. Looking at images like candles stimulates your lower temporal lobe, where you process some visual stimuli.
3. Chanting stimulates the connection where your temporal, frontal and parietal lobes meet; this can stimulate relaxation.

4. Feelings of joy or awe mean your temporal lobe (regulates emotion) is active.
5. When you transcend a sense of separation from your surroundings and feel "at one with the universe," the top part of your parietal lobe (processes sensations) is quiet.

Thus, meditation has a physical effect on how and where your brain reacts and processes information. It is not quackery, magic, or just a figment of imagination.

Meditation also can boost parts of the immune system. Researchers at the University of Wisconsin-Madison enrolled 41 people in a trial of so-called "mindfulness" meditation. Participants were administered a flu vaccine. Eight weeks later, those who meditated had *higher* levels of antibody against the flu.[67]

If meditation and other mind-body therapies, like biofeedback and prayer, can slow the heartbeat, then they probably do so by stimulating the vagus nerve. The vagus nerve, which slows the heart rate, also transmits signals that inhibit both the immune system and the production of a cytokine TNF, or tumor necrosis factor. TNF causes local pain and redness and activates a chain of immune activity related to inflammation, as occurs with the swelling of the brain in response to injury or brain tumor. Therefore, it is possible that mind-body practices have a beneficial effect on the immune system.[68]

PRAYER AND SPIRITUAL HEALING

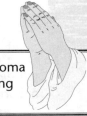

Prayer and spiritual healing are widely used. Most practitioners believe that their inner intentions become manifest through love, energy, or a Higher Power.[69] However, the conventional community attributes benefits from these interventions to the patient's hope, expectation, or support from a practitioner.[70] In either case, the patient's experience is usually a positive one.

> NIH-sponsored clinical trial for glioblastoma patients tests if prayer and distant healing might promote longer life.

When individuals are diagnosed or treated for cancer, spiritual counseling can be helpful. It accentuates the notion of a divine force greater than oneself, and thus, helps cancer patients to cope, focus, and maintain a sense of purpose. Furthermore, prayer (associated with spiritual counseling) permits the patient to express his or her inner emotions and thoughts.[71]

Based on the possibility of healing energy, the National Institutes of Health sponsored a clinical trial for *glioblastoma multiforme* patients. It is a double blind, randomized, controlled clinical trial of "distant healing intentionality." This study assesses whether distant healing affects survival time and loss of function under conditions where hope and expectation are controlled. The study will include approximately 150 patients who have *glioblastoma multiforme* and are beginning radiotherapy. Patients will be photographed and assessed for quality of life, psychological status, and physical symptoms as well as health habits and attitude toward distant healing.

"Healers" from diverse schools and backgrounds from communities across the United States are assigned to patients by rotation; each patient in the distant healing group will be treated for two weeks by 10 different healers over the 20-week intervention. Healers will have photographs of subjects and send "mental intention for health and well being" to subjects for one hour daily, three times per week. The healing intervention is performed at a distance; patients and healers will never meet, nor will patients know their group assignment. The study's findings will provide the basis for developing a larger, definitive trial. For location and information, contact Andrew Freinkel, M.D. 415-600-1294 (e-mail freinkel@cooper.cpmc.org); or Marianne Yeung 415-600-1295; e-mail myeung@cooper.cpmc.org).[72]

HYPNOTHERAPY

In one study of pain and survival, cancer patients who received hypnotherapy experienced 50 percent less pain and lived an average of one year longer than a control group.[73] Hypnotherapy has a powerful effect on reducing pain from procedures like spinal taps and bone marrow samples in children.[74] It is effective for reduction of chemotherapy-related nausea and vomiting.[75]

Hypnosis affects anxiety, depression and pain by changing the mind's ability to control bodily processes, like sensing discomfort. It may also enhance immunity.[76,77] In a study of self-hypnosis, 61 percent of patients claimed that they were benefited, with 11 of 41 patients reporting more optimism, less anxiety, and improved sleep.[78] With heightened relaxation and decreased anxiety, one may be able to assume more control and adopt better coping strategies.[79]

EDUCATION THERAPY

One interpretation of the lesson of Adam and Eve in the Garden of Eden was that the desire for knowledge (good and evil) met with loss of power, shame, pain and banishment from the Garden. A recent study offering knowledge to patients with cancer came to the opposite conclusion: educational information sessions enhanced coping and quality of life. Dr. Elena Farace gave a manual of instructions to caregivers on more effective care giving for people with malignant brain tumors. She found not only *decreased* stress in the caretakers, but also *increased* quality of life in the patients![80]

Information can alleviate the stress related to feeling ignorant and uneducated about your medical condition. In another study of 94 patients with newly diagnosed leukemia, patients received a one-hour educational session with a nurse, reviewing information about the disease and instructions for taking medications. Those who attended the sessions had a decreased rate of death and increased survival time; they were also more compliant about taking their medication.[81] The National Institutes of Health (NIH) does not consider patient education to be CAM therapy. I have included it here because of the positive effects that it can have on health... and survival.

These studies show that for people with cancer, knowledge is power! Learning about your disease, not hiding from it, can increase the quality and possibly length of life. This book, or others like it, is educational therapy!

SUPPORT GROUPS

Support groups were discussed in Chapter 3: Getting Organized. Here, I would like to provide the reasons why joining a support group can

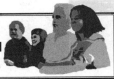

Both education and support groups have contributed to better length and quality of life for patients with cancer.

help you live longer. They provide more benefits than just education. Even so, the NIH and National Center for Complementary and Alternative Medicine (NCCAM) do not classify support groups under CAM.

Support groups usually concentrate on five major areas: 1) telling your story; 2) managing medical advice; 3) seeking and exchanging information; 4) preparing for the "long haul"; and 5) addressing family life changes. The support group provides a safe and specific therapeutic place for brain tumor patients and their families to

□**Bottom Line** CAM therapies can make you feel better and enhance your quality of life. That may help you live longer and enjoy more of life.

discuss the difficulties of survival and maintaining quality of life after treatment.[82] At least three major studies have shown a benefit in mood, depression, and quality of life for those attending a support group. Attendees demonstrate longer survival and improved immunity.[83]

A series of six-week, psycho-educational group therapy sessions for melanoma patients resulted in important benefits for the mind and immune system. Compared to pre-therapy assessments, this program lowered levels of confusion, depression, fatigue, and mood disturbance; it increased strength, coping ability, and optimism. In addition, the group participants showed an increase in the number of their immune cells (lymphocytes). Six months later, there was a continued increase of lymphocytes and an increase in interferon alpha-augmented natural killer cells. Only 20 percent of the tumors recurred in the experimental group (compared with 38 percent of control group). Only 8 percent of the experimental group died compared with 29 percent of control group.[84,85] Effect of the group support lasted up to 10 years![86] A similar story occurred with breast cancer groups.[87]

PSYCHOTHERAPY

Psychotherapy is based on the premise that distress stems not just from your brain tumor. It also is affected by thoughts and feelings about your disease and situation, your ability to cope with and take control of a situation in which you may feel powerless.

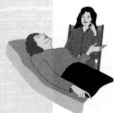

"Fighting spirit" was induced in patients with all stages of cancer, using a cognitive-behavioral therapy program. The program encouraged patients to express their emotions, plan activities associated with pleasure or control and challenge negative thinking. About 57 patients comprised two groups: 1) the problem-focused, cognitive behavioral treatment program, or 2) eight weeks of supportive counseling.

After eight weeks, the cognitive behavioral treatment group reported significantly greater "fighting spirit," less helplessness and anxiety, and better coping with cancer compared with the counseling only group. Four months later, the treatment group continued to experience greater improvements than the counseling group. Moreover, patients with advanced disease showed as much improvement as those with local disease.[88]

RELAXATION TRAINING AND GUIDED IMAGERY

Progressive muscle relaxation (a "tense and release" exercise with controlled breathing) coupled with guided imagery (peaceful visualization) reduces pain, anxiety, and emotional distress. Guided imagery allows individuals to enter a relaxed state of mind and then focus their attention on positive, pleasing, *successful* images associated with the issues they are confronting. Guided imagery reduced pain and need for medication in 67 percent of cancer patients; 92 percent reported a more relaxed state. Such a non-invasive treatment might allow you to assume more control over your life and therapy.[89]

AROMATHERAPY

Aromatherapy lessens anxiety and vomiting in cancer patients. In this traditionally European practice, essential plant oils are absorbed through the skin or diffused through the air and inhaled into the nose. From there, a chemical scent message goes to the brain's limbic system. Two English studies measured the physical and psychological effects of aromatherapy on the cancer patient and both concluded that most patients have reduced pain, depression, anxiety, and tension [90,91] For more information refer to the web sites in Table 18-6.

MUSIC THERAPY

Music can be relaxing and make people less anxious during chemotherapy.[92] It is inexpensive and easily performed. Particular variations reduced anxiety and increased relaxation in 47 adults given a personalized, taped message accompanied by music during chemotherapy. The 50 patients in the control group showed no change. In another study, 15 cancer patients received a choice of seven types of music to listen to over a period of three days, alternately listening to a 60-cycle hum. Seventy-five percent of patients found the music pleasant and relaxing. Eighty-six percent reported that it enabled them to take their mind off their pain.[93]

SUMMARY

CAM methods are complementary to healthful living. There are many stories of long-term survivors of highly malignant brain tumors who used complementary methods along with western medicine.[94] I personally know of two survivors who feel that these methods were at least partially responsible for their survival (ER and Ben Williams [94]). Certainly, this practice has had a positive effect on their state of health, mind, mood, and function. Given the inseparability of mind and body, these effects potentially can be quite powerful.

Having good information is the first step for people who would like to see if CAM therapies are helpful. Search out and evaluate the resources provided in this chapter. Are all these good sources? Unfortunately, there is no guarantee that questionable, false, or outdated information won'tbe found on the Internet. However, you can compare what these sources have to say and empower yourself with knowledge.

Bottom line There is one overriding theme from all the CAM research – your actions put you more in control of your life.

Table 18-6 Internet Resources for Complementary and Alternative Medicine (CAM)

Subject	Web Site or Contact Information
CAM and clinical trials	http://www3.cancer.gov/occam/
CAM information	http://nccam.nih.gov/health; (government sponsored)
Common herbs- uses for symptom relief	http://www.aafp.org/afp/981001ap/zink.html (American Academy Physicians www.cancersymptoms.org http://www.braintumor.org/pservices/conference2002/wallacetext.pdf
Herbs-General	http://www.mcphs.edu/si/sl/subject_guides/herbdrug.html (Longwood Herbal Task Force) http://www.ars-grin.gov/duke (U.S. Dept. Agriculture- plant database)
Herbals-supplements	http://www.mayoclinic.com/invoke.cfm?objectid=AA08B116-819D-4B5A-B1762D54761490D9 http://www.mdanderson.org/departments/cimer http://www.mcp.edu/herbal/. http://www.braintrust.org/resources/therapies.html http://www.nutritional-solutions.net/Articles/BestSupplementsJeanneWallace.pdf http://www.holisticcancersolutions.com/braintumorsarticle.htm

Supplements and Nutrition

Subject	Web Site or Contact Information
Antineoplastons	http://cis.nci.nih.gov/fact/7_43.htm http://www.weeklyuniverse.com/2003/burzynski.htm http://www.heall.com/body/altmed/treatment/antineoplastons.html) http://www.cancermed.com/ The Institute web site http://www.mcphs.edu/herbal/antineoplastons/antineoplastons.cis.pdf www.virtualtrials.com http://www.quackwatch.org/01QuackeryRelatedTopics/Cancer/burzynski1.html
CanCell/ Entelev/ Protocel	http://www.1uphealth.com/alternative-medicine/cancell-entelev-3.html http://www.danielwoods.com/cancell.html. http://altcancer.silvermedicine.org/protocel.htm

89

Table 18-6 Internet Resources Continued

Coenzyme Q10	http://cis.nci.nih.gov/fact/9_16.htm http://www.mcp.edu/herbal/
Copper chelating drugs and anti-angiogenesis	http://www.cancerprotocol.com/role_of_copper.html. http://www.medscape.com/viewarticle/417732 http://www.coldcure.com/html/anti_ang.html
Drug interactions- Side effects,	http://www.quackwatch.org/index.html http://seattlepi.nwsource.com/local/22927_cancer14.shtml http://www.fiery-foods.com/dave/capsaicin.asp http://www.marinol.com/patient/pat01.html
Essaic tea	http://www.cancer.gov/cancerinfo/pdq/cam/essiac
Laetrile	http://www.1uphealth.com/alternative-medicine/laetrile-amygdalin-2.html
Macrobiotic therapy	http://www.kushiinstitute.org/whatismacro.html http://www.quackwatch.org/01QuackeryRelatedTopics/kushi.html http://www.holisticmed.com/www/macrobiotics.html
MedWatch safety alert	www.fda.gov/medwatch
Natural Immune stimu-lants	http://www.furrykids.net/impower2.htm) See www.virtualtrials.com for a list of these.)
Supplements for Cancer treatment, advice	http://www.dietcancer.com/index.html http://www.holisticcancersolutions.com/CancerTextPage.htm http://www.holisticcancersolutions.com paid information http://www.braintumor.org/pservices/conference2002/wallacetext.pdf www.toweracupuncture.com
Yunnan Paiyao effects on platelets	http://www.dr-zhang.com/index.htm www.simplesherbs.com/chinese.htm

Alternative Medical Systems

Aromatherapy	http://www.heall.com/body/altmed/treatment/aromatherapy/index.html
Ayurvedic institutes [95]	American Institute of Vedic Studies P.O. Box 8357, Santa Fe, NM 87504. (505) 983-9385 Ayurveda Holistic Center. Bayville, Long Island, NY. (516)759-7731 mail@Ayurvedahc.com mail@Ayurvedahc.com http://www.Ayurvedahc.com The Ayurvedic Institute. 11311 Menaul, NE Albuquerque, New Mexico 87112. (505)291-9698. info@Ayurveda.com http://www.Ayurveda.com Center for Mind/Body Medicine. P.O. Box 1048, La Jolla, CA 92038. (619)794-2425. National Institute of Ayurvedic Medicine. (914)278-8700. drgerson@erols.com http://www.niam.com The Rocky Mountain Institute of Yoga and Ayurveda. P.O. Box 1091, Boulder, CO 80306. (303)443-6923.
Ayurvedic practices	http://www.findarticles.com/cf_dls/g2603/0000/2603000014/p1/article.jhtml?term=%2B%22Ayurvedic+medicine%22 http://www.findarticles.com/cf_0/g2603/0003/2603000321/p6/article.jhtml?term= (detoxification) http://www.Ayurvedahc.com http://www.Ayurveda.com
Massage	http://www.mskcc.org/mskcc/html/11997.cfm.
Scams	http://www.quackwatch.org/index.html
Traditional Chinese medicine (TCM) and herbs	http://www.tcmstudent.com/ http://tcm.health-info.org www.acupuncture.com http://www.healthepic.com/accupuncture/static/Acupnhistory.htm

Joya Tillem, MD, Mona Patel and Terry Williams provided research assistance for this section.

CHAPTER 19

Cancer-Fighting Drugs – Chemotherapy, Antibiotics, Marrow Stimulants and Their Side Effects

The Brain Tumor List has been of great importance to me through my 7 years of this oligo tumor; 3 years and 2 months on Temodar. The list made me aware of Temodar when it was in clinical trials. I was eager to select it over other chemo drugs when I had to make a decision. Fortunately, my tumor has the receptive genes for chemotherapy.

Gladys, a New Jersey Lady

Key search words

- nausea
- side effect
- drug interaction
- neupogen
- chemotherapy

- white cell
- blood count
- antibiotic
- drug safety
- intrathecal therapy

- anti-seizure drug
- steroid
- marrow stimulant
- medication error
- red cell

This book and its companion[1] both contain a chapter on medications. This chapter highlights medications that fight cancer, control or eliminate nausea, and help maintain normal levels of blood cells and clotting factors. Chapter 9 contains medications most people may take around the time of diagnosis and initial treatment, such as steroids, anti-seizure drugs and medicines to control fatigue and pain.

ERROR PREVENTION

CHEMOTHERAPY: EFFECTIVE...AND DANGEROUS

The *greatest* danger in taking chemotherapy or other medication for your brain tumor is not the side effects of the drug. Rather, it is the possibility of an inadvertent medication error. Medical errors are a public health problem. Collectively they are one of the nation's leading causes of death and injury. From 44,000 to 98,000 people die in United States' hospitals each year as the result of medical errors. This

> Medication errors occur when critical information is missing from the medical record.

means that more people die from medical errors than from motor vehicle accidents, breast cancer, or AIDS.[2] Preventing errors, basic precautions, and questions to ask are discussed more fully in Chapter 9, Medications.[1]

To protect yourself, you should ask your doctor five simple questions each time you receive a prescription for chemotherapy or other medication:
1. Why am I on it?
2. What does it do?
3. What are the side effects?
4. Who is responsible for monitoring me while I am on this medication?
5. To whom should I direct inquiries, day or night, if I have side effects?

When you are at home, before you take your medicine:
- Make sure that you are taking the right pills at the right dosage.
- Double-check each prescription. Make sure the medicine has *your* name on it.
- Learn what the tablets are supposed to look like. If they are a different size, color, or shape from what you have had before, Do Not Take Them before consulting your pharmacist.

Cancer is one disease in which being proactive in monitoring medication can save your life! Table 19-1 outlines an overall plan to prevent medication-related errors and enhance your care. Read the following story about a patient whom I had seen once in consultation for a second opinion:

Marlene, a 41-year-old married, executive secretary had a Grade 3 oligodendroglioma and was taking 160 mg of Temodar five days each month, by combining a 100 mg. tablet with three 20 mg. tablets. For her fifth course, she was mistakenly given four 250 mg tablets by the pharmacist and she took them as directed before. One month later, she developed liver failure and died. Neither she nor her husband questioned the changed shape or size of the tablets. Don't let this happen to you.

Table 19-1 Prevention of Medication-Related Errors[3]
1. Be an active member of your health care team.
2. Ensure all your doctors know your weight & all medications (prescription, over-the-counter meds, supplements, vitamins, herbs).
3. Inform your doctor about allergies or reactions to any medication.
4. Make sure you can read the prescription your doctor writes.
5. Ask the pharmacist, "Is this the medicine my doctor prescribed?"
6. Ask for information about drugs in terms that you understand – from your physician and pharmacist.
7. Ask about directions on your medicine labels, if you don't quite understand them.
8. Ask your pharmacist for the best device to measure your liquid medication. Ask questions if you are not sure how to use the device.
9. Ask for written information about medication side effects.

DANGEROUS DRUG INTERACTIONS – FINDING INFORMATION

This section is near the beginning of the chapter, because knowing about these resources can save your life!

Find out if your drugs are incompatible with any over-the-counter or herbal agents you may be taking, or if there are possible reactions that you could experience. These avoidable, sometimes life-threatening drug-drug interactions cost nearly $130 billion each year! Most often, if you receive all your medications from one pharmacy, this will be done for you... but better to be safe than sorry. Your pharmacist may be in the best position, having all your drug records available, to assist you.

▸**Bottom Line** If your new prescription pills are a different size, color, or shape from what you have had before, DO NOT TAKE THEM

Use the web sites below, as well, to research your prescribed medications and find possible interactions or incompatibilities they might have with other products.

- http://www.nowfoods.com/index.php/Drug-Safety-Check/Home/cat_id/2534
- http://health.discovery.com/encyclopedias/checker/checker.jsp?&jspLetter=B
- http://www.drugstore.com/pharmacy/drugchecker/default.asp?aid=333158&aparam=MSNFS_discount_prescriptions

For example, Dilantin can have the unexpected side effect of inactivating your chemotherapy. It has nothing to do with drug safety. Rather, the anticonvulsant stimulates your liver to degrade important drugs, such as the topotecan family of chemotherapy (CPT-11, Irinotecan).The effectiveness of CPT-11 chemotherapy was compromised in patients with brain tumors who were also taking anticonvulsant medication.[4] It is altogether possible that in patients who took Dilantin-like drugs, serum levels of CPT-11 never reached effective concentrations. That study[4] is now being analyzed comparing the blood levels of chemotherapeutic agents in patients who are on, or off Dilantin-like drugs. Many newer chemotherapy trials will not allow patients to be enrolled if they are on Dilantin-like drugs.

> Dilantin can inactivate your chemotherapy

Even some herbal medications like curcumin (the Indian spice called turmeric) can also inactivate chemotherapy (see Chapter 18: Complementary and Alternative Therapies.).

SYMPTOM-RELIEF MEDICATIONS

Symptom relief is my first topic, rather than jumping right to chemotherapy. Why? Let me tell you about the first patient whom I cared for as an oncology fellow in 1978.

Jimmy G was an 18-year-old Chinese-American student, who had a very supportive, extended family. He had a malignant germ cell tumor, which in 1978 was curable with intensive chemotherapy and radiation. He received outpatient, intravenous cisplatin for two months. We used the best anti-nausea medications available at the time: Benadryl, Compazine and Decadron. X-rays showed that his tumor had disappeared in response to the medication.

Bottom Line You are the CEO of your medical team. Your goal is to get the best care, make the wisest treatment choices and prevent mistakes.

Before he began the third monthly course, he announced that the nausea and vomiting was more than he could stand. "Death could not be more cruel," he said to me, and he refused any more chemotherapy. His parents said that they would talk to him at home about his decision. He died four months later of recurrent tumor.

> Symptom-relief medicines are not optional. They are critical to your success.

Cisplatin is one of the most nausea-producing drugs that we use to treat cancer. In 1990, Zofran became available and reduced nausea/vomiting by 80 to 100 percent. I have no doubt that Jimmy would be alive today if Zofran had been available. These medicines are not secondary or optional. They are essential to your success.

Table 19-2 Brain Tumors: Reasons for Taking Medications
Relief & prevention of nausea, vomiting.
Fighting cancer.
Stimulating the bone marrow.
Controlling infection with antibiotics.

The sections in this Chapter are organized according to the headings in Table 19-2.

NAUSEA AND VOMITING

Why Should I Take Anti-Emetics (to Prevent Nausea)?

Jimmy's experience taught me, first hand, how devastating symptoms can be. Many doctors neither understand nor witness the discomfort that their patients experience. That is why you must be vigilant and demand appropriate anti-

> Anticipatory nausea occurs at the thought of the drug; before getting to the clinic.

emetics. We now have at least three medications in a class called "5-HT receptor antagonists": Zofran, Kytril and Anzmet. Their use has profoundly changed the patient's experience of cancer treatment. Nonetheless, many people will experience *anticipatory* nausea and vomiting. Anticipatory means they vomit at the thought of the drug, or even on the way to the clinic or hospital. This affects compliance with taking the drug and can mean the difference between life and death.

The following post on the Temozolomide web site by Isabel illustrates how a change in chemotherapy drugs can completely change one's outlook and quality of life:

Kytril or Zofran? I can speak of Zofran. It has been awesome for me. I take 300 mg. of Temodar and used to be very sick with just compazine, and then I switched to Zofran. It has worked great for me. No constipation, but I eat prunes, high fiber diet, etc. The nurses I talk to say Senokot and Colace work great for the constipation, too.

Isabel, Jackson, MS. Oligo, diagnosed May 1, 2002.

Why Must I Be Proactive About Getting Effective Anti-Emetics?

There are two FDA-approved chemotherapy drugs for brain tumors: oral CeeNU (the intravenous form is called BiCNU); and Temodar. Nausea and vomiting occurred in more than 80 percent of patients who took them. The older anti-emetics, Thorazine and Compazine by pill or suppository, do not work for most patients. High-dose metoclopramide (Reglan) was used with better results in the way of nausea, but it frequently caused severe muscular spasms, particularly in those less than 30 years of age.

Health insurance companies prefer that their doctors prescribe older, less effective drugs because of cost – $0.50 to $1.00 per dose instead of $7.00 to $15.00 per dose. They require physicians to fill out additional forms and make a "special" request. Insurance and HMO administrators do not understand that nausea is not a *comfort* issue.

How Do Anti-Emetics Work?

Anti-emetics block the chemical-binding sites in the nausea and vomiting centers of your brain, called the "trigger zones" and in the nerves inside the intestine that give us a sickly feeling. No binding = no vomiting. People may have better results with one particular brand. Anti-emetics are effective in pill or intravenous form taken 30 to 60 minutes *before* chemotherapy. Sometimes a second pill is needed 12 to 24 hours after. Side effects can include headache (10 percent), constipation (4 percent) and rarely, allergy.

> Anti-emetics are effective in pill or IV form taken 30-60 minutes before chemotherapy.

The most common reason why the anti-emetics do not work is that people forget to take them! Some may not feel they are unnecessary, particularly if they had no side effects with the first round of chemotherapy. Do you really need to put your hand in the fire to see if it is hot? Enough said.

□Bottom Line→ You must demand that you receive the correct anti-emetic before your chemotherapy.

Who Is Responsible to Prevent Nausea and Vomiting?

Your oncologist or radiation therapist will usually be responsible for recommending and prescribing the anti-emetic medication. Your primary physician may participate, too. Make sure each doctor knows what he or she is responsible for and what your expectations are for effective treatment. The more you know and ask, the better off you will be. But even medication advice from medical professionals can sometimes be inaccurate or not up to date, as in the example below:

> Who will monitor you is important. HMOs may require test pre-authorizations.

The oncologist indicated that my dad had gotten sick (nausea/vomiting) during the last two five-day rounds of Temodar because he hadn't taken the Decadron with it. (He had been tapered off of Decadron after six weeks of radiation.) The doc said he should take the Decadron (not sure of the dosage) when he takes the Temodar. Dad was using Compazine for rounds two and three, but still got sick on day one of each round. I suggested that they ask about Zofran for the next round, but then they brought up this Decadron issue. Any input would be appreciated. Round four starts in a few weeks. Thanks.

> Anti-emetics often "do not work" because people forget to take them!

Eugene L., Visalia, CA

FATIGUE

See Chapter 9.[1]

PAIN

See Chapter 9.[1]

> Preventative anti-nausea medications can mean the difference between life and death.

STEROIDS

See also Chapter 9.[1]

ALLEVIATING SIDE EFFECTS OF CHEMOTHERAPY

Receiving chemotherapy often makes for a close partnership with your team physician. You must be in contact to report positive as well as negative, unwanted side effects. I have summarized six treatment suggestions that many patients have used to diminish or eliminate unwanted effects. You should discuss these actions with your physician *before* starting any (see Table 19-3).

Table 19-3 Strategies for Managing Chemotherapy Side Effects
1. Change the time of day that drugs are taken.
2. Spread intake throughout the day.
3. Switch medications: For nausea, try Zofran or Kytril. (Some people advocate lemon juice or fresh ginger root as well. Many physicians may not be acquainted with "alternative" methods. (See Chapter 18: Complementary, Alternative Therapies.)
4. Try "cold caps", to reduce hair loss. This may reduce blood flow to the scalp; and we do not know if this also reduces blood flow to the tumor. If so, it may inhibit the effectiveness of chemotherapy.
5. Be proactive. Join local or on-line discussion groups and get honest information from people who have been through chemotherapy.

FREQUENTLY ASKED QUESTIONS ABOUT CANCER AND CHEMOTHERAPY

Of the 1.2 million or so people in the United States who are diagnosed with cancer each year, 400,000 will undergo chemotherapy. Traditional chemotherapy medications can cure, heal, or injure. They are often accompanied by side effects – nausea, vomiting, fatigue, low blood counts, and hair loss. The good news is that both modern and ancient techniques can minimize these side effects; or in the case of nausea and vomiting, they can prevent them from occurring at all.

There is some overlap between this section and Chapter 17: Traditional Approaches to Treatments. This section stresses the administration, effects and side effects of common chemotherapy medications, while Chapter 17 discusses their applications and reasons for treatment.

WHAT IS A CANCER CELL?

Let us start with the basics about the cancer cell – the reason that you need to know about chemotherapy in the first place. A cancer cell is built like any other cell in your body (see Figure 19-1). It has an outer "skin" called the *cell membrane*. The cell communicates with the outside world through "receptors" on the membrane, in this case the lock and key for Transforming Growth Factor-β (TGF-B) is illustrated. There is an inner "sea" called *cytoplasm* in which proteins are made (from RNA) and later broken down, and energy is generated or used. Inside the sea is a "nucleus" and inside its *nuclear membrane* is the instructional programs for the genes (DNA) for activating cell division when it will split into daughter cells.

What is unique about a cancer cell? Its control signals (brakes) to stop dividing are not working; and its program to die is turned off. Thus, it becomes immortal.

How Do Chemotherapy Drugs Work?

Chemotherapy drugs interfere with cell functions at special locations inside the cell. Until recently, most chemotherapy was designed for other cancers and only belatedly tested with brain tumors. Drug developers are designing "smart" drugs that take advantage of unique targets on the brain cancer cell. For example, new drugs like Iressa and Tarceva bind to the epidermal growth factor (EGF) receptor on the glioma cell surface, which could stop its "grow and divide" message inside. Other drug combinations, like "P-C-V" and now Temodar, work well for grade 3 gliomas and oligodendrogliomas. However, we still do not know why.

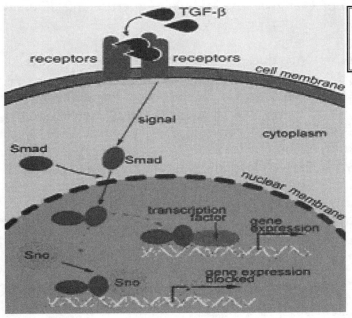

Iressa and Tarceva bind to the epidermal growth factor (EGF) receptor on the glioblastoma, which may stop the "grow and divide" message.

Figure 19-1

Bottom Line A cancer cell – control signals to stop dividing are not working; its program to die is turned off – it becomes immortal.

103

See Table 19-4 for the characteristics and challenges of ideal chemotherapy drugs that are specific for brain cancers (see also *Table 19-10* on Internet Resources.)

Table 19-4 Eight Major Challenges for Drugs to Be Effective in Brain Cancer
1. Being absorbed into the bloodstream
2. Binding to carriers in the blood
3. Reaching the tumor by blood flow
4. Crossing the blood tumor barrier (BTB)
5. Crossing the cell membrane into the cell
6. Not getting pumped out of the cell
7. Hitting the target inside the cell
8. Not damaging normal cells

WHAT IS DIFFERENT ABOUT MEDICATIONS FOR BRAIN TUMORS?

New symptoms or problems during treatment are a challenge. This is all the more reason to have a coordinated team, as described in Chapter 5: Doctors and other Team members.[1] Below are four examples of why broad expertise and different specialists are necessary:

1. Are changes in my symptoms due to the tumor or a side effect of treatments?
   • You become drowsy or have a seizure while taking Procarbazine and Dilantin. <u>It could be due to tumor, scar tissue, change in steroids or the chemotherapy.</u>
2. Was it a stroke, or weakness, or trouble thinking?
   • <u>It could be due to low platelets, a bleed into the tumor, growing tumor, or changed steroid dose.</u>
3. What is responsible for my low blood count during chemotherapy?
   • <u>It could be due to an anticonvulsant, the antibiotic Bactrim, other medications, infection, or foods.</u>
4. If an MRI scan shows a new "spot," does this mean tumor progression or necrosis?
   • <u>It could be due to a lowered steroid dosage, ineffective chemotherapy, bleeding, progress of tumor, or some other cause.</u>

Who Is Responsible for Supervising Your Chemotherapy?

Your (neuro)oncologist is responsible for schedules, blood monitoring, managing side effects, and prescriptions. Other doctors will often take direction from the oncologist during this time. The exception is the neurosurgeon who can place Gliadel wafers inside your tumor.

> Make sure each doctor knows for what he/she is responsible in your treatment.

What Medications Are Affected by Steroids?

You might be on steroids when you are taking chemotherapy. Steroids affect the blood levels of many drugs. Before you take any drug, tell your doctor which prescription and non-prescription medications you are taking, especially the following:
- Aspirin, arthritis medication.
- Anticoagulants ("blood thinners"), diuretics ("water pills").
- Female hormones (such as birth control pills), diabetes medication.
- Antibiotics, anti-seizure medications.

Do not start or stop taking any medicine without your physician's or pharmacist's approval. See also Chapter 9.[1]

Can You Receive Financial Assistance for Medications?

Frequently, your insurance will pay for part, if not all, of your bills. Major drug companies, worldwide, provide assistance in getting medications to those in need (Table 19-10). Many people are able to obtain medications free of charge by enrolling in a clinical trial (see also Chapter 23: Manging costs, benefits, and your healthcare with Insurance, HMOs and more...).

Chemotherapy May Affect Your Blood Counts. What Does This Mean?

Your chemotherapy doctor routinely will order several tests to monitor your blood cell counts, as a measure of your bone marrow reserve. Without these results, your therapy cannot be well managed. Know which physicians are keeping track of your blood

> Know which physicians are keeping track of your blood counts. Assign responsibility to one physician to discuss results with others.

counts. As chief executive officer (CEO) of your body, assign responsibility to one physician who will discuss the results with you and others. You can keep track of your blood counts in your notebook (see Chapter 3).[1]

Blood Count Guidelines: What Do I Need to Look Out for?

White Blood Cells (WBC)

These are the body's main defense against infection. You need not worry about increased risk of infection, unless your WBC count becomes very low. A special WBC, called a *neutrophil*, fights off bacteria. If the neutrophil cell count is "less than 500," you are *neutropenic* and at increased risk of infection. If this is the case, you may be treated with a medication, Neupogen, to raise the neutrophil count. And your chemotherapy may be stopped until the counts come back to normal.

> If the neutrophil cell count (ANC) is "less than 500," you are neutropenic & at increased risk of infection

Neutrophils, polys: You can calculate your Absolute Neutrophil Count, called ANC, by looking at your blood count results form (see Figure 19-2 for a sample CBC report).

In the example in Figure 19-2, the WBC = 5.2, which is 5,200 and your poly count is 40.1 percent.

The ANC calculation is 5,200 x 40.1 percent = 2085, so you are not neutropenic and could receive chemotherapy.

Figure 19-2   Sample Clinical Laboratory Report

Pt Name Smith, Jon Q.	Date Drawn 01/03/04	Date Received 01/03/04	Date of Report 01/04/04
TEST NAME	RESULT	UNITS	REFERENCE RANGE*
COMPLETE BLOOD COUNT W/ DIFFERENTIAL			
WBC	5.2	thous/cu.mm	3.9-11.1
RBC	3.51 L	Mil/cu.mm	4.20-5.70
HGB (HEMOGLOBIN)	14.5	g/dL	13.2-16.9
HCT (HEMATOCRIT)	41.2	Percent	38.5-49.0
MCV	117H	fl	80-97
MCH	41.4H	pg	27.5-33.5
MCHC	35.3	percent	32.0-36.0
RDW	11.8	percent	11.0-15.0
PLATELET COUNT	172	thous/cu.mm	140-390
MPV	7.6	fl	7.5-11.5
DIFFERENTIAL			
TOTAL NEUTROPHILS, %	40.1	percent	38.0-80.0
TOTAL LYMPHOCYTES, %	46.1	percent	15.0-49.0
MONOCYTES, %	12.9	percent	0.0-13.0
EOSINOPHILS, %	0.6	percent	0.0-8.0
BASOPHILS, %	0.3	percent	0.0-0.2
TOTAL NEUTROPHILS, (ANC) ABSOLUTE	2085	Cells/cu.mm	1650-800
TOTAL LYMPHOCYTES, (ALC) ABSOLUTE	2397	Cells/cu.mm	1000-3500
MONOCYTES, ABSOLUTE	671	Cells/cu.mm	40-900
EOSINOPHILS, ABSOLUTE	31	Cells/cu.mm	30-600
BASOPHILS, ABSOLUTE	16	Cells/cu.mm	0-125

ANC = [% neutrophils x your white cell count (WBC)].

Lymphocytes

These are another type of WBC and are listed under the differential count. Lymphs fight viruses and fungi. If these are low ("lymphopenic"), you can have infections that spread, like *shingles* or *pneumocystis pneumonia*. The calculation is performed the same way as in the ANC above. Some doctors will calculate your absolute lymphocyte count.

> Steroids incapacitate lymphocytes & weaken your immune system.

Red Blood Cells (RBC)

RBCs contain hemoglobin that carries oxygen to all parts of the body. If you have too few RBCs, your body may be oxygen-starved, and you may feel tired or nauseated. This condition is called *anemia*. We measure RBC levels by monitoring your hemoglobin or hematocrit (see Figure 19-2). If your hemoglobin is less than 8.0 or hematocrit is below 25 percent, you may need an RBC transfusion or RBC stimulant, like Epogen or Procrit, or wait for your counts to come up spontaneously before receiving more chemotherapy.

> Bactrim (2-3/week) prevents pneumonia if lymphocyte counts are low.

Platelets

These cells in the blood plug holes and help form a clot in response to injury. Without enough platelets, you may bruise or bleed easily. When platelet counts are less than 25,000-50,000, your doctors *might* consider giving you a platelet transfusion.

WHY MUST I AVOID ASPIRIN WHEN TAKING CHEMOTHERAPY?

Aspirin paralyzes blood platelets so that they do not plug holes that prevents bleeding. If other clotting factors are low, this compounds the problem even more. Tylenol is a safer alternative to aspirin, and Advil is usually considered safe as well.

> Aspirin paralyzes blood platelets so that they do not plug holes to prevent bleeding.

FIGHTING CANCER

CAUTIONS ABOUT RECEIVING THE NEWEST DRUG TO TREAT YOUR TUMOR

The Internet is buzzing with the latest "amaze-ocillin" that is curing cancer. Why won't your doctor prescribe it for you?

Some doctors may work work with you in using new or "off label" medications and complementary or alternative therapies. Other physicians are more conservative and reluctant to use untried methods (see example below). Many people with brain tumors are desperate for a solution, particularly if their tumor has recurred. But the latest new treatment may have a darker side. See the recent headline about Thalidomide below.

> *Thalidomide Associated with Blood Clots*
> *Thalidomide, used increasingly as an adjunct in cancer treatment because of its potent angiogenesis inhibitor activity, is being linked to a significant number of blood clots in cancer patients receiving the drug. Clots traveling to the lungs occurred approximately two months after starting thalidomide and at rates as high as 43 percent of patients. Thromboembolic events were much higher when thalidomide was given in combination with other types of chemotherapy.[5]*

CHARACTERISTICS OF COMMON CHEMOTHERAPY DRUGS

Table 19-5 condenses critical information that cannot be found easily in any one source. Supplemental information can be obtained from your doctor, brain tumor foundations or the web sites listed in Table 19-10. The common and trade names are presented as well as major side effects and important interactions with other drugs. A discussion of the individual medications follows the chart and are represented in order of the route of administration.

> Chemotherapy slows repair of mouth & intestinal tract & lowers neutrophil counts.

DIFFERENT WAYS OF ADMINISTERING CHEMOTHERAPY

Systemic – the pill or injected form travels through blood (system) to the tumor.

Regional – the drug is placed directly in or around the tumor.

Intrathecal – a form of regional therapy injected through the spine via a thin needle or into a small reservoir under the scalp that connects to the brain's ventricles via a thin tube.

Table 19-5   Chemotherapies Commonly Used for Brain Tumors

Generic name	Trade name, (strength)	Major side effects	Interactions
Carboplatin	Paraplatin intravenous	Low blood count, liver, hearing abnormalities	
Carmustine (intravenous) See Lomustine	BiCNU	Lung damage, serious, especially in patients treated as children	
Cisplatin	Platinol iv	Nausea, Vomiting Kidney damage Hearing loss Peripheral neuropathy Low white & red cell counts Low sodium, potassium levels	Radiation
Cyclophos-phamide	Cytoxan	Low blood counts Bladder irritation & bleeding, Sterility	
Cytosine Arabinoside	Cytosar-U	Low blood counts Brain-cerebellar inflammation	
Etoposide VP-16	Vespid	Leukemia Low blood pressure	
Irinotecan, CPT-11*	Camptosar	Diarrhea	Dilantin family antconvulsants Spices
Lomustine	CeeNU pills 10, 40,100 mg	Nausea Delayed low blood count Lung damage	Suspected interaction with Tagamet
Methotrexate	Mexate 2.5 mg	Low blood counts Brain damage if given after radiation Mouth & Intestine ulcers and sores	Radiation

			Foods Alcohol, Cheese, Yogurt, Bananas, Chocolate Medications: Amphetamines, Antihistamines, Isocarboxazid (Marplan), Phenelzine (Nardil), Tranylcypromine (Parnate), Selegiline (Eldepryl)
Procarbazine	Matulane 50 mg.	Nausea, Vomiting Fatigue, Rash Neuropathy, Tremors Coma, Seizures, Low blood counts Lung inflammation Interferes with Monamine Oxidase (MAO) inhibitors used for depression, Parkinson's Disease	
Tamoxifen	Nolvadex	Raised cholesterol levels Bloating	Blood clotting and thinning agents
Temozolomide	Temodar /Temodal 5,20,100,250 mg.	Fatigue Constipation Nausea Low blood counts	Suspected similarity to procarbazine, unproven
Vincristine	Oncovin 1mg liquid	Pain in arm, leg, jaw Constipation Paralysis	
PCV-procarbazine, CCNU, vincristine		See individual medications	See individual medications

* For on line information: http://www.nlm.nih.gov/medlineplus/druginformation.html

SYSTEMIC CHEMOTHERAPY DRUGS

WHAT IS PCV?

"P-C-V," is the abbreviation for a combination of three chemotherapy medications: <u>P</u>rocarbazine, <u>C</u>CNU, and <u>V</u>incristine. It is effective therapy for people with anaplastic astrocytomas[6] and oligodendrogliomas,[7] but not for glioblastoma multiforme (see Chapter 17:Traditional Approaches to Treatment). The three component drugs are discussed individually, below.

What Is Important to Know about Procarbazine?

1. For dosages not equal to whole tablets, either the 50-mg tablet can be split or whole pills can be taken on alternate days.
2. It penetrates well into the brain and cerebrospinal fluid.
3. For nausea, see anti-emetics earlier in this chapter.
4. It should be taken at the same time each day.
5. Doses for each course should be adjusted by preceding blood counts.
6. Blood cell toxicity appears in 7-14 days; cells can remain low for 14 to 28 days (see Table 19-7).
7. Dilantin and similar anticonvulsants in combination with Procarbazine may increase risk of allergic reactions.[8] This combination may also reduce key enzymes in the liver that detoxify certain "amines" (see below).
8. Foods that contain tyramine, such as red wine, veined cheeses, bananas, vanilla, and so forth, should be avoided because procarbazine prevents them from being broken down. Typical reactions after eating these foods include headache, flushed face, palpitations, nausea, vomiting, or a rise in blood pressure. (See Table 19-6 and references[9,10] for an extended food-avoidance list.)
9. Procarbazine can cause an unusual lung allergy that resembles pneumonia.

Table 19-6 Procarbazine: Foods to Avoid

- Cheese and cheese spreads (except: cottage or cream cheese, farmer's cheese)
- Dry or fermented sausage (including bologna, salami, & pepperoni)
- Meat or yeast extracts (such as Marmite, Vegemite, Bovril, Oxo, Brewer's yeast, miso)
- Broad beans (such as fava beans & Chinese pea pods)
- Alcoholic beverages (such as red wine, vermouth, & port)
- Smoked or pickled meat or fish
- Meat or fish that is not fresh (that may have started to spoil)

What Is Important to Know about CCNU, BCNU?

These two medications are FDA-approved in North America. BCNU, also known as BiCNU, is the intravenous form; CCNU (CeeNU) is the oral form. There has been limited comparative testing of these forms; CeeNU may be more potent and BiCNU may result in more lung toxicity. Many clinical trials have used BCNU, possibly because its use could be reimbursed under insurance and MediCare guidelines. The precautions below apply equally to both drug forms:

1. The dose should be prescribed for only one course at a time.
2. Both CeeNU and BiCNU cross the blood-brain barrier and enter spinal fluid.
3. Nausea and vomiting can be prevented by taking anti-emetics. (See discussion of anti-emetics earlier in this chapter.)
4. All pills should be taken at once, at the instructed time.
5. The second month's dose should be adjusted to blood counts after the preceding dose. Table 19-7 is a sample guide to dosage adjustment after the initial dose, according to white and platelet counts.
6. Toxicity to blood cells shows up in three to six weeks. Counts can remain low for six to twelve weeks after several courses.
7. Lung function tests should be performed after every other course.

Table 19-7 Sample Guidelines for Blood Count & Dosing Changes During Chemotherapy			
Lowest Count After Previous Dose			Percentage Of Prior Dose To Use For Next Dose
White cells	(ANC) Absolute Neutrophil	Platelets	
4000	> 2500	100,000	100
3000-3999	> 1000	75,000-99,999	100
2000-2999	Between 750-999	25,000-74,999	50-75 or Physician judgment
Less than 2000	Between 500-749	Less than 25,000	25-50 or Physician judgment
Less than 1000	Less than 500	Less than 10,000	Physician judgment

What Is Important to Know about Vincristine?

1. It must be given intravenously. The maximum dose is usually 2.0 mg.
2. It can cause a severe burn, loss of skin & pain if it leaks into the skin.
3. It rarely causes nausea or vomiting.
4. It is not toxic to blood cells or bone marrow.

5. It can produce significant constipation. A high fiber diet, lots of liquids and daily Colace can help. No bowel movements for five to 10 days are common.
6. Doses after the initial course should be adjusted by blood count levels, degree of constipation or pain in the jaw, arm, leg, and abdomen.
7. Neuropathy (pain, weakness, paralysis) in legs takes months for recovery.

What Is Important to Know about Temozolomide (Temodar)?

1. FDA-approved for new and recurrent grade 3 astrocytomas and oligodendrogliomas and Glioblastone multiforme.
2. Penetrates well into the brain and cerebrospinal fluid.
3. Pills come in four strengths: 5, 20, 100, and 250 mg. Be careful to check that you are receiving the right dose when you pick up your medications.
4. Take the pills at once, whole, on an empty stomach, preferably at bedtime.
5. For young children or anyone with a feeding tube, place the contents of the capsule in water or applesauce and give immediately. Use gloves when handling broken pills. (Chemotherapy is toxic; can be absorbed in your skin!)
6. Major toxicities: nausea, vomiting, constipation, fatigue, low blood counts in 5-10 percent of patients.
7. Nausea and vomiting are more than 95 percent preventable.
8. Low blood counts are dose-limiting but predictable.
   • White cell and platelet counts bottom out in three weeks on a five-day-per-month schedule.
   • Dose-limiting low platelet counts persist for 7-42 days.
9. Forty-one percent of patients will have low lymphocyte counts and 15 percent of patients will show dangerously low lymphocyte counts on a five-day-per-month schedule. Low lymphocyte counts correlate with dangerous types of pneumonia like *pneumocystis*. Bactrim antibiotic is recommended if lymphocyte count is low.

> Check your lymphocyte counts on Temodar. Take Bactrim/Septra if they become low.

10. Doses after the initial 28-day course are adjusted according to blood counts.
11. Lethargy and fatigue occur in 32 percent of malignant glioma patients.[11]
12. Allergies with Procarbazine have not been reported with Temodar.
13. One report of Dilantin toxicity in patients on Temodar.[12]

Bottom Line → Temodar comes in strengths of: 5, 20, 100, and 250 mg. Check that you are receiving the right dose.

What Is Important to Know about Platinum-Based Drugs (Cisplatin, and Carboplatin)?

1. Cisplatin combinations with etoposide, ifosfamide or bleomycin, have been valuable in the treatment of medulloblastoma, primitive neuroectodermal tumors (PNETs) and metastatic germ cell tumors.
2. Cisplatin and carboplatin are given intravenously.
3. Carboplatin-vincristine combination has been used for low-grade gliomas and PNETs.
4. Cisplatin causes major hearing toxicity. Hearing tests or "brain stem evoked potentials" should be performed before every (other) course.
5. Cisplatin causes major kidney damage. Kidney function tests should be taken before each course.
6. Carboplatin penetrates the blood-brain barrier better than cisplatin. There is no proof whether or not it is more effective.
7. Cisplatin is a nausea-producing drug; nausea can be alleviated or prevented. See anti-emetics above. Delayed nausea occurs days later
8. Doses to be adjusted to blood counts, kidney function, & hearing tests.
9. Low blood cell counts show up at 7-14 days, remaining low for four weeks.
10. Carboplatin doses are predicted according to a special (Calvert) formula that uses a measure of kidney function.
11. Hydration before / after cisplatin, with added mannitol will promote urine flow and partially protect the kidneys.
12. Evening, not morning, cisplatin may have less kidney damage.
13. Amifostine, glutathione, and thiosulfate *may* protect against cisplatin toxicity.

> Cisplatin has serious kidney and hearing side effects.

What Is Important to Know about the Mustard Drug Family: Thiotepa Cyclophosphamide, Ifosfamide, Melphalan, Nitrogen Mustard?

1. Nitrogen mustard was a poison gas in World War 1.
2. Most are administered intravenously and become activated after passing through the liver. They penetrate well into brain and cerebrospinal fluid.
3. They are used in treatment of PNETs and recurrent childhood tumors.
4. Cyclophosphamide and ifosfamide can cause severe hemorrhage in the bladder. Large amounts of intravenous and oral fluids, and sometimes a bladder-protectant called *acetylcysteine*, can prevent this complication.
5. Mustards produce significant nausea. See discussion of anti-emetics earlier in the chapter and Chapter 9.[1]
6. Doses after the initial course are adjusted according to blood counts.
7. Toxicity to blood cells shows up in 7-10 days. Counts remain low 2-4 weeks.
8. They can cause sterility, second cancers, and scarring of the lung.

What Is Important to Know about Methotrexate (Mexate)?

1. Methotrexate is FDA-approved for treating choriocarcinoma and lymphomas.
2. Methotrexate (and Ara C, and possibly VP-16) have increased the five-year survival rate for lymphoma to about 50 percent.
3. It comes in both pill (2.5 mg.) and injectable forms.
4. Take the pills at once, on an empty stomach, preferably at bedtime.
5. It usually does not cause nausea.
6. Low doses (12-30 mg per week) penetrate poorly into the brain and cerebrospinal fluid.
7. Brain toxicity is unique. If given *after* radiation to the brain, it can cause damage and poor mental functioning. Methotrexate given before radiation usually is not a problem.
8. Major toxicities at low doses can cause mouth and anal sores, lowered blood counts, and liver damage.
9. For central nervous system lymphoma, methotrexate is given at 100-1000 times the usual dosage (3000-15,000 mg intravenously. This dosage penetrates the brain and cerebrospinal fluid and requires blood level monitoring for 3-5 days. An Infusion of the drug leucovorin (similar to the vitamin folic acid) "rescues" the normal cells.

> For central nervous system lymphoma, methotrexate is given at 100-1000 times the usual dosage.

10. Doses after the initial course are adjusted according to blood counts.
11. Blood cell toxicity occurs in 7-14 days. Counts are low for 2-4 weeks.
12. Methotrexate can be given regionally (via intrathecal route). See section under intrathecal therapy.

What Is Important to Know about Cytosine Arabinoside (Ara-C)?

1. Given by intravenous or intrathecal route.
2. Treatment of leukemia, lymphoma, spinal metastases, and germ cell tumors.
3. Penetrates well into the brain and cerebrospinal fluid.
4. Can cause nausea and vomiting. See section on anti-emetics.
5. Doses after the initial course are adjusted according to blood counts.
6. Blood cell toxicity occurs in 7-14 days. Counts remain low 2-4 weeks.

What is Important to Know about Etoposide (VP-16)?

1. Comes in 50 mg pills or in a liquid that can be swallowed or injected.
2. Used to treat germ cell tumors of the testicle and ovary, CNS lymphomas, recurrent oligodendrogliomas, and childhood PNETs.
3. Penetrates poorly into the brain and cerebrospinal fluid.

4. Can cause vomiting. See discussion of anti-emetics in this chapter.
5. Doses after the initial 14 days are adjusted according to blood counts.
6. Toxicity to blood cells shows up in 7-14 days.
7. Intravenous administration can cause a drop in blood pressure, if there has not been prior adequate liquid intake.

What Is Important to Know about the Campothecin Family (Topotecan, Irinotecan?

1. Includes topotecan (Hycamtin) and irinotecan (Camptosar, CPT-11) which are administered intravenously.
2. Irinotecan is being studied to treat adult gliomas and colon cancer.
3. Penetrates well into the brain and cerebrospinal fluid.
4. Can cause nausea and vomiting. See discussion of anti-emetics.
5. Toxicity to blood cells shows up in 7-14 days.
6. Doses after the initial course are adjusted according to blood counts.
7. Dilantin and related chemotherapy can *interfere* with drug effects.
8. Toptecans can cause delayed diarrhea.
    • Early onset of diarrhea can be prevented by premedication with atropine at 0.25-1.0 mg by intravenous injection.
    • Later onset diarrhea is treated with loperamide (Imodium) as 4 mg, then 2 mg every 2 hours until the problem ceases.

Anti-Estrogens (Tamoxifen) and How They Work

Tamoxifen (Nolvadex) is an anti-estrogen drug designed to reduce or stop the action of the female hormone, estrogen. Think of this process as a "lock and key" mechanism. Cell surface receptors are the locks and the female hormones are the keys. When hormones come into contact with receptors, they unlock or activate the cancer cells' message to divide. Tamoxifen imitates hormone activity and fits into the lock, but the key does not turn and the cells do not divide. The tamoxifen key remains in place, so that estrogen is prevented from reaching the cancer cells. This results in slowing or stopping cancer cell growth. The effect of anti-estrogens on brain tumors like meningiomas may be different than that for gliomas, however.[13]

REGIONAL CHEMOTHERAPY

In regional or local chemotherapy, drugs are placed inside or around the tumor. This approach is designed to overcome the major disadvantage of "systemic" delivery to the tumor – toxicity to blood, liver, and kidneys.

Gliadel Wafers

Gliadel is a BCNU impregnated wafer. Neurosurgeons place BCNU-impregnated biodegradable wafers (the size of a quarter) into a tumor cavity without need to consult with a (neuro) oncologist. Up to eight wafers can be placed at one time.

> Gliadel is a local therapy placed inside the tumor at the time of surgery.

1. FDA-approved for recurrent and newly diagnosed *glioblastoma multiforme*.
2. BCNU leeches out of wafer into the tumor over 2-14 days; wafers are later resobsorbed.
3. BCNU concentration in the tumor area is 5-10 times that reached by intravenous routes.
4. Gliadel does not cause systemic symptoms: nausea, low blood counts, or lung toxicity.
5. For practical purposes, it is a one-time therapy.
6. Delayed healing, brain swelling, and skin infections are reported.
7. Gliadel wafer increased survival time about eight weeks.[14]

INTRATHECAL (IT) CHEMOTHERAPY

Intrathecal chemotherapy is a regional therapy injected either through the spine via a thin needle or into a small reservoir under the scalp which is connected to the brain's ventricles through a thin tube. It is used in the treatment of primary or metastatic brain tumors, which have leptomeningeal spread (along the coverings of the spinal cord) or are floating in cerebrospinal fluid (CSF). This condition, also called "neoplastic meningitis," occurs in 2-7 percent of all adult cancers.[15]

> Intrathecal therapy is injected through a spinal tap or into a reservoir under the scalp.

Useful drugs for intrathecal chemotherapy include methotrexate (Mexate), thiotepa (Thioplex in the mustard family), cytosine arabinoside (Ara-C or Cytosar), and DepoCyte. The latter is a long acting form of Ara-C, approved for the treatment of nervous system leukemia and lymphoma.

What Is Important about Intrathecal Methotrexate (Mexate) and Cytosine Arabinoside (Ara-C or Cytosar)?

1. Both are liquids injected though a spinal needle or into a reservoir.
2. Adult intrathecal therapy doses are 12-15 mg methotrexate, and 25-100 mg cytosine arabinoside, given in 5-10 cc. volume (1 to 2 tsp.) twice a week. A steroid may be included to reduce inflammation.

3. Combination of methotrexate, steroid and Ara-C is called "triple intrathecal therapy."
4. The drugs circulate and penetrate around the brain and cerebrospinal fluid and later diffuse into the blood stream.
5. This therapy has been successful in treating nervous system leukemia and lymphoma. It is also effective for neoplastic meningitis from melanoma and cancers of the breast, lung, colon, and ovaries.
6. Forty percent of patients will experience side effects such as sterile *meningitis* (inflammation reaction of the coverings of the brain and spinal cord). It occurs two-24 hours after injection and includes nausea, fever, stiff neck, backache, headache, and rarely convulsions.
7. Cytosine arabinoside can also cause cerebellar inflammation, resulting in difficulty in walking and standing.
8. Methotrexate can be toxic to blood cells because it diffuses back into the blood stream. Should this occur, oral folinic acid, also called leucovorin "rescue," is usually prescribed?
9. Ulcers can appear in the mouth or anus 3-7 days after administration.
10. With previous radiation therapy to the brain, careful consideration of intrathecal methotrexate therapy is warranted, with informed consent, because of the increased risk of degenerative brain disease.
11. The side effects of cytosine arabinoside are similar to those of methotrexate except that its effects on radiated brain are less likely.

What Is Important to Know about DepoCyte?

DepoCyte is FDA-approved for treating neoplastic meningitis caused by lymphoma or leukemia. It is cytosine arabinoside encapsulated in small fat-like droplet *micelles* that cause a "slow release" and minimize toxicity. It can be given once every two weeks instead of twice a week.

> DepoCyte is a treatment for neoplastic meningitis of lymphoma. It is a long acting form of Ara-C.

1. DepoCyte comes in ready-to-use vials: 50 mg Ara-C at 10 mg/mL.
2. Patients receiving DepoCyte should receive dexamethasone to lessen symptoms of "sterile meningitis" (see above). These symptoms occur in 100 percent of cycles without dexamethasone versus 33 percent of cycles with dexamethasone. If untreated, "sterile meningitis" can be fatal.
3. There is a survival advantage of people treated with DepoCyte compared with cytosine arabinoside.

What Is Important to Know about Intrathecal Thiotepa (Thioplex)?

1. It is approved for neoplastic meningitis caused by the most common carcinomas, such as lung, ovary and breast.
2. Common adult dose is 10 mg in 5-10 cc. (1 to 2 teaspoons) weekly.
3. Administration and side effects are similar to those of Ara-C.
4. Patients receiving thiotepa should also receive dexa methasone.

Prevention of Problems With Regional Intrathecal Chemotherapy

The major side effects of regional intrathecal chemotherapy are a) chemical meningitis or arachnoiditis (inflammation) and b) infectious meningitis. There are simple guidelines that will lessen the chance of chemical (sterile) meningitis.[16] You should discuss these with your doctor before the drugs are administered:

1. Be monitored by a skilled nurse or physician during the drug infusion.
2. The drugs *must* be mixed/diluted properly before injection. If not dissolved, it causes irritation. The diluting liquid (saline and water) must not contain preservative that can cause inflammation.
3. Slow injection (5-15 min.) is preferable to one less than 5 mins. The reasons for rapid injection, whether through spinal tap or intra-ventricular pathways, are mainly economic: the cancer center or physician can see more patients, rather than sitting with you for 20-30 minutes. Once the needle is in, there is no additional pain by taking a longer time for infusion (5-10 minutes versus one minute).

> Slower intrathecal injections (5-15 min.) are preferable to quick ones (< 5 minutes).

4. Infection prevention requires meticulous attention to scrubbing the injection site (skin over the reservoir or backbone). That means applying anti-bacterial soap or iodine-containing scrubs, wiping with alcohol to remove any residue, and letting the area dry before a needle for anesthetic is used. A less-experienced individual may not adhere to these techniques of sterilization.
5. This should not be a painful procedure. There are anesthetic creams (ELA-Max) that are applied to the skin 30 minutes before the injection. This should dull or eliminate the needle-stick pain. If the doctor or nurse does not know about this (it has been available since 2001), ask them to obtain it for you.

Responsibilities During and After Intrathecal Chemotherapy

The doctor who orders and injects the medication is responsible for the effects of the drug and any of its side effects: infection, pain, fever, and so forth. One can have a painful reaction or an infection as a complication, even with the best of techniques. Nonetheless, to increase the odds in your favor be proactive. Before

Bottom Line ▶ The doctor who orders and injects the medication is responsible to care for the effects of the drug and any of its side effects.

you have the procedure, ask these questions (see Table 19-8):

Table 19-8 Questions to Ask about Intrathecal Therapy
1. How many intrathecal therapy infusions has the doctor performed?
2. Which sterile technique will he or she use?
3. Whom do you call, if there are any side effects?
4. How can you reach that person 24 hours a day?
5. When you will get blood counts? Who will order and authorize them?
6. Are steroids being used to reduce inflammation?
7. What pain medications can you have for headache or backache?

BONE MARROW STIMULANTS

FREQUENTLY ASKED QUESTIONS

How Do They Work?

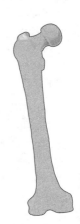

The bone marrow is the factory inside long bones and the spine where most blood cells are born and released. Marrow stimulants are natural or synthetic chemicals that signal the early marrow cells (red cells, neutrophils, or platelets) to divide and multiply into mature cells. This causes their levels in the blood to rise.

What Benefit Do Marrow Stimulants Offer Me?

Chemotherapy treatment can cause a drop in levels of red and white blood cells and/ or platelets because of slower marrow (factory) production. Which cells may be affected is not always predictable for the individual patient, although certain drugs may cause more white cell versus platelet effects. Toxicity occurs more frequently after several cycles of chemotherapy; it is cumulative. Marrow stimulants could prevent complications of anemia, infection or bleeding. See Table 19-9 for a summary of indications and side effects.

> Marrow stimulants signal early marrow cells to divide into mature red cells, neutrophils, or platelets.

Only red cells and platelets are available for transfusion,

Only red cells and platelets are available for transfusion, but this brings its own dangers, albeit rare, of infection (AIDS, hepatitis) and allergic reactions. Marrow stimulants avoid these dangers from occurring, because no transfusion is needed.

Who Is Responsible for My Care While I Am on Marrow Stimulants?

The oncologist or neurooncologist who prescribes chemotherapy and marrow stimulants usually will be responsible for monitoring blood counts, side effects and regulating dosages.

Table 19-9 Indications and Side Effects of Blood and Marrow Stimulants		
Indication/ Condition	Product	Side effects
Low neutrophil counts (white blood cells that fight infection and eat bacteria)	G-CSF Neupogen Neulasta (a long acting G-CSF)	Bone pain Difficulty breathing Rupture of spleen
Low neutrophil count	GM- CSF Leukine (used in marrow harvesting for transplantation)	Fever Chills Swolen feet/ lower legs Sudden weight gain Rapid or irregular pulse
Anemia-low red cell count (affects oxygen delivery to tissues)	Epogen Procrit (both raise red blood cell levels)	High blood pressure Blood clots
Low platelets/ Bleeding (plug holes in blood vessels and form the initial clot)	Neumega (IL-11) can raise platelet levels	Swollen feet or hands Difficult breathing Irregular heart rhythm Stroke
Lymphocytes make antibodies or kill viruses, fungus, and tumor cells.	No stimulant available at this time.	

RED BLOOD CELL STIMULANTS

People with anemia feel tired, sleep more, have decreased energy, become short of breath or have headaches.

Procrit and Epogen (erythropoietins) are red blood cell stimulants and are injected intravenously or under the skin. Their strength is expressed in the number of (U)nits. In two large trials (more than

5000 people), one weekly dosage increased hemoglobin levels, improved quality of life, and decreased transfusion needs.[17,18]

WHY DO WE NEED THEM?

People who have lower red blood cell (RBC) levels are anemic. They may feel tired, sleep more, have decreased energy, become short of breath, have headaches, or notice heart pounding.

AVOIDING PROBLEMS WITH RED BLOOD CELL STIMULANTS

Major side effects of red blood cell stimulants are high blood pressure and blood clots in the legs, but these are relatively rare (less than 1 percent of all patients treated). Erythropoietin therapy is used only with hematocrit levels below 36 percent; treatment is stopped when levels become greater than 40 percent during therapy.

> Side effects of red cell stimulants are high blood pressure and blood clots.

WHITE CELL STIMULANTS

WHY DO WE NEED THEM? WHAT DO THEY DO?

Chemotherapy drugs harm all cells, particularly actively dividing ones. A neutrophil, also called "poly" [short for *poly-morphonuclear leukocyte*] is one type of white cell, lives for only 6 to 12 hours, and poof! Gone. It is the most rapidly dividing of all cells and, if the factory slows down, is the first to be affected. Polys are the major defense system against bacteria that penetrate skin and linings of the mouth and intestines.

The chance of serious infection increases as neutrophils levels drop "below 500." "*Neutropenic*" means that your absolute neutrophil count (ANC), or percentage of neutrophils multiplied by the total white cell count, is less than 500. Below 250, the danger of infection is even greater.

> Neutrophil white cells are a major defense against bacteria.

Until the development of G-CSF, Neupogen, there was no medical way to increase white blood cell levels; it was not practical to transfuse them. The "G" CSFs stimulate the early marrow cells to make a "decision" to become neutrophils.

Currently, three drugs stimulate white blood cells: G-CSF (granulocyte-colony stimulating factor) or filogastrim (Neupogen), a longer acting Neupogen (Neulasta), and GM-CSF or sargramostim (Leukine). G-CSF is usually recommended because it has fewer side effects.

AVOIDING PROBLEMS WITH WHITE BLOOD CELL STIMULANTS

The major side effect of white blood cell stimulants is bone pain. Cells are made in the bone marrow and when the marrow space enlarges to produce the cells, it puts pressure on the bone covering (periosteum) that has pain-sensitive nerve fibers. Less frequent side effects are joint ache, chills and fever, rash, and muscle aches. Ibuprofen (Advil) or acetaminophen (Tylenol) usually relieves the discomfort.

> A major side effect of white blood cell stimulants is bone pain.

EVIDENCE FOR EFFECTIVENESS OF WHITE CELL STIMULANTS AND PAYMENTS

The American Society of Clinical Oncology (ASCO) guidelines state:

> ...routine use of CSFs in all neutropenic patients is not recommended, but preventative use in neutropenic patients _may_ reduce hospital stay and possibly increase cost savings.[19]

This waffling on the issue with "may" is contradictory to scientific proof of the effectiveness of white blood cell stimulants in patients with fever, neutropenia, and a risk factor: pneumonia, hypotension, fungal infection, or multi-organ system dysfunction. It is also a reason that insurance companies use to deny coverage.

BENEFITS AND INSURANCE COVERAGE FOR WHITE BLOOD CELL STIMULANTS

There is no question that G-CSF raises the blood neutrophil count. It also mobilizes marrow cells for re-transfusion after powerful chemotherapy.[20] What is less clear is its benefit on survival. Few studies have been done regarding their effectiveness, specifically with brain tumor patients.[21] The major problem has been knowing when to use it, managing side effects, and its high cost. If cost were not an issue, these drugs would be used more, even when their benefit may not be

> G-CSF can raise the neutrophil count. Less clear is its benefit on survival.

so clear. Once these issues are addressed, G-CSF holds the promise of saving tens of thousands of lives every year from the infection-related side effects.

The American Society of Clinical Oncology (ASCO) guidelines are used by some insurance companies as the basis for their reimbursement policies.[22] One guideline states:

> *Primary administration of CSFs is NOT recommended for previously untreated patients receiving most chemotherapy regimens. Primary administration of CSFs should be reserved for patients with an expected incidence of febrile neutropenia of 40 percent or greater.*

The problem is that patients are almost always in the "gray zone" – where things are not clear-cut. Insurance companies and HMOs are asking your doctor to guess whether his or her treatment has a 40 percent (39 percent Vs 41 percent) chance of resulting in low white cell counts and fever! On the contrary, your physician does not want to take a chance that could cost you your life. He (or she) either will want you to have the treatment or not; in other words, you will not

> Insurance companies/HMOs ask your doctor to guess whether treatment has a 40% chance of low white cell counts and fever!

be regarded by your physician as a 40 percent risk. You will be treated as either a 0 percent or 100 percent risk.

You may want to use the following information with the references to fight an insurance denial, if that occurs:

> *Adding G-CSF to antibiotic therapy in high-risk, chemotherapy-induced, febrile neutropenic patients significantly reduced the average hospital stay, median cost of hospital stay, duration of antibiotic therapy, and duration of grade IV neutropenia, compared with patients who received antibiotics alone.[23] In another study, continuous G-CSF reduced hematologic toxicity in 22 patients receiving vinorelbine and carboplatin for brain metastases.[24]*

PLATELET STIMULANTS

THE PROBLEM OF THROMBOCYTOPENIA (LOW PLATELET COUNTS)

A devastating side effect of chemotherapy is poor platelet production. Traditional replacement for platelets has been by transfusion of individual units from blood donors or one large transfusion extracted from one donor. The latter is called a "pheresis," or machine extraction of *single-donor* platelets. This method provides platelets but has significant disadvantages to the recipient: possible allergic (transfusion) reactions; potential infection; and shorter platelet survival.

Pros and Cons of Platelet Stimulants

IL-11(Oprelvekin, Neumega) an FDA-approved platelet stimulator, is an artificially produced hormone, similar to normal IL-11, which is derived from skin cells called fibroblasts. Neumega can definitely stimulate the body's own production of platelets, but its use has been moderated by the severity of its side effects.[25,26] Given that it causes fluid retention and can increase a clotting protein in the blood called fibrinogen, it would seem a higher-risk drug, specifically for brain tumor patients who already are prone to blood clots.

There are no studies on the use of platelet growth stimulants with brain tumor patients. The decision to use it, or not, should be between you and your physician.

INFECTIONS AND ANTIBIOTICS

Frequently Asked Questions

Why Are You Susceptible to Infections?

All of us have been on antibiotics for upper respiratory, sinus, skin, or urinary tract infections. When the immune system is depressed by chemotherapy, the decisions about antibiotics take on a new and more serious context. The reason is that our relationship with the germs in our environment has changed. In the "healthy" state,

- Our skin barriers are intact.
- Our neutrophils can gobble up bacteria that penetrate our gums or skin.
- Our lymphocytes (white cells) make antibodies to protect us against new infections.

Chemotherapy changes all this. It slows the repair of skin in our mouth and intestinal tract and can lower our neutrophil count. Furthermore, steroids make our lymphocytes less effective or make them leave the circulation. That is why we are more susceptible to infection. In addition, after you take one antibiotic to clear an infection, the "good" bacteria in your gut and on your skin are reduced. This allows the more resistant and dangerous ones to multiply, such as "staph" and fungi.

Why Are You Taking Antibiotics?

The simple answer is that you have an infection from which you may not recover without them, and the "bug" is sensitive to the antibiotic. Most frequently, antibiotics are prescribed when you have a fever or are neutropenic (low on neutrophils) and you are at risk of septicemia or sepsis ("blood poisoning"). Many different and effective antibiotic combinations are available, depending upon your doctor's experience and choice. This chapter will not discuss specific antibiotics.

When Should You Take Prophylactic (Preventive) Antibiotics?

A prophylactic antibiotic is given to prevent an infection. This is not useful most of the time and leads to the development of resistant bacteria that have become more difficult to treat. For example, antibiotics like penicillin and amoxicillin have been prescribed in the treatment of colds and viral respiratory infections, even though they are ineffective against viruses. The consequence of this practice is that now common forms of bacteria, such as *pneumococcus*, staph, and strep, have become resistant and require increasingly stronger antibiotics to control them.

Some people with brain tumors will have the need for prophylactic Septra or Bactrim (sulfamethoxazole/trimethoprim). Those at higher risk for infection have one or more of the following: radiation therapy, steroids, a low lymphocyte counts, or chemotherapy. Several people taking Temodar contracted a dangerous type of pneumonia called *pneumocystis carinii*. This is a protozoan (one-cell germ) infection that rapidly progresses in hours, and is not responsive to most antibiotics. In adults and children with cancer, Bactrim or Septra two to three times a week can prevent it.

Anticipating and Avoiding Problems with Prophylactic Antibiotics

Remind your doctor if you have any risk factors for its use:
1. Radiation therapy
   - Steroids
   - Low lymphocyte counts
   - Temodar or other chemotherapy
2. Bactrim or Septra can make you sensitive to sunlight. Use sun block.

3. There is a significant interaction of Septra/ Bactrim with Dilantin
   • This can cause liver function tests to become elevated.
   • The combination lowers neutrophil counts/causes vitamin B6-like anemia.
3. Get frequent blood counts to monitor your ANC.
4. Monitor Dilantin levels regularly (monthly) to check if in therapeutic range.

You may want to review Chapter 17: Treatments, for information specific to your type of tumor. Chapter 20 reviews the side effects and late effects of the treatments. Lastly, the web references are a rich source of information (see Table 19-10).

Table 19-10 Web Sites for Medication Information

Blood test interpretation	http://web2.iadfw.net/uthman/lab_test.html
Drug information	http://www.nlm.nih.gov/medlineplus/druginfo/uspdi/203051.html http://www.bccancer.bc.ca/pg_g_05.asp?PageID=22&ParentID=4 (Canada) http://www.bccancer.bc.ca/PPI/CancerTreatment/CancerDrugsGeneralInformationforPatients/DrugsWork.htm http://www.bccancer.bc.ca/HPI/DrugDatabase/DrugIndexPt/default.htm www.virtualtrials.com http://brain.mgh.harvard.edu/ChemoGuide.htm www.chemocare.com
Drug Interactions between drugs	http://health.discovery.com/encyclopedias/checker/checker.jsp?&jspLetter=B http://www.drugstore.com/pharmacy/drugchecker/default.asp?aid=333158&aparam=MS NFS_discount_prescriptions http://www.nowfoods.com/index.php/Drug-Safety-Check/Home/cat_id/2534 http://www.drugstore.com/pharmacy/drugchecker/default.asp?aid=333158&aparam=MS NFS_discount_prescriptions
Interactions between drugs, herbal, and dietary supplements	http://my.webmd.com/medical_information/drug_and_herb/default.htm http://www.nowfoods.com/index.php/Drug-Safety-Check/Home/cat_id/2534
Marrow stimulants	http://www.biologictherapy.org/aboutbiotherapy/about_cytokines_hema_gcsf.html
Medication access and cost-reduction	http://www.helpingpatients.org
Medication error prevention	http://www.ahrq.gov/consumer/20tipkid.htm http://www.ucp.org/ucp_channeldoc.cfm/1/11/54-54/4276
Morphine drug doses	http://www.stat.washington.edu/TALARIA/table10.html
NIH drug information site	http://www.nlm.nih.gov/medlineplus/druginfo/uspdi/203051.html

Table 19-10 Web Sites for Medication Information (continued)

Pain & other symptoms-discussions	http://www.cancernetwork.com/journals/primary/p9511e.htm http://www.cancersymptoms.org http://www.wellnessweb.com/pain/pain.htm
Pain ladder	http://www.wellnessweb.com/pain/who_ladder__of_pain_control.htm
Pain treatment	http://www.wellnessweb.com/pain/pain.htm http://www.acponline.org/public/h_care/3-pain.htm http://www.drugs.com/percodan.html
Patient Safety Institute	www.ptsafety.org
Seizures	http://www.intelihealth.com/IH/ihtIH/WSIHW000/9339/10075.html

CHAPTER 20

Early & Later Side Effects of Treatment, or of the Brain Tumor

There comes a time when we have to pick up the pieces, do damage control, and move forward- living with the emotional and financial consequences of the diagnosis.

John, a brain tumor survivor, Burlington, VT.

Tumor necrosis: Why is this a problem?
Neuropsychological effects: Memory and personality
Overcoming the effects of radiation on memory

THE DISGUISED DISABILITY

SURVIVOR'S GUILT

WILL LIFE EVER RETURN TO NORMAL?
"Was" and "Is"
Help with care giving
Coping with lingering side effects

⚿ Key search words

- blood clot
- frontal lobe
- paralysis
- steroid
- hypothyroidism
- late effect

- brain damage
- cerebellar mutism
- seizures
- hormones
- quality of life
- side effect

- dementia
- hydrocephalus
- necrosis
- sexual function
- hospice

Your brain is not just a collection of nerve cells and neural networks. It defines who you are in a distinctive way – your interests, personality, mood and outlook. Treatments to the brain uniquely affect each person. The effects can make some

> Treatment for brain tumors can have dramatic after-effects on daily activities & quality of life.

of your simple daily activities more difficult: choosing what to wear, dressing yourself as quickly as you used to, making a cup of coffee without having to think about it, understanding a friend's joke or even recognizing your loved ones. These may be short term, but some might last. Thus, it is important to really understand choices and risks so that you will not wish later that you had done something differently.

Each of us faces issues about aging and recognizing limitations, a scary journey by itself. But often it is life that is the scary journey and not just one particular challenge. This uncomfortable journey about brain tumors and serious side effects is just a part of the life challenge that with knowledge and help can be less scary!

Patricia McGrath, Ontario, Canada

This chapter includes information about common, short-term, and usually reversible side effects that you might experience in addition to the late effects that can develop months to years after treatment and may be more permanent. I will also be candid about items such as sexuality and quality of life, which are often not discussed between patient and physician. For listings of specific drug side effects, including chemotherapy, see Chapter 19: Cancer-Fighting Medications, and Chapter 9:Medications for Pain, Fatigue, Brain Swelling and Seizures in the companion book.[1] Let's start with the most frequently asked questions about side or after effects of treatment.

FREQUENTLY ASKED QUESTIONS

SHOULD YOU MAKE TREATMENT DECISIONS BASED ON ADVERSE SIDE EFFECTS?

We are incredibly lucky to live at a time when so many previously life-ending diseases, like cancer, can be treated so we can continue to live longer and better. In a strange way, it is a luxury to be alive to experience the after-effects of cancer therapy. Fortunately, symptoms like skin swelling from radiation or low blood counts from chemotherapy occur and resolve within days to months. They are truly reversible and will not persist after treatment. Some late side effects in your functions, while unavoidable, also can also be helped with rehabilitation.

Many physicians and medical textbooks describe all side effects as either "acute" (meaning short-term) or "chronic" (meaning long-term) and leave it at that. They seem to ignore the impact of the effects on you and your life. This level of information is inadequate when you and your doctor need to discuss what to do next. From your point of view as the patient, it is essential to consider not only what might happen but how long it may last. You might want to ask the following nine questions about how treatment side effects might affect you personally (see Table 20-1).

Table 20-1 Questions to Ask Your Doctor about After-Effects of Treatments
1. What are the known side effects of this particular treatment?
2. What are the odds that I will be affected?
3. How might my everyday functioning be changed?
4. Will my quality of life be affected temporarily or permanently?
5. How might these changes affect the people I live with or love?
6. How can I avoid or minimize these side effects?
7. How do I distinguish *treatment* effects from *tumor* effects?
8. Will I get these side effects from the cancer, even if I do not receive the treatments?
9. What else should I know and where should I look for more information?

CAN YOU AVOID LONG-TERM SIDE EFFECTS?

Most of the time the answer is, no. After making the decision that you want to live, the next major choice was to accept what might happen to you, after cancer treatment. Now, your challenge becomes how to avoid as many long-term side effects as possible.

Asking questions at the time of treatment decisions will also allow you to decide against a treatment that you do not want, because of the *risk* for side effects. It also can be very helpful to simply ask your physician in the follow up phase of your treatment, whether or not your symptoms are late (long-term) effects of treatment.

Do You Have a Side Effect of Therapy? Why Is It Important To Know?

If you feel different and act differently, it may be a side effect of treatment. For example, you feel so tired that you need to rest all day, while before treatment you were active. Then the fatigue might be a side effect. Unfortunately, we don't always know whether a change is a side effect, unless it goes away. Long after treatment, we may still not know whether a particular symptom was an after effect or not. The best thing to do is discuss these symptoms during visits with your physician. Reading and having discussions with your Internet groups can be helpful, too.

Anything from depression to a secondary cancer *could* be an after-effect. This has financial implications, because if the problem is treatment-related, then it will more likely be covered under your health insurance. Individual side effects are discussed in the sections below.

Mental Depression – Can It Be a Side Effect of Your Disease or Treatment?

The answer is yes. After all, you have been through a lot. Depression can be a direct function of a brain injury, an hormone imbalance, or medication side effect. Also, it can come about in response to residual disabilities, ranging from memory problems to paralysis resulting from tumor or treatment.

Unfortunately, patients often report that their friends or doctors will ask, "How can you be depressed? You are so lucky to be alive." Depression is a physical illness, not "something in your mind." It can be related to the tumor or surgery or after brain injury and is increasingly recognized as a common problem. It is not the same as a *depressive mental disorder.*

Psychologists, social workers, and other cancer center professionals should be able to assist you. Treatment could include joining a support group, art or music therapy, individual or group psychotherapy, or a consultation with a psychiatrist to see if medication might be needed to get you over a rough patch. It is important to discuss your experiences and feelings with your supporters and family members as well as your physicians.

WHERE CAN YOU OBTAIN INFORMATION ABOUT SIDE EFFECTS?

You should let your health-care specialists (below) know about what you are experiencing during each phase of your therapy. They are your most likely resources for answers to questions in Table 20-1. Because both training and individual experiences can differ, you might get conflicting information, depending on whom you ask.

- Your treating physician – your most likely resource.
- Your pharmacist can advise about potential side effects of your medications and reactions that you should report immediately to your doctor.
- Your nurse might give you written materials and guide you to specialists within your health-care system.
- Your social worker can link you with community resources during all stages of therapy.
- A neuropsychologist can help identify your weak and strong areas and help you to develop strategies to compensate for weaknesses.
- Psychologists can help with strategies for dealing with the stress of treatment and its potential side effects.
- Friends and patient support groups.
- Internet groups.

(Table 20-5 at the end of this Chapter summarizes additional Internet resources.)

EARLY SIDE EFFECTS - AROUND THE TIME OF DIAGNOSIS

INITIAL DIAGNOSTIC EXAMINATIONS

The side effects that you could experience during this period are related to the different medications and tests that you might undergo. None has long-term consequences for you, except possibly radiation from the CT scanner.

The Scanner

MRI and CT scans by themselves are painless and may take 10 to 60 minutes to complete. The CT scan uses X-rays while the MRI employs magnetic energy. Some people experience claustrophobia (a sense of being closed in or feeling as if they are in a coffin) after sliding into the MRI scanner. Also, the MRI scanner makes a loud, jackhammer-like noise. To counteract these effects, the following have been helpful:

- Meditation and relaxation exercises
- Counting
- Listening to music or stories with headphones
- Anti-anxiety medication 30 minutes before the test (which allows some people to sleep through the scan)
- Aromatherapy
- There are "open" MRI scanners. However the fine detail obtained by these is inferior to the regular scanner. I recommend them only as a last resort.

The Contrast Liquid

Frequently, the CT scan will be performed with iodine "contrast" medication that is injected into your vein over a few minutes. This technique enables doctors to see the blood flow to the area of the tumor. Some people experience a warmth or fullness in their belly after this procedure. Reactions are rare, except in those who are allergic to iodine (see Table 20-5, MRI and CT scans).

Radiation and CT Scans

The radiation dose in CT scans is calibrated for adults. This dose can be six times that needed by a smaller adult or child. Before your scan, check with the radiologist as to whether or not the machine is calibrated for a minimal dose (to a child). If not, request re-calibration to a minimal dose if you are a small adult or the tests for your child. Radiation effects are cumulative and are a rare, but preventable cause of later-developing secondary cancers (see Table 20-5 for more information on CT scans and radiation dosage).

Blood Tests, Injection of Medications

These require a needle stick in a vein. If these will be frequent and are uncomfortable for you, there is relief in two new medications: Topicaine or Ela-Max. These are creamy salves that can be put on a skin patch, like toothpaste, 30 to 60 minutes before the "stick," and it will numb the skin. They can be used with young children, too.

Electroencephalograms (EEGs)

The EEG measures electrical activity in the brain and is often used to diagnose seizures. A cap with many wires is placed on the head. You will usually lie still or sleep while the electrical "activity" is being recorded. If your scalp is sensitive, an ice cap or skin anesthetic can be placed first so that you do not feel any needle sticks into the scalp.

SURGICAL PROCEDURES

Surgery for a brain tumor is often an emergency, life-saving procedure, and there may not be time to seek opinions about lessening side effects. Also, too much time spent "shopping" for different opinions can lead to damage from growing tumor. The neurosurgeon will advise the patient that paralysis, death, seizures, visual changes, speech-arrest, balance, or walking problems can occur, depending on the tumor's location.

Long-term, permanent after-effects might be lessened (if surgery is not an emergency) by having the surgery done by an experienced neurosurgeon who removes 50 or more tumors per year. See Chapter 5: Doctors and Other Team Members, for questions to ask your neurosurgeon.

Stereotactic Biopsies and MRIs

These involve the placement of a metal or plastic frame, or coin-like markers, on the head in order to identify the tumor's location prior to surgery. In some centers, the frame will be attached to your head either with adhesive or screws, which can be uncomfortable. Ask for anesthetic cream or another form of local anesthetic to lessen the pain of this procedure. (See Chapter 17, Traditional Approaches to Treatment: and Table 20-5 for more information about the role of neurosurgery and stereotactic biopsy.)

Functional MRIs

These are MRIs that are combined with a question and answer test in order to localize activity in different areas of the brain. For example, the frontal and temporal lobes are the locations for memory of objects that we recognize and place pictures together with words. We may "see" an artichoke, but the word for it may be found in either the *main* or *accessory speech* areas. Most of the time the *language* areas are on our dominant side, but not always. Experienced neurosurgeons will request a "functional MRI" (fMRI) prior to surgery to find out where it is safe to operate and how much tumor can be removed while staying away from these important areas. This preparation will usually leave these functions intact. (See Table 20-5 functional MRI.)

Brain Mapping

Also called *cortical mapping*, this can be critical to preserving brain function; this also depends upon the exact location of the tumor and extent of surgery. Tumors can actually push the motor strip and move it away from its classical position on

> Functional MRI and brain mapping pre-operatively may prevent some loss of functions.

the pre-central gyrus, making mapping all the more crucial. The motor control part of the frontal lobes can be "mapped" by electrical stimulation during surgery. This enables the surgeon to avoid resecting this area, thus minimizing the risk of face, arm or leg paralysis. (See Chapter 2: The Basics for brain anatomy and functions.[1]) You will not experience pain during surgery with this procedure. There is one web site that has an illustrated lecture with good quality pictures, while others describe this process in words (see Table 20-5 for web sites).

SIDE EFFECTS AFTER SURGERY

Weakness, paralysis, or any of the problems mentioned below can occur after surgery. Expert management, sometimes in the Intensive Care Unit (ICU), can control and sometimes prevent them. Surgery alone may not be the cause for these problems. It is reasonable to ask the neurosurgeon whether it was the surgery, presence or swelling of tumor, or a blood supply problem after the surgery that was the cause. The effects also could begin or become magnified during or after a course of radiation therapy (see Table 20-2).

Table 20-2 Side Effects After Surgery	
1. Blood clots	6. Fatigue and sleep
2. Steroid effects	7. Changes in personality or frontal lobe
3. Hydrocephalus, (water on the brain)	syndromes
4. Cerebellar mutism (CM)	8. Poor appetite regulation
5. Seizures	9. Paralysis or stroke

1. Blood Clots

Blood clots can occur in up to 20 percent of people with brain tumors. They can be due to either a pre-existing blood circulation problem or the tumor that activates the body's blood clotting system. Often they can be prevented with tight stockings and massage of the thighs before and after surgery. Usually clots start in the leg with symptoms of (painful) swelling in the calf. Their danger is that blood clots can loosen and travel to the lungs and heart. Blood thinners (heparin followed by coumadin) are used to treat this. If needed, a special (Greenfield) filter can be placed in the body's main vein (vena cava). It is inserted through a vein in the groin. This prevents clots from traveling to the heart and lungs (see Table 20-5 for information on blood clot prevention).

> Blood clots are not predictable but can be prevented and treated effectively.

2. Steroid Effects

Steroids, like dexamethasone, are used to prevent or treat brain swelling. They have both short- and long-term effects: weight gain, fluid retention, acne, calcium loss, sugar diabetes, osteoporosis, pancreatitis, and so on. You must know which doctor is both responsible and knowledgeable about adjusting your steroids. The goal is to lower and stop them as soon as possible. (See Chapter 9 in the companion book that describes symptoms that occur as a result of steroids.[1])

The following excerpt is from a woman whose husband did not have positive experiences with Decadron management. Her husband's doctors were neither communicating with nor keeping close oversight of her husband.

> *Is anyone else sick to death of hearing about doctors who mismanage Decadron? Bart was left on steroids for four months, because no one doctor was in charge. I have heard so many stories of people left on high doses for way too long without beginning weaning, and then lots of stories…where the Decadron was weaned too quickly. I feel…all doctors who prescribe Decadron should have to go to a brain tumor class taught by the survivors!*

> Susan, wife of Bart, Akron, OH

Steroids can also affect the mind in the same way that a recurrent tumor can. At the worst extreme are changes in personality – difficult-to-manage aggressive and combative behavior. The effect is not predictable and can last as long as the person is on higher doses of steroids. Knowing that this can occur and lowering steroid levels as soon as possible may lessen the chances of disrupting family life. Sometimes psychiatric medications may be helpful to control steroid-induced behaviors.

> Steroids are valuable but have major side effects. Know who is responsible for monitoring your dose.

3. Hydrocephalus (Also called "Water on the Brain.")

Tumors that connect with or are adjacent to the ventricles can cause increased pressure in the head due to the release of proteins that clog the cerebrospinal fluid re-absorption system. Treatments include waiting, steroids, an external drainage tube, or a permanent shunt of fluid from the ventricles to the abdomen to bypass the obstruction. (See Figure 20-1, and Chapter 17: Figure 17-3.)

4. Post-Operative Cerebellar Mutism (CM)

It is increasingly recognized that surgery in the back area of the brain, near the cerebellum and fourth ventricle, is associated with a peculiar series of events, called cerebellar mutism (CM) or posterior fossa syndrome (PFS). The patient, often a child, wakes up from surgery speaking and moving, but shortly afterward stops speaking, has difficulty hearing, swallowing, and sometimes walking. The exact cause is unknown, but the nerves controlling these functions are in the area of the operation. Recovery with intensive rehabilitation can be complete or partial over months to years. There no known way to prevent it at this time. (See Table 20-5 for more information on cerebellar mutism.)

> Recognizing side effects can be difficult. Ask physicians, nurses, pharmacists, Internet groups for info.

A parent, Lois, weighs in with her perspective:

- Parents might not have been warned that CM is a possibility.
- Not all physicians treating kids who have had surgery for brain tumors are aware of CM - e.g., PICU/hospital docs. Even if they are, they do not fully understand its complexity nor the long-term issues related to it.
- Many view it as a short-term condition, and while "mutism" is, problems are not over when speech returns and they don't all get this. Parents need a lot more information than they get from their docs.
- My daughter endured hours of speech therapy that was not really appropriate. She was asked repeatedly, day after day, to speak into a microphone to make a computerized dog jump. But she wasn't really able. I think the point is that speech therapy can be helpful, but should take into account the neurological aspects of CM and recovery. For kids feel like they are failing or disappointing others by not being able to speak, therapy can be counterproductive.

5. Seizures

Seizures usually do not occur after surgery, if they were not present beforehand. However, they may occur, particularly if the tumor is in or near the frontal or temporal lobes. Many neurosurgeons place their "at risk" patients on anti-seizure medications just before and after surgery. Often patients are on these medications for at least six months, since state motor vehicle licensing bureaus require drivers to be seizure-free for six months in order to qualify as a licensed driver. Seizures also can mean a recurrence of tumor. A new seizure is an important reason to talk with your doctor. Blood levels of anti-seizure medication need to be monitored to prevent under- and over-medication.

> Seizures require medication & blood level monitoring.

6. Fatigue and Sleep

It is common to have lack of energy, sleep 14+ hours a day, or have difficulty getting to sleep after major surgery. This is a cumulative effect of anesthesia on the body's metabolism, physical stress, brain injury, and abnormal cycles of melatonin or thyroid stimulating hormone (TSH) secretion within the brain. It may take weeks, months, or longer to get back to a normal waking-sleeping cycle. See also Chapter 9: Medications-Pain, Fatigue, Brain Swelling and Seizures, for more information about fatigue and its treatment.[1]

7. Changes in Personality or Frontal Lobe Syndrome

Surgery to remove tumors in the frontal lobes bears additional risks for brain function that might be progressive and permanent. The questions to the operating surgeon and radiation oncologist in Table 20-1 are relevant here. This part of the brain controls wakefulness, memory, impulsiveness, personality characteristics, and "executive functions" (see Chapter 2, The Basics). It also allows you to start and organize activities like getting dressed, planning a trip to the market, making coffee, operating a TV remote control, or telling a joke. It is the part of your brain that makes you unique (your "personality"). Removal of tumor and brain in this location can literally change the person that you are. Symptoms may include sleeping more, responding to but not starting activities, reduced inhibition, poor judgment and not recognizing family. Similar effects also can occur following radiation therapy to the frontal lobes.

> Surgery to remove a tumor in the frontal lobes bears additional risk for brain function.

A professional associate of mine whose husband had such a surgery made the following suggestion, based on her experience:

Have a family discussion about dealing with potential abnormal behaviors, just to minimize stress and prevent an additional sense of crisis, if side effects develop. This allows the person with the brain tumor to help resolve the situation as a contributing family member before problems emerge. Everyone follows the plan rather than have to react without knowing which options there may be. Plans anticipate abusive behavior, impulse spending, whatever might be anticipated depending on the tumor location. So if things crop up later on, they can say, "look at this list, some of these problems from the tumor are happening to us."

> Have a family discussion about dealing with potential abnormal behaviors *before* surgery.

See how the changes are described in a letter about one of my patients below:

Craig had tests for his brain and he started off very smart, evidently. He has changed. What I miss most is his sense of humor...he was always so quick, so funny, and that is gone. He sits a lot and is tired, and so much falls on me that I am tired too. But then brain cancer is not a pretty disease. What is more important than your mind? I remember when Craig realized something was wrong with him he said, "Please, don't let it be my brain."

Julie, wife of Craig, Pontiac, MI.

Craig has a frontal lobe tumor that responded well to multiple therapies. He continues to work as a sales representative. Both he and his wife knew ahead of time of the potential for the damage that occurred. It would have been more devastating to Julie, his wife, had it come as a surprise.

Personality changes can be subtle and are often missed in a physician's examination.[2] Often, changes can be recognized only with reference to previous behavior and not with a routine clinical examination. Moreover, abnormal behaviors may fluctuate from one testing occasion to another. A standard neurological examination or psychological test, such as the Wechsler Adult Intelligence Scale, often yields a "normal" finding. Thus, special neuropsychological techniques, interpreted by an experienced professional, are required to examine frontal lobe *function*. These methods assess current behavior and how this compares with previous behavior. (See Table 20-5 for more information about frontal lobe syndromes.)

> Changes in personality can occur with brain injury, swelling, tumor, or medications.

Question: *My sister had surgery for a primary brain lymphoma in the falx cerebri in 1996, followed by 6 weeks of radiation to her entire brain and later, chemotherapy. Once she arrived home, she recovered slowly – learning to walk with a cane and climb stairs. In the last three years, she has regressed and is not walking or standing on her own. MRIs and all other tests show no tumor recurrence, yet she can't seem to find a doctor who knows how to treat her problem. Is she suffering from effects of the radiation or chemotherapy? She is 58 years old and desperately needs help if it's still possible.*

> Short-term memory problems can be due to radiation-induced inflammation, steroid changes, necrosis, tumor progression, or brain damage.

John, Omaha, NE

Answer: Your sister needs to go to a major (university medical) center with a rehabilitation department. More than likely, a neurological and physiatrist (rehabilitation) consultation is necessary. It is impossible to diagnose over the Internet, but this scenario is consistent with radiation effects. Other causes are also possible.

8. Paralysis or Stroke

Paralysis or stroke can occur even in the best of circumstances. Discuss reasons and treatment for them with your neurosurgeon.

9. Appetite Regulation

Changes in appetite can be due to many causes: radiation, chemotherapy, depression, and tumors in areas of the hypothalamus. Also, some tumors release substances that give a feeling of satiety or fullness, with no motivation to eat. Medications like Megace can stimulate the appetite. Steroids can induce an insatiable appetite. Food restriction or substitution would be needed in order to avoid weight gain.

SIDE EFFECTS DURING & SOON AFTER RADIATION THERAPY

Radiation therapy delivers high-energy to the tumor and surrounding brain. Brain-related side effects are a result of the *location* and *amount* of energy received. Mental side effects will be greater for the frontal lobes than for a small part of the occipital (back) lobe. The X-knife, GammaKnife, proton beam therapy, and possibly brachytherapy (Gliasite) pose a greater risk for more inflammation and necrosis (dead tissue) than standard radiation because of their high energy (see later in this chapter).

The American Brain Tumor Association (ABTA) has an excellent primer, which details most side effects of common radiation therapy and their treatments (see Table 20-5 and http://www.abta.org/radiationtherapy.php). Most other general radiation web sites talk about radiation, but not specifically to the brain.

Skin Effects and Hair Loss

These are common and are usually short-term. The skin becomes red and the scalp itches. When radiation is administered to the brain for longer than three to four weeks, most people begin to notice hair loss. If a small area is treated, loss is confined to that spot. If the entire brain is treated, hair loss occurs over the whole head. However, the degree of loss, areas of re-growth and permanence may vary.

Hearing Loss

This can be a permanent side effect of radiation treatment, albeit infrequently, and this is most likely to occur when platinum chemotherapy (cisplatin) is used simultaneously, as it affects the sensitive nerve endings in the inner ear. The following passage illustrates another common side effect that causes temporary hearing loss – fluid buildup in the middle ear:

> *Stephen had severe hearing loss in his right ear, post radiation, which lasted eight months. Some of you suggested that it may be hardened earwax due to radiation. Well, in his case, we had a surprise! It was due to fluid build-up from radiation. The ear, nose, and throat surgeon made a very small incision in his eardrum, drained the fluid, and placed a tiny tube in his eardrum to allow drainage. The tube will fall out on its own in 6-12 months. As soon as the fluid was drained, he could hear again! This was a huge positive step in helping him to feel "normal. He goes to work full time, drives, rides a bike, etc., so we are living our lives as best as we can.*

> Sheila, wife of Stephen, survivor extraordinaire, Boston, MA

Behavior and Memory Problems

These are the most serious effects about which you may not be advised. On the minor end of the spectrum, many patients complain of sleepiness, minor confusion, or disorientation for several hours after daily radiation treatment to the brain. This condition may last for four to eight weeks and is due to inflammation, swelling, in the brain. A short nap is usually beneficial; medications and vocational rehabilitation also can help.[3] More severe side effects can be major brain swelling, paralysis, and psychotic behaviors. The latter can also be a side effect of steroids. Thus it may not be easy to sort out the cause; this requires expert help from your team. (See Chapter 9: Medications for pain, fatigue, brain swelling and seizures.[1])

LATER EFFECTS OF TREATMENT

The late (long-term) effects that I discuss here are not intended to be comprehensive but are ones that you are less likely to find via the Internet or from other sources (see Table 20-3). They may occur months to years after completing therapy. I also include emotional responses to treatment as a side effect.

Table 20-3 Major Later Effects of Brain Tumor Treatments
1. Endocrine – thyroid dysfunction, mineral loss, sugar imbalance, diminished sexual function or development
2. Bones – osteoporosis, fractures
3. Neurological – weakness, paralysis, seizures, fatigue, sensory loss
4. Gastrointestinal – persistent vomiting
5. Visual – impaired vision, cataracts
6. Psychological – depression, loss of inhibition, memory loss, impaired information processing, dementia, reduced job-related capabilities
7. Secondary cancers (Chapter 24)

Usually the causes are multiple and difficult to separate. However, the end results can be described under a few sub-categories:

- Destruction of sensitive areas of the brain by the tumor.
- Removal of the tumor by surgery (previous section).
- Radiation effects to tumor and/ or narrowing of blood vessels.
- Combined effects of tumor and therapy.
- Steroids, chemotherapy, and other drugs.

First to be discussed are the combined effects. This will be followed by a separate section describing those effects usually attributable to the radiation.

COMBINED EFFECTS OF TUMOR AND THERAPY

Sugar Diabetes

> Diabetes can be caused by steroids and may improve when medication is stopped.

This can be unmasked by steroid treatment, while the latter is relieving temporary swelling before and after surgery or during radiation. It is not unusual to have high blood sugar levels after starting steroids. Sometimes this requires a change of diet or insulin supplementation to control blood sugar levels. The sugar intolerance often disappears when steroids are discontinued. Radiation itself is not responsible for diabetic conditions.

Osteoporosis (Thinning of Bone)

This usually occurs months or years after initial therapy with chemotherapy, inactivity or radiation. It can lead to the collapse of the backbones (vertebrae) as well as the long bones of the hips and arms. It results from the loss of calcium, reduced mobility and exercise, medications like steroids, and vitamin A.

> Osteoporosis (bone thinning) can be lessened or prevented by early detection and treatment.

Osteoporosis can be lessened and possibly prevented by early detection and treatment. Twice yearly monitoring using a CT bone scan (DEXA bone density test) of the hip can detect the problem. Lowering doses of steroids and vitamin A, if possible, and taking bone-building medications like calcium supplements and vitamin D-like drugs (Fosamax) can build new bone. Graded exercise also will help. Radiation to the spine may contribute but is not the only cause.

Infertility

This can be due to ovary or testicular damage from chemotherapy or pituitary malfunction induced by tumor, surgery, chemotherapy or radiation.

"Chemotherapy Brain"

In the early phases of chemotherapy treatment, patients have experienced memory problems, "fuzzy" thinking, commonly known as "chemo-brain." It probably is caused by multiple sources including chemotherapy, sleep deprivation, anxiety and depression. Many patients have reported that these symptoms continue long after the treatment ends. Until very recently there has been little research in this area.[4,5] Oncologists are aware of this problem and can suggest medication and exercises to counteract it.

Effects on the Pituitary Gland

The pituitary gland lies almost directly behind the nose and is sensitive to radiation at doses over 2400 cGy (cGy is a unit of radiation dosage). Taking instruction from the brain's hypothalamus, it is called the "master gland" because it produces more than eight hormones that regulate such functions as:

- Sugar: energy storage and conversion of sugar into carbohydrate storage.
- Salt: mineral balance for proper cell function (sodium and water balance).
- Sex: sexual function (desire, testicular and ovarian function, fertility, and menstrual cycle).
- Metabolism: activity level, thyroid function.
- Growth.

In the pituitary gland region, the tumor, surgery or radiation can cause irregular or absent menstrual periods, infertility, lack of sexual desire, milk secretion from the breast in men and women, tiredness, and weight gain. (See Chapter 2: Basics about Brain Tumors.[1])

Growth hormone deficiency also occurs in adults but does not have such obvious effects as in children who have not reached their adult height or gone through puberty (see also Chapter 22A: Children with Brain Tumors: Special Considerations in Diagnosis and Treatment, and Chapter 22B: Children and Brain Tumors: Longer Term Psychological and Social Issues).

Children with midbrain tumors who have received surgery or radiation often exhibit hormone deficiencies causing stunted growth, delayed or *early* puberty, and problems with salt and water balance. Learning disabilities are also common in children with brain tumors as a result of the tumor or radiation treatment.

Milk Secretion

This can be a side effect of surgery, the tumor, or radiation-induced damage to the base (stalk) of the pituitary gland. This can result in the persistent secretion of prolactin hormone, which stimulates the male and female breast to make milk. Unfortunately, this condition usually does not improve with time.

Thyroid Effects

These can occur as a result of either "scatter" from head or neck radiation or a central effect on the pituitary or "master gland." The thyroid is an H–shaped gland attached to your "Adam's apple" in the center of your throat. It secretes hormones that control your body's metabolism. Low thyroid activity can mimic recurrent tumor, radiation-induced brain damage, or steroid withdrawal. Symptoms include slow thinking, sleepiness, weakness, ankle swelling, dry skin, or hair loss.

> Low thyroid activity can mimic recurrent tumor, radiation-induced brain damage, or steroid withdrawal.

Avoidance of direct damage to the thyroid depends on accurate aim and shielding of the gland by the radiation oncologist. If radiation to the thyroid or pituitary gland cannot be avoided, then regular testing of thyroid blood levels every 6-12 months can diagnose a problem. About 35-50 percent of children treated for medulloblastoma will develop low thyroid function. The frequency of reduced thyroid activity in adults is not well known, but could be 50 percent or higher.[7] Treatment with thyroid hormone (L-thyroxine) will reverse all symptoms.

> Low thyroid activity can be effectively treated, if recognized.

SEXUAL FUNCTION

Problems with sexual function can occur before or after tumor removal or radiation; few studies document the frequency of this as a side effect. Almost all of my male patients have said that they had difficulty with erections and lacked sexual desire for weeks to months after surgery and then radiation. Little data exists on female sexual response after a brain tumor diagnosis.[6]

The cause of sexual dysfunction is usually attributed to hypothalamic (32 percent) or primary testicle/ovary damage (10 percent) from spinal radiation. In one study, half of the male patients, compared to only 6 percent of controls, reported erectile dysfunction at one to 11 years after treatment. About 30 percent of women patients experienced breast milk secretion and half reported irregular or few menstrual periods.[7] The impact of radiation therapy on sexual function is not "psychological." Hormone replacement therapy, for example, may help.

◻Bottom Line▶ The impact of therapy on sexual function is not "psychological." It is a gland malfunction that might be helped with hormone replacement therapy.

OVERCOMING SEXUAL PROBLEMS

At times, lack of sexual attraction or desire may get you down and make you irritable, frustrated and angry. A perfect solution may not exist for every problem. The following poignant yet candid vignettes reflect creative ways in which three couples adapted to changes in their sexual relationship caused by brain tumor treatments.[8]

Margaret and I had some physical sex problems while she was suffering with the brain tumor. Some of these also arose with our being in our 50s and from her medication. There were also problems arising from thrush infection. There is also a tendency for us all to go very coy and proper when a person is in a hospital bed, standing by, smiling blandly. Tell the person under the covers that his/her body is still loved, and that you still want to touch. What can be worse than to feel remote, untouchable? What does come to the fore is the need to be generous and understanding and to read responses to tiny touches well.

It seems to me that at the core of dealing with this is the status one gives to the penetrative sex act and orgasm itself. There are a thousand and one things to do which produce sexual pleasure and reward and satisfaction other than…"jump 'n' hump" penetrative intercourse. If you have your eyes-wide-open, life-sharing, skin sharing, a warm and understanding relationship; if you accept change, exploit opportunities in life,… accept that the biggest sex organ is the brain, you can cover a lot of miles together in an afternoon, evening, night, or morning.

You need to ration energy and make decisions to allocate time when energy is available… at least to make room for spontaneity outside what may have been past patterns of 'standard spontaneity.' Evenings after full days… are not the ideal. Location: there are corners in hospital corridors that come in handy, if you are prepared to live a little dangerously. Seek opportunities, enjoy every moment of life.

David, spouse to Margaret, Melbourne, Australia

It went from 4-5 times per week down to maybe 3-4 per month. As the patient, it has not been all my fault. My wife lost interest last year when I started to show signs of the tumor recurring. With multiple seizures and left side weakness, it was difficult to do much of anything.

I am now in a clinical trial with Temodar and VP-16, and I am far too weak to do anything 2-3 days after I start a chemotherapy cycle; so I try to plan for when I am off the chemo during a 12-16 day recovery time and hope my wife's time of the month does not fall in that time frame. I also think that you take it slow and don't expect the poor guy to get it up in a flash. That's one of our problems; when my wife rushes it, I have a hard time keeping it going. There is an old saying that 'It's not the size of the ship in the sea as much as it is the motion in the ocean.'

I agree that sex is secondary in our minds while dealing with side effects from tumor(s) and medications. Our last experience with sex wasn't pleasant for him. And believe me SEX was a very important expression for the both of us. We often talked of how much we missed that wonderful part of our lives. It became less of a priority for us since we spent so much time together, talking,

Advice on post-treatment sexual function issues may be obtained from support groups and physicians.

listening to music, watching movies, traveling etc...I believe we both just came to grips with sex not being the most important issue at the time. Our love for one another was demonstrated in other possible ways.

In the later stages (weeks) personality changes, mood swings, anger, frustration seemed to take center stage. I could only imagine how he felt with the frontal lobe tumor affecting so many of these symptoms. John was such a fighter. His main concern (looking back on it) was fighting and staying active until the end. He kept his family from suffering along with him while he died. He gave in to the cancer only days before he died. How strong he was! I miss him.

Emily, proud wife of John, Southampton, England

RADIATION THERAPY AS A CAUSE OF LATE EFFECTS

RADIOSURGERY – THE POSITIVES AND NEGATIVES ABOUT SIDE EFFECTS

GammaKnife or X-Knife is focused, high-energy radiation treatment given in one or several sessions. These provide excellent tumor control for one to six small areas of tumor. They can even be a better choice than whole brain radiation, with less potential for generalized brain damage and dementia, although it is important to remember that your doctor first approve this type of treatment for your case. The most frequent side effects include swelling of brain tissue and the development of necrosis (dead tissue) over months to years that the body's "clean-up" systems cannot remove (see also Chapter 17: Traditional Approaches to Treatment).

TUMOR NECROSIS. WHY IS THIS A PROBLEM?

Necrosis (dead tissue) can be misdiagnosed as *live* tumor. If this happens, the patient may wrongly receive a dismal prognosis or unnecessary toxic therapy that leads to serious side effects or possibly death. The necrosis also can act like "tumor," causing increasing swelling, and putting pressure on vital areas with accompanying weakness, headache, and psychological changes. Even our most sensitive tests (such as MRI, PET, thallium) distinguish between live and dead tumor only 80-90 percent of the time. To make matters more complicated, necrosis may actually contain tumor cells.

When the most likely diagnosis is necrosis, steroids are prescribed for weeks to months. No other medical treatment (examples: oxygen, hyperbaric chamber, heparin) has a proven record of effectiveness, although they are often tried and seem to work in some cases. Complications, like seizures and weakness, sometimes necessitate the surgical removal of necrosis.[9]

The e-mail message below describes such side effects following external radiation and implantation with GliaSite (a concentrated, local form of radiation that can cause necrosis like GammaKnife or X-Knife. (See also Chapter 17: Traditional Approaches to Treatment.) Remember this is a side effect. The therapy may be very effective in killing the tumor.

> Necrosis can be misdiagnosed as live tumor & the patient can receive a dismal prognosis.

> *About three years ago, my adult son Jeff completed one year of Temodar and a few months of PCV, radiation, and Gliasite treatments. He was doing great until recently when he had some seizures. They operated and found no tumor but lots of necrosis and they removed 90 percent of it. He has not had any seizures since and was just weaned off decadron. He is now back to work as an engineer at General Motors in Detroit. His only problem now is a sensation in his left cheek area. But even that has diminished.*
>
> Chris, Father of Jeff, Chicago, IL

Bottom Line You must receive answers to critical questions before radiation starts. Only then can you can make the most informed decision possible.

NEUROPSYCHOLOGICAL EFFECTS: MEMORY AND PERSONALITY

The following are generally accepted truths about brain tumors and the more serious effects of radiation therapy.

1. A younger adult will usually tolerate whole brain radiation better than people over 60 years old, a group who will have more memory or personality effects. The risk may be greatest for those more than 60 years of age.[10,11]
2. Whole brain radiation is associated with more loss of mental functions (dementia) than localized and/or limited field stereotactic radiation.[12]
3. Symptoms can change with steroid adjustments. Increased swelling from tumor growth or too rapid a tapering from dexamethasone can cause identical symptoms of confusion, weakness, paralysis.
4. Growing tumor as well as its treatment can sometimes cause the same unwanted harmful effects, making choices more difficult.
5. In patients older than 70 with *glioblastoma multiforme,* chemotherapy and whole brain radiation may be equally effective.[13]
6. Moderate to severe memory impairment is common in children. Its effects are worse in children younger than age three. The extent of dysfunction depends on which part of the brain receives radiation.

Longer lasting memory problems can occur as a result of tumor, surgery, or radiation. Here is an example of someone who was unprepared for his wife's change in memory and personality:

I have read that there are risks with radiation and now I'm thinking that Diana is far enough out to where I'm starting to see side effects. She has done extremely well since her glioblastoma multiforme diagnosis and treatment. Lately, she seems to be getting kind of 'spacey' or 'out of it,' especially when she gets fatigued or tired. For example, she will ask the same questions repetitively. This weekend my son spent the night at a friend's house and, prior to his leaving, she must have asked him seven times if it was OK with his folks.

She also seems to be more forgetful. She will be 50 in May, so perhaps that could be part of it, but I'm not sure. There have been several instances where I have asked her for something. She is at a complete loss for remembering where the item is, when she had just had it a short time before. None of these things are show-stoppers by any means. However, I find myself getting short-tempered with her because of this. I know that I should be asking Donna's doctors this

154   **Bottom Line** → Radiosurgery could be a better choice than whole brain radiation with less potential for brain injury and dementia.

stuff, but she is usually with me, and it is very difficult to speak about this with her in the room.

George, hubby to Diana, Aurora, CO

This is not a trivial problem. It is serious. Diana is having memory problems, and her spouse does not know how to deal with it. Memory loss could be due to several causes: radiation-induced inflammation, necrosis, steroid changes, and progression of brain damage. When the caretaker cannot speak privately with the doctor, it understandable to seek advice on the Internet. On the other hand, it is possible to make a separate consultation appointment so the physician who has the closest working relationship with the family can deal directly with the caretaker over these important issues.

> Symptoms can change with decadron adjustments.

The most significant memory and personality changes will typically appear after six to 12 months of treatment. When this occurs, many caregivers feel isolated and unable to understand what is happening. Getting support from others from the local support network or via the Internet can be enormously helpful:

Thanks so much for your words of encouragement as I so need them right now...I am finding Rob's personality truly unnerving on some days. He changes so drastically from one minute to the next, and I don't know how to handle it. One of our many therapists keeps telling me to 'externalize' it and remember that it is not always he who is talking. That's so easy for someone to say. When he is swearing at me, telling me to f*#% off and get the hell out of the house, it is not so easy to externalize it. Sometimes I get scared that he is exhibiting signs of a multiple personality disorder of some kind. It's so hard. They say you treat the ones you love the worst because you know they'll be there for you. His behavior is so totally inappropriate, some days I am in shock. Trying to explain to him is pointless, too, because then he just says he will do whatever he wants.

One of the parts of his brain that is affected is reasoning, empathy, logic, ability to comprehend unreasonable behavior and such things...I wonder if it is always just the tumor. I am so frustrated these days, even though everyone keeps telling me how strong I am. I am so tired...that some days I don't think I can handle it anymore. Things may get harder instead of easier and I am terrified. ... I don't know...I guess I just had to get that out. Thanks again to you all for your kindness and education. I have already gotten some great information from you.

Lorraine, Beverly Hills, CA

The neuropsychological consequences of brain radiation do not appear on most of the otherwise comprehensive brain tumor sites. Even information booklets about the side effects of radiation from the American Cancer Society do not include discussion of serious neuropsychological deficits. They talk about decreased libido, memory loss, and intolerance of cold weather (see references in Table 20-5). The following note shows how advance knowledge can make life easier and prevent a loved one from feeling cheated, misled, or lied to:

> *We had excellent medical care, but no one prepared or warned us how the last surgery and radiation would change John – irrational, impulsive about spending, quick to anger, and close to being physically abusive. We still don't know the causes, but had we known it might happen, while he was in his right mind, we would have dealt with finances. I wouldn't have been so reluctant to tell someone how mean and frightening he had become. Then there is the aftermath, where you learn to live in a new normal life but may have lost the full person that you had known.*
>
> *I didn't realize until last year that I was grieving for the loss of the John I had married and finally let myself feel sad. I was also frightened and saddened that I was grieving too for the person whom I am now married to. At some times he is not a person I like, but he can't help it. I am lucky because at other times there are such glimpses of himself.*
>
> Paula, wife of John, Hamilton, OH

Paula is not angry at the whole world. Rather, she laments not having been informed about what to expect. With forewarning, she could have proactively developed a durable power of attorney and avoided financial complications. Is this difficult information to hear? Yes. Is it a difficult statement for doctors to make? Yes. That is why you must ask about these possibilities.

Difficult choices have to be made between a compromised mind and life itself. The course of treatment-associated memory and personality problems is not predictable; it may stabilize or get worse over time. Without information, you cannot make an informed choice: The following web site reflects the anger of not being told what the downside of treatment may portend.

> *We were never informed by any doctor involved with my wife's chemotherapies or radiation therapies about the possible late or delayed side effects of treatment, nor the alternatives to treatment. Ann and I were corralled into*

believing this was the only thing to do – no other choice, and no mention of the late side effects.

I saw my soul mate being slowly tortured to death because of what I did not know before. I spent two years of sleepless nights finding out what the oncologists didn't tell us. I never realized a patient had to be just as knowledgeable as or even more knowledgeable than the oncologists. Not having the knowledge beforehand resulted in the death of my wife. She really wanted to live...with me.[14]

> Long-lasting memory problems can occur as a result of tumor, surgery, or radiation.

Some serious problems may not be avoidable, but at least you can prepare in advance and be aware of treatable side effects. Many times, it will be up to you to ask the right questions.

OVERCOMING THE EFFECTS OF RADIATION ON MEMORY

The decreased ability to remember new information (short-term memory) is a side effect of radiation therapy on the brain that may emerge after months or even years. Through neuropsychological testing, strategies to compensate and help can often be designed specifically for you. (See Chapter 5: Doctors and Other Team Members.[1]) These might include one or more of the following aids (see Table 20-4):

Table 20-4 Useful Aids to Compensate for Short-Term Memory Problems
1. Written or audible instructions.
2. Reminders on the refrigerator.
3. 3 x 5 cards on which daily tasks can be written.
4. Weekly organizer boxes for medications.
5. Pre-programmed cell phone.
6. Yoga, massage or complementary (herbal) medications for anxiety.
7. Numbered communicator board for those who have lost speech (See Table 20-7).
8. Newer drug therapies like Aricept that may protect the brain from further injury, or attention-enhancing drugs like Ritalin & Provigil.

Major medical centers would most likely have access to newer cognitive therapy and drug treatments for the affected brain functions. The following Internet exchanges capture not only the value of compensating strategies but also the worth of Internet-based support groups:

Sean: *"We suffer internal symptoms that others cannot see – It's called executive function. I saw a speech therapist for a few months after my surgery,*

> Decreased ability to remember new information (short-term memory) is a side effect of radiation that can appear after months or years.

and she got me hooked on doing simple crossword puzzles. 'Look up the answers if you get stuck, or you'll go nuttier than you are already,' she told me. She also gave me stacks of sheets with simple mathematical problems - arithmetic, geometric, and word problems. You can't believe how much good it did. I still can't remember what 2 + 2 is; but the rest has improved."

Jeanne: *"My dad, too, has similar difficulties. I think it is a response to the injuries that are posed on the brain, such as surgery, radiation, and chemotherapy. We recently learned from a physical and occupational therapist that my dad's difficulties are a result of motor planning difficulties — the process of combining, ordering, and prioritizing complex tasks. Without this skill, many daily tasks become what my dad calls "tedious." He has trouble making instant decisions as well as using the TV remote control, any electronic equipment, and the stove. It's because he can't order the steps in his mind about what to do. My dad's tumor is in his right frontal lobe.*

Martha: *It's not exactly short-term memory and not exactly judgment. I don't know the exact word. I'll give you a very simple example. I'll be driving along and say "Steve, is this our exit?"...He freezes and cannot answer. It's sort of that split-second decision-making that is missing. That's the thing I have relied on for 30 years; unfortunately, my split-second decision-making is also a bit atrophied, so I'm struggling here and missing a lot of exits.*

THE DISGUISED DISABILITY

I learned about a new type of disability from Sheryl and Patty. Both articulate their experiences about living with brain tumors, and each shares an enlightening view of the world. Sheryl coined the phrase "disguised disability" to describe the problem:

> *That's part of the problem – most of us look well, but we HATE hearing, 'Oh you look great!' Why? Because you can't SEE our disabilities. Unlike a stroke patient, we are expected to 'get over it.' Many of our problems are cognitive or visual...you can't see that, can you?*

◻**Bottom Line**▸ For memory issues, use reminder notes, refrigerator messages, writing daily tasks on 3 x 5 cards.

Patty elaborates on her experience:

> The one thing that I hate is when people mention that I look great, and then I see a puzzled look on their face. I didn't really know how I was supposed to act or look when having a brain tumor. I feel like telling them, 'Gee, I'm sorry that I look great.'
>
> If I hear that someone was diagnosed with something that I don't know about, I go home and look it up in my medical book. I feel it is better, as a friend, to understand what is wrong. People should not assume anything. I think it would be nice if you could have a small section on how to deal with situations like this; it happens every day.
>
> I had a weird thing happen at a bridal shower for my niece. I joked that I was Dana's aunt, and I'm the one 'with a hole in her head.' She laughed and finally opened up to me. After the shower was over, the bridesmaids had told my niece that they…were in awe of my having a brain tumor. I really don't know what advice you could give on this, but other brain tumor survivors go through the same thing.

What do you do about this? You cannot change the world while you are living with a brain tumor. You can let people know what is going on inside you and how they can best respond to you. My patient Jack put it this way: "When all is done…talk to me."

SURVIVOR GUILT

As strange as it may sound, many long-term survivors ask, "Why was I pulled out of line? It was *my* turn," knowing that others have died of a similar disease. It is helpful to discuss and acknowledge these normal feelings, if you have them. The longer that one survives, the more intense those feelings may become after losing friends in support groups, for example.

> It is helpful to discuss and acknowledge normal feelings of survivor guilt.

> I was the one with the terrible seizures, the lousy memory…yet I'm still on this journey, full of day-to-day struggles. I always believed it was MY turn – and so did he. I will never understand why Paul was taken instead of me. I think about him all the time…dream that he is alive and angry with me…won't tell me where he is…

> Sheryl, Boca Raton, FL

159

WILL LIFE EVER RETURN TO NORMAL?

Yes...and no. Returning to work and family reflects the sum total of your lingering side effects and the power of rehabilitation. The patient, the caregiver, and family all want a return to *normal* – the way things were *before* the tumor. For most families with brain tumors, however, there will be a *new* normal. A friend with a *glioblastoma multiforme* put it aptly:

> For most families with brain tumors there will be a new normal.

My biggest issue was acceptance – an understanding of the real limitations that came...some quickly, some long-term, some still occurring. This is my new "self," someone I never was, finding new things to make me feel whole and productive. I am sure there's much more laying around in me somewhere. Sometimes it just has to be found through chatting.

Ada, Beverly Hills, CA

"WAS" AND "IS"

You can spend time mourning the loss of what was, but that *was* is now different from *is*. How different? What *is* will depend on your tumor location and type, and the quality of care that you received during the treatment pathway.

Things are different during and after the time a serious illness becomes a way of life. People change. Families change. Jobs change. Opportunities change. Children change. Lives change.

Laura, wife of Henry, Baton Rouge, LA

In the following passages, the wife of a patient of mine reflects upon the challenges of reintegrating into the world with a husband who has a new "self":

In retrospect, the hardest thing is losing someone who was 100 percent your life partner. Some days he seems so much like himself that you talk as if he was the old Jim and other days you see him not really there – more emotionally labile but not emotionally real. I said to the social worker that he does care about and for me – it's just that his capacity for caring is very different now. Sometimes he responds more to how I affect his immediate activities than having an actual awareness of me. Maybe there is no way to adequately prepare families...but I think you need to touch on these things in your book.

Things here have been very difficult. We wondered about many of the symptoms in the past couple of years (e.g. impulsivity, irritability, anger out of proportion to the provoking situation, poor judgment about money), and thought that they resulted from frontal lobe damage in the '95 craniotomy. I had been hoping that the serenity of December would last. Basically, we don't know if the problems are related to tumor, pituitary function, radiation damage, drugs, etc., nor is there any assurance that they will go away.

There have been increasingly intense rage outbursts directed at me. I know I am difficult at times, but these are provoked by minor incidents – such as my accidentally disconnecting the phone. I have twice been afraid for my safety and it is still unbelievable that I am saying this about a man who is so kind and good and would never hurt anyone. I keep hoping that it will be better, but the incidents are increasing and today one happened in the car immediately before I parked. I went to the desk after he went into the Radiation Oncology suite and asked to speak with someone to help me understand what is happening.

Penelope, Toronto, Canada

HELP WITH CARE GIVING

Sometimes the neuropsychological effects of the tumor or its treatment take their toll on the caregivers. Help in the home or even transfer to an assisted living center or skilled nursing facility may become necessary temporarily or for the longer term. A caregiver who asks for help is acting courageously – not selfishly. Neither is it a sign of "giving up."

> Social worker or case manager from your health-care team can assist in deciding if a home helper is needed.

The first avenue of approach is for family and close friends to organize themselves and share in domestic responsibilities. Whether it is feeding the dog, paying bills, or cooking an occasional meal, everyone can help. Stepping in for a morning or afternoon can give the regular caregiver a much-needed break. (See Chapter 5: Doctors and Other Team Members, regarding the important role of the caregiver.[1])

The social worker or case manager from your health-care team often can be the best help for assistance outside the home. Their experience can help you decide if home help is needed for feeding, giving medications, bathing, and so forth. Special equipment – such as an electronic bed, a feeding apparatus, a chair to facilitate sitting and standing – could make life easier.

If working within the confines of home proves not to be a feasible choice, then a skilled nursing facility or hospice may be the best option.

COPING WITH LINGERING SIDE EFFECTS

The problems are real, but their solutions are not easy, quick, or sometimes possible. My belief, though, is that a competent health-care team will increase your odds of being "the best that you can be." In short:

- If low thyroid is a problem, treat it.
- If paralysis limits movement, use the best rehabilitation you can find to build maximal strength and mobility of your functioning parts.
- If you suffer from pain, depression, or rage, then try medications, daily activities, medication changes, massage, yoga, or other complementary therapies.
- If you have memory loss, try using reminder notes, refrigerator messages, 3 x 5 cards on which daily tasks can be written, a preprogrammed cell phone, and possibly medications.
- If speech is affected, perhaps try the "50 help phrases-communication board" developed by a loving caregiver, Teresa.[15] (See Table 20-7 for a model of the board.)

□**Bottom Line** ► Life is sometimes good. It isn't always fair.

Table 20-5 Internet Resources for Side Effects

Blood clot prevention	http://www.greenfieldfilter.com
Brain mapping and loss of function	http://www.radiology.wisc.edu/Med_Students/ neuroradiology/fmri http://www.uscneurosurgery.com/glossary/m/mapping.htm http://seizure.health.ufl.edu/clinical/mapping.htm.
Cerebellar mutism	http://www.childhoodbraintumor.org/02cerebellarmutismlo ice.htm http://health.groups.yahoo.com/group/cerebellarmutism http://www.braintumorkids.org/Medical_News/Cerebellar_ Mutism/posterior_fossa_syndrome.pdf
DEXA Scan (osteoporosis)	http://www.radiologyinfo.org/content/dexa.htm http://www.hss.edu/Departments/Centers/Osteoporosis-Prevention-Center/FAQs/
EEG	http://health.yahoo.com/health/encyclopedia/003931/ 0.html
Frontal lobe syndromes	http://www.ect.org/effects/lobe.html. http://www.chiroweb.com/archives/13/14/05.html
Functional MRI	http://www.radiologyinfo.com/content/functional_mr.htm
Hydrocephalus	http://www.nhfonline.org/page7.html http://www.patientcenters.com/hydrocephalus/news/ differences.html http://www.nyneurosurgery.org/hydro_shunt.htm http://www.hydroassoc.org
Radiation side effects	http://www.abta.org/radiationtherapy.php http://www.abta.org/buildingknowledge5.htm. http://content.health.msn.com/content/article/4/1680_ 50264 http://www.cancer.org/docroot/CRI/content/CRI_2_4_4X_ Radiation_Therapy_3.asp?sitearea http://www.mdadvice.com/topics/radiotherapy/info/ radside.html
Scans- CT and radiation dosage	http://www.eurekalert.org/pub_releases/2003-05/arrs-sr5042403.php, http://www.safety.duke.edu/radsafety/ct_ed and http://www.injuryboard.com/view.cfm/article=891/?ref=ink

Scans- MRI and other scans	http://www.imaginis.com/mri-scan http://health.yahoo.com/health/dc/003791/0.html
Seizures	http://www.emedicine.com/neuro/topic106.htm http://www.nlm.nih.gov/medlineplus/seizures.html http://www.vh.org/adult/provider/familymedicine/ fphandbook/chapter09/04-9.html
Sex and brain tumors	http://www.virtualtrials.com/faq\Sex.cfm
Stereotactic biopsy	http://www.yna.org/new%20pages/sbb.html http://www.mssm.edu/neurosurgery/stereotactic/ biopsy.shtml
Word and speech recognition	http://www.radiologyinfo.com/content/functional_mr.htm http://en2.wikipedia.org/wiki/Magnetic_resonance_ imaging http://www.radiologyinfo.com/content/functional_mr.htm

Table 20-7 Help Phrases for Home or Hospital [15]

1. I AM HUNGRY

2. I AM THIRSTY

3. I WANT WATER

4. I WANT COFFEE/TEA

5. I WANT COLD SODA/JUICE

6. I WANT SOME ICE

7. TOO HOT / TOO COLD

8. I HAVE PAIN HERE

9. I HAVE A BED SORE HERE

10. PLEASE TURN ME

11. I NEED THE BEDPAN

12. PLEASE FIX MY PILLOW

13. FIX/CHANGE MY BED

14. I WANT TO SLEEP

15. PLEASE OPEN THE DOOR

16. PLEASE CLOSE THE DOOR

17. THE LIGHT IS IN MY EYES

18. CALL THE DOCTOR

19. CALL THE NURSE

20. CALL SON/DAUGHTER

21. CALL MY WIFE/HUSBAND

22. CALL MOTHER/FATHER

23. CALL PRIEST/MINISTER

24. I WANT PAPER & PENCIL

25. PLEASE READ TO ME

26. I WANT BOOK/ MAG.

27. PLEASE BRING MY MAIL

28. I WANT MY GLASSES

29. I WANT MY TEETH

30. HOW IS MY CAT/DOG/PET

31. PLEASE TURN TV OFF

32. PLEASE TURN TV ON

33. TURN RADIO ON/OFF

34. I WANT A TISSUE

35. SWAB MY MOUTH

36. BRUSH MY TEETH

37. PLEASE COMB MY HAIR

38. GET ME A MIRROR

39. GET MY PURSE/WALLET

40. WHAT TIME IS IT?

41. WHAT DAY IS IT?

42. WHAT IS THE WEATHER?

43. I WANT ANOTHER PILLOW

44. I WANT A BLANKET

45. WHO IS COMING TO SEE ME, WHEN?

46. I FEEL WORSE

47. I FEEL BETTER

48. THANK YOU

49. PLEASE SMILE!

50. I LOVE YOU VERY MUCH!

CHAPTER 21

Clinical Trials – What Is in It for Me?

There are risks and costs to a program of action. But they are far less than the long-range risks and costs of comfortable inaction.

John F. Kennedy (1917 - 1963)

⚷ **Key search words**

- clinical trial
- Belmont report
- IRB
- Orphan drug
- guinea pig
- informed consent
- costs
- FDA
- Tuskegee Experiment
- institutional review board
- insurance
- experimental therapy

Obtaining honest, factual and complete information helps you overcome the normal anxiety associated with participating in a clinical trial. Here are the rules on how they work, where you can get specific information about them, and what advantages or disadvantages they might offer you.

INTRODUCTION

By the time you are reading this chapter, you may be considering surgery. Or you have made it through surgery and know the name of your tumor, medications, and other conditions. You may be wondering if an experimental therapy may be better that the standard available medical treatment. Or you have been told that your tumor has recurred, and there is no standard therapy for you.

Every potential clinical trial subject must weigh the pros and cons of participating based on the types of treatments that are available, the potential that they will be effective, and the risks of participating in the research treatment.

With that said, most people want to know more about a clinical trial. In terms of enrollment, it is interesting that about 3 percent of adult cancer patients participate compared with more than 75 percent of children. A recent study showed that the main barrier to participation in clinical trials is not the attitude of patients; rather, it is the reluctance of physicians to tell their patients about possible trials and the lack of available clinical trials.[1] I have summarized the concerns that people may offer (see Table 21-1). Do any of these apply to you? The answers are discussed in the rest of this chapter.

> Most people want to know more about a clinical trial. Many have concerns.

Table 21-1 Concerns about Clinical Trials	
Concern	Effect on Fears, Feelings & Emotions
• Will I be a "guinea pig?"	• Loss of control, pain
• Is this the next step to dying?	• Dying, suffering
• Will I be told everything that I need to know?	• Choice, control
• How far must I travel to receive treatment?	• Convenience, expense
• What are the advantages for life, quality of life?	• Control, suffering, cure
• Can I withdraw if I do not like it?	• Control
• How much will it cost me?	• Expense

Let me inform you of my own prejudices regarding trials for people with brain tumors. I am not impartial – I am pro-trial! I make no apologies for this. In my opinion, clinical trials are the best way to get the most advanced, state-of-the-art therapy, when your doctors do not know what is best. The pharmaceutical manufacturers test and the FDA approves more drugs today than at any other time in our history.[2] As a bonus, the average person treated on early phase clinical trials did have improved survival compared with those on "best available" conventional treatments.[3] This finding is all the more remarkable considering that most of the Phase 1 studies do not show increased tumor response rates. It could be that more careful monitoring and prevention of complications occur in the trials.

Revisiting the interpretation of Eve and Adam in the Garden of Eden (Chapters 1 and 2),[4] I believe that seeking knowledge can lead you toward consciousness and understanding, and away from fear.

WHAT IS A CLINICAL TRIAL?

A clinical trial is a method designed to study, scientifically, the effectiveness of a specific treatment. In the area of brain tumors and cancer, it can evaluate chemotherapy, radiation therapy, biologic therapy, a surgical technique, a device, and/or quality of life (QOL). The outcome could be the effect on length or quality of life, or how well a drug or device works.

> A clinical trial is a method to study the effectiveness of a specific treatment.

WHAT IS A PROTOCOL?

A *protocol* is the "recipe" for how the trial will be performed: eligible types of tumors, age and health of the participant, drug amount and timing, type and frequency of required tests, and so forth. These variables are all defined by the researchers initiating the clinical trial. The protocol and trial undergo oversight and monitoring at each institution or hospital by an Institutional Review Board. (IRB). The role of the IRB is discussed in detail below.

> A protocol is the "recipe" for how the trial will be performed.

WHAT ARE PHASES OF A TRIAL?

There are at least three types of clinical trials, detailed below. These reflect advancing stages in development of the drug, device, or technique under study.

Phase 1: Determination of safe drug doses and schedules

- The main goal is to find the safe dose of medication or safety of the instrument or technique.
- Animal studies or results with other cancers suggest the drug, device, or technique being tested could be a promising treatment.
- The treatment possibly has not been evaluated before in people with brain tumors.
- Eligible patients need *not* have a documented tumor in a specific site.
- Patients are carefully observed for side effects (toxicity) and for any indications of anti-cancer effectiveness.
- Patients must be able to perform daily living activities independently (Karnofsky score).[5]

> Phases of a trial reflect advancing stages in development of the drug, device or technique.

Phase 2: Determination of effectiveness

- The safe dose of medication has already been determined (Phase 1).
- The study question is, "Does the treatment shrink or stabilize the tumor?"
- Eligibility:
   The trial is open to patients who have relapsed on initial therapy.
   It can be designed for newly diagnosed patients as well.
- It is usually a single treatment (it is not being compared with something else).
- The tumor stage and amount of tumor need to be documented.
- No placebo or comparison control group is used.

Phase 3: Comparison with an existing, effective standard therapy

- The patient may receive either the experimental or the standard treatment.
- A computer assigns the person to a treatment: a process called "randomization."
- The investigator does not know which treatment is best.
- Sometimes, no treatment, standard treatment or placebo can be the comparison group.
- Most cancer trials do *not* use placebos.

WHY AM I UNEASY ABOUT CLINICAL TRIALS?

As a patient you want the best treatment available for your tumor – period! For many brain tumors, however, other than surgery and radiation therapy, we do

Bottom Line The average person on early phase clinical trials had improved survival compared with "best available" conventional treatments.

not know the *right* treatment for initial therapy or recurrence. The clinical trial is a method of determining that information.

Many of the treatments that you have received so far were developed with clinical trials in which other patients participated. These include surgical approaches, instruments used during surgery, the amount of dye necessary to visualize a tumor with an MRI scan, and chemotherapy drugs (such as CeeNU, Temodar, Gliadel), and Gliasite radiation implant for recurrent gliomas. Therapies continuously evolve, based on knowledge of collective experience, not just opinion.

MY PROTECTIONS AND RIGHTS

What is unknown can make you feel uneasy, as if you are a guinea pig. The significance of the Tuskegee experiment described below, as reported in 1973, has had lasting effects on everyone considering a clinical trial. In part, based on that unethical study, there are more protections today for persons considering participation in a clinical trial in the United States than at any other time in history.

The Tuskegee Study

The following passage from a news release highlights the ethical violations (underlined) that today all Institutional Review Boards protect against.

> *This experiment symbolizes medical misconduct and blatant disregard for human rights that took place in the name of science. The study's principal investigators were not mad scientists; they were government physicians, respected men of science who published reports on the study in the leading medical journals.[6]*

> *In 1932, the Public Health Service, working with the Tuskegee Institute, began a study in Macon County, Alabama, to record the natural history of syphilis…It was called the 'Tuskegee Study of Untreated Syphilis in the Negro Male.' The United States Public Health Service, in trying to learn more about syphilis and justify treatment programs for Blacks, <u>withheld adequate treatment</u> from a group of poor black men who had the disease, causing <u>needless pain and suffering</u> for the men and their loved ones.*

> *What Went Wrong? In July 1972, a front-page New York Times story about the Tuskegee Study caused a public outcry that led the Assistant Secretary for Health and Scientific Affairs to appoint an Ad Hoc Advisory Panel to review the*

study. The panel found that the <u>men had "agreed" to be examined and treated</u>. However, there was <u>no evidence that researchers had informed them of the study or its real purpose.</u> In fact, the <u>men had been misled</u> and <u>had not been given all the facts</u> required to provide <u>informed consent.</u>

The men were <u>never given adequate treatment</u> for their disease. Even when penicillin became the drug of choice for syphilis in 1947, <u>researchers did not offer it</u> to the subjects. The advisory panel found nothing to show that subjects were ever given the <u>choice of quitting the study</u>, even when this new, highly effective treatment became widely used.

The advisory panel concluded that the Tuskegee Study was "ethically unjustified"—the <u>knowledge gained was sparse when compared with the risks</u> the study posed for its subjects. In October 1972, the panel advised stopping the study at once. A month later, the Assistant Secretary for Health and Scientific Affairs announced the end of the Tuskegee Study. In the wake of Tuskegee and other studies, government took a closer look at research involving human subjects and made changes to prevent the moral breaches that occurred in Tuskegee from happening again.

THE BELMONT REPORT

The Federal government responded to the critique of the Tuskegee Study. Five years later in 1978, the National Commission for the Protection of Human Subjects of Biomedical and Behavioral Research finalized its report entitled, *The Belmont Report*: *Ethical Principles and Guidelines for the Protection of Human Subjects of Research*. This was the result of a conference at the Smithsonian Institution in Washington, D.C. where the discussions took place. The report sets forth the basic principles of acceptable conduct for research involving human subjects:

> The men in the Tuskegee study were never given treatment for their disease, even when penicillin became the drug of choice in 1947.

Respect for persons – recognition of the personal dignity and autonomy of individuals, and special protection of those persons with diminished autonomy.

Beneficence – an obligation to protect persons from harm by maximizing anticipated benefits and minimizing possible risks of harm.

Justice – the fair distribution of benefits and burdens of research.

□ **Bottom Line** ▶ As a result of the Tuskegee experiment, there are more protections today for persons considering participation in a clinical trial in the U.S. than at any time in history.

These three principles are now accepted as the three quintessential requirements for the ethical conduct of research involving human subjects.

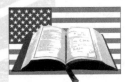

The *Report* also describes how these principles apply to the conduct of research. Specifically:

- Principle of respect for persons underlies the need to obtain <u>informed consent</u>;
- Principle of beneficence underlies the need to engage in a <u>risk/benefit analysis</u> and to <u>minimize risks</u>; and
- Principle of justice requires that <u>subjects be fairly selected</u>.

As was mandated by the congressional charge to the Commission, the *Report* also provides a distinction between *practice* and *research*. The Belmont Report is now used by almost every biomedical institution carrying out clinical research. It defines basic ethical principles and the boundaries between practice and research.[7]

HOW DOES THE IRB PROTECT MY INTERESTS?

The Institutional Review Board (IRB) at a hospital or university is a group of medical professionals, lay people, and clergy who review and discuss every study, periodically monitor each one, and receive reports of side effects or unexpected adverse events. This board supplements any oversight that a sponsoring pharmaceutical company or medical device manufacturer might have. The IRB reviews a clinical trial to ensure that it has safeguards to protect those who participate and to prevent or minimize significant risks. The 11 points asked of each study closely follow the omissions in the Tuskegee experiment and put into action the recommendations of the *Belmont Report* (see Table 21-2).

> Belmont Principles: • Informed consent
> • A risk/benefit analysis to minimize
> risks. • Fair selection of subjects.

Bottom line The Belmont Report sets forth basic principles for acceptable research conduct with human subjects.

Table 21-2 IRB Criteria for Evaluation, Approval, & Monitoring of a Research Study
1. Clear information will be given to the patient about the purpose of the study through informed consent.
2. A clear description of the drugs or devices to be tested will be given to all participants.
3. There will be absence of pressure or inappropriate incentives to enroll in the study.
4. Patients will be given assurance of minimal risks (if any).
5. A risk-benefit analysis shows that personal benefits outweigh the risks.
6. Freedom to withdraw is clearly stated and equally available to all patients.
7. Selection of subjects will be equitable; minorities will not be over- or under-represented.
8. Conduct of the study will be monitored. Participants will be informed who is responsible and to whom the study will be reported.
9. Patient comments and complaints will be reviewed.
10. Privacy and confidentiality will be maintained. Release of any personal information will be clearly stated in advance of the agreement to participate.
11. Responsibilities of each affiliated investigator will be clearly defined.

CAN I WITHDRAW FROM THE STUDY?

Yes! Your rights as a study participant are secured by both State regulations and the Code of Federal Regulations CFR:Title 45, part 46.116 General requirements for informed consent.[8,9] The underlined words address issues that were learned from the Tuskegee study and are now incorporated into law. The Institutional Review Board's responsibility is to ensure that the law is upheld for clinical trial participants. (See Table 21-2 for a list of IRB criteria for the evaluation and approval of a research study.)

The law accomplishes the following on your behalf:

1. It safeguards the welfare of humans and assures that subjects are given enough information about the research to make informed decisions whether or not to participate.
2. Federal and state laws mandate the establishment of an Institutional Review Board (IRB). The IRB is responsible for: a) initial and continuing review; and b) approval of research that involves subjects in an institution; or c) conduct of research by an individual (affiliated with the institution) who agrees to assume responsibility for the study.

3. The laws require that specified information be given so that a person may give <u>informed consent</u> and <u>that this consent process be documented</u>.

4. Federal Policy for "protection of human subjects" governs human research funded or conducted by a Federal department or agency. Under federal and state law, "No investigator may involve a human being as a subject in medical research, unless the investigator has obtained the legally effective <u>informed consent</u> of the subject or the subject's legally authorized representative."

> Local IRB is responsible for putting *Belmont Report* protections into action for your safety.

5. Requirements for informed consent
   - There must be sufficient opportunity to consider whether or not to participate in order to minimize the possibility of coercion or undue influence.
   - Information about the study must be presented in a language understandable to the person giving consent. California law states <u>that the information must be given in a language in which the person giving consent is fluent. (Other states have similar provisions.)</u>
   - No informed consent may include any language that frees the investigator from blame or responsibility for negligence.
   - The end of this chapter details the complete basic elements of the "Patient's Bill of Rights" (see Table 21-11).

Federal government oversight has been unforgiving, even with leading cancer centers. Potential conflicts of interest that ethicists believe might pose risks to patients and to the integrity of scientific studies have been made public. (An example of a publicized ethical violation can be found on the following web site: http://www.washingtonpost.com/wp-srv/national/daily/may99/duke12.htm; the legal responsibility of the IRB is illustrated at: http://www.sskrplaw.com/gene/robertson/complaint1.html).

Experimental Subject's Bill of Rights

The (California) Protection of Human Subjects in Medical Experimentation Act requires that all subjects be given a copy of the "Experimental Subject's Bills of Rights" before consent to participate in any medical experiment is obtained (most other states have similar legislation). The Bill of Rights <u>must be in writing</u> (in a language in which the subject is fluent), and <u>must be signed</u> and <u>dated by the subject</u>. A sample copy appears at the end of this chapter in Table 21-11. Other states may have similar provisions.

HOW IS A CLINICAL TRIAL DEVELOPED AND CONDUCTED?

The clinical trial is developed by an individual or team at a hospital, academic center, institute, or commercial company. The goal of a clinical trial is to improve treatment or diagnosis for the benefit of patients. The biomedical company that develops the drug or device may sponsor or pay for (part of) the trial costs, such as:

- Nurses to obtain data and follow-up with patient contact.
- Secretarial costs, costs of submission for Institutional Review Board approval.
- Your Laboratory or transportation expenses.
- Administrative time for the Principal Investigator, the one responsible for the trial.

Depending upon the stage of research, the clinical trial will conform to criteria for Phase 1, 2, or 3.

The physician (Principal Investigator, or PI) writes a protocol using ethical, scientific, state and federal guidelines. The PI is responsible for the conduct of the trial as well as any updates or changes made during the trial.

Each clinical trial follows a treatment plan or protocol, the "recipe" for drug amount, timing, type and frequency of tests required, costs to patient, and so on. Most trials must be approved at each outpatient clinic, hospital, university, or other institution by an Institutional Review Board (IRB). Ask if yours is approved.

> Principal Investigator (PI) writes a protocol using ethical, scientific, state, and federal guidelines. PI is responsible for conduct of the trial.

TO JOIN OR NOT TO JOIN A CLINICAL TRIAL

WHY WOULD I CHOOSE A CLINICAL TRIAL?

This is an individual decision and people voice many different, personal reasons (see Table 21-3).

Table 21-3 Reasons to Enroll in a Clinical Trial	
Personal Objective	Example of Possible Reasons
To try a new treatment and increase hope for a cure and longer life	The current treatment is not what you wish. Side effects of the standard treatment could outweigh the benefits. Example: someone with a GBM may think side effects of BCNU (standard therapy) are not worth the possible benefits.
To feel better	The tumor is causing troubling effects on your function that is not being helped by the current therapy. A new therapy may shrink the tumor.
To assist in helping others in the future.	Participation is consistent with your philosophy of life and would represent a legacy to your family or community. Example: A drug study for pain control that can benefit you as well as others.

HOW AND WHERE DO YOU FIND A CLINICAL TRIAL FOR YOUR TUMOR TYPE?

The first and easiest way is to ask your specialist physician what clinical trials he or she may have available to you. Most brain tumor specialists will have access to clinical trials. If there are none being conducted locally, perhaps he or she can call another center or refer you to another physician.

Some Web sites allow you to search by your tumor type and situation.

In the uncommon situation where your physician cannot help, it is time to become adventuresome and use other resources (see Chapter 4: Surfing the Web" and Table 21-4, that list other resources for finding clinical trials).[4] Academic centers, universities, institutes with formal neurooncology programs, and large neurosurgical and radiation centers offer the greatest number of all phases of clinical trials. (See also Chapter 7: Tables 7-8, 7-9, and 7-10)[4] This does not mean that their studies are best for you, however.

Nationwide, Phase 2 and 3 clinical trials take place both in local oncologists' offices and in large medical centers. The most up-to-date information can be obtained on web sites or by telephone. Clinical trials, especially a Phase 1 study, can be intermittently closed. So a call to the principal investigator's (PI)'s office will confirm its status.

Table 21-4 Resources for Finding Clinical Trials

1. Primary physician, physician friends, or specialist experts.

2. Support groups at your hospital, in your community.

3. Television stories on the news, Discovery and Health channels.

4. Local library and health magazines, references books, Time and Newsweek.

5. Commercial advertisements in the newspaper.

6. Friends.

7. Brain Tumor Organizations, such as the American Brain Tumor Association, Brain Tumor Society, National Brain Tumor Foundation, NCI, and so forth.

8. The world wide web (Internet) using "key search words" and the last table in each chapter of this book (see also Chapter 4: Searching the Web).

9. Web site Examples

General information on finding a clinical trial	www.virtualtrials.com
	http://cancer.gov/clinicaltrials
	http://www.nabtt.org
	http://cancer.gov/clinicaltrials/finding
	https://www.veritasmedicine.com
	https://www.veritasmedicine.com/d_index_
	    tc.cfm?did=3&cid=0
	http://www.emergingmed.com (78 listed clinical trials as of
	    February 16, 2005)

Glioma, Meningioma trials	www.virtualtrials.com
Neurofibromatosis trials	http://www.nf.org/clinical_trials
Pituitary Trials	http://www.virtualtrials.com/pitlst.cfm http://www.pituitary.org http://www.braintumors.com http://capstoneclinic-dl.slis.ua.edu/patientinfo/ endocrinology/pituitary.html
Acoustic neuroma trials	www.ANAusa.org/list.htm http://www.acousticneuroma.neurosurgery.pitt.edu
Germ cell tumor trials	http://www.emedicine.com/med/topic863.htm http://www.emedicine.com/med/topic759.htm http://www.centerwatch.com/patient/studies/cat564.html

Using the world wide web sometimes can be daunting. You begin by not knowing about one study, and then you find too many from which to choose! Some web sites allow you to search by your tumor type and situation (recurrent or newly diagnosed tumor). The www.virtualtrials.com and http://www.emergingmed.com sites allow a search by type of tumor. You can search for "less toxic" or complementary and alternative types of trials on www.virtualtrials.com .

Narrow your choices down to only clinical trials for which you are eligible (see Table 21-5). If, for example, a trial is for *newly diagnosed* patients with meningiomas and yours is a *recurrent* tumor, do not bother. It is not for you! If there is any question, most sites have a phone number or e-mail address for your inquiry. Often, eligibility rules are posted on the web site (see Table 21-10).

Table 21-5 Facts You Need to Know for Clinical Trial Eligibility
1. Type of tumor and histological grade (e.g., astrocytoma, grades 3 and 4).
2. Whether the tumor is new or recurrent.
3. Size or spread of tumor (localized or metastatic).
4. Age (some trials are for adults or children).
5. Previous treatments (radiation; types of chemotherapy)
6. Quality of functioning (Karnofsky score of 60% or more).
7. Distance from home (convenience).
8. Location where treatment must be given (near home or only at treating institution).

WHAT IS A KARNOFSKY SCORE?

The Karnofsky score is a rating of your ability to perform activities of daily living (ADLs), such as getting dressed and feeding yourself. It is used to assess your eligibility for enrollment in a clinical (experimental drug) trial, your response to treatments, or even eligibility for hospice care (see Table 21-6).

▭▸ **Bottom Line** The Karnofsky score is a rating of your ability to perform activities of daily living.

Table 21-6 Karnofsky Performance Scale	
Description of Function/Activities/Needs	Index
Normal, no complaints; no evidence of disease	100%
Able to carry on normal activity; minor signs of disease	90%
Normal activity with effort; some signs of symptoms of disease	80%
Cares for self; unable to carry on normal activity or to do active work	70%
Requires occasional assistance but is able to care for most of own needs	60%
Requires considerable assistance with ADLs and frequent medical care	50%
Disabled; requires special care and maximum assistance	40%
Severely disabled, although death not imminent	30%
Gravely ill; unable to swallow; totally dependent	20%
Actively dying	10%
Death	0%

WHICH IS THE BEST TRIAL FOR YOU?

Deciding on the best trial is a personal decision based on your search results, possible benefits to you, potential side effects, phase of trial, location of the trial, number of visits and tests required, and your comfort with the treatment team.[10] I have prepared a list of questions to help you make this decision (see Table 21-7).

WHAT IS IMPORTANT TO KNOW IN CONSIDERING A CLINICAL TRIAL?

Considering a clinical trial can be an emotionally charged experience, as your life may be at stake. It is important not to overlook critical questions before enrollment. Some people become disenchanted with their choice of clinical trial, when they experienced unwanted (unexpected) side effects, for example. Age should not be a factor in enrollment. A recent study showed that older brain tumor patients had no worse survival on a clinical trial than younger counterparts.[11]

Here are 14 questions that will help you to assess whether or not a specific clinical trial is for you. There are no right or wrong answers here. The questions are designed to help you determine how comfortable you are with the treatment team and plan.

Table 21-7 Questions to Ask About the Clinical Trial		
General		
1. Who is conducting the study? Is it an individual institution or a national trial?		
2. In which phase is this clinical trial?		
3. Has the treatment been tested on people with brain tumors before?		
4. Where will I receive my treatment?		
5. Is there an institution close to home where I can receive the treatment?		
6. Does the center have a special neuro-oncology (or brain tumor) program?		
Treatment–related		
7. Who will be the physician directly responsible for my care, while I receive experimental therapy? Will my local doctor be involved?		
8. What tests, treatments, hospital stay, and time will be required?		
9. What other choices are available?		
10. Are there other competing studies at this institution?		
11. How do the study treatments compare?		
12. Which potential side effects may occur? How could they affect my daily life?		
13. What does the treatment cost? Is any part provided free of charge to me?		
14. Which treatment, tests, and physician visits are paid for by the study? For what am I responsible? (See Chapter 23: Managing Costs and Benefits: Insurance and HMOs.)		

You need to know who will be responsible for your care (#7) for important and practical reasons. The principal investigator in charge of the study may not be the one answering your anxious phone calls on Friday evening, when you have a fever or forgot yesterday's dose of medication. Large institutions (#10) may have several oncology groups or studies coming from different departments that do not always communicate with each other. These questions will ascertain that you have in your possession the maximum information from the institution.

WHAT PRECAUTIONS ARE NEEDED TO EVALUATE CLINICAL TRIALS ON THE INTERNET?

Web sites that provide listings of clinical trials are growing in popularity (Tables 21-4, 21-10), but a new United States government report reveals a potential danger for patients. At least 60 percent of sites did not indicate the phase of the clinical trial, making it impossible for a patient to distinguish a Phase I trial that is designed strictly to test the safety of an experimental drug from a Phase III trial comparing two or more treatments. While 12 sites generate revenue, half of them fail to disclose how they do so. Financial relationships can affect which trials are offered and how a site's information is presented and interpreted. None of the sites disclosed the risks of participating in a study, and less than a third give the names of the trial sponsors. Such omissions undermine the goal of the informed consent process.[12]

FREQUENTLY ASKED QUESTIONS ABOUT CLINICAL TRIALS

WHY CAN'T I JUST GET THE NEW TREATMENT "OFF STUDY" IF I DO NOT QUALIFY?

Many people feel uncomfortable with being *randomized* to one alternative. They

> There are good reasons not to accept "experimental" therapy without being in a clinical trial.

want the "latest," not the standard option, and may ask the investigator for permission to use just the experimental therapy "off study." Does it ever happen? Yes. Should it? No. Here is why:

1. Safety reasons

This is not treatment; it is an experimental, unproven therapy. Initial results may be promising, but it still is not an approved drug, combination, or device. There is a real possibility that it might not be beneficial or that it can cause unexpected side effects. Who is responsible for the harmful side effects? Such effects are illustrated in the 2002 news report below on a hot new anti–EGF receptor therapy:

> Gefitinib (Iressa) has been taken by at least 10,000 cancer patients since it was cleared for use in Japan in July 2000. In October 2002, Astra-Zeneca issued a safety warning to doctors after the company received reports of severe side effects in 26 patients, including 13 (with lung cancer) who died.

Although the drug did not necessarily cause the deaths, it was investigational in the United States for brain tumors. Therefore, all patients enrolled in any trials had their records evaluated carefully. Without being in the study, no such notification would have taken place.

2. Ethical reasons

A patient who is not formally enrolled in the study, who has not given written consent for the experimental drug but still sees this as treatment, drains the financial and administrative support for the other patients who are formally enrolled in the study.

3. Scientific reasons

The "off study" patient's data cannot be used in the study; therefore, it does not help the study meet its intended goals. Information that is obtained "off study" (tumor response or serious side effects) are not reported as part of the study. (The side effects may be included in an individual case report.)

4. Legal reasons

The principal investigator (PI) must respond to the Institutional Review Board, study sponsor, and federal oversight agency regarding the reasons why a participating patient was not enrolled in the study. The way they see it, if the patient was ineligible for the study, then he/she should not have received the drug. Thus, the institution's status is called into question; the PI's research reputation and ability to serve in this capacity again are at risk; and his or her license to practice medicine may be jeopardized.

5. Burden of responsibility reasons

Another approach is for you to petition the principal investigator (PI), institution, or National Cancer Institute (NCI), in order to get "compassionate exemption" for use of the experimental treatment. There are reasons why the PI of a study might shy away from doing this, in addition to items #1 through 4 above. If they reject your request, it is because of the burden of added responsibility, not because they are unkind or unfeeling for your critical situation. If the physician agrees to administer the drug to a patient who is not a registered participants, he/ she must make a complex, formal proposal for each case to the NCI oversight board, provide documentation for the exemption, and promise to provide individual follow-up reports to the NCI of all toxicity for the life of the patient.

What Are the Latest Approaches Being Tested in Clinical Trials?

Up to the 1990s, the vast majority of (the few) clinical trials for brain tumors were aimed at testing radiation therapy doses or chemotherapies useful for other cancers. There are now at least 140 trials using novel strategies for brain tumors. (For web resources regarding clinical trials, see Tables 21-4 and 21-10, and the list on http://www.emergingmed.com.) As results accrue, successful approaches will be moved up to larger Phase 2 and 3 trials. Sometimes a news release will highlight a promising therapy,[13] but many of these do not work out over time. Table 21-8 summarizes 10 new approaches that target people with brain tumors. The underlined key word examples in Table 21-8 can be used in your Internet search for even more new therapy options.

After deciding on a clinical trial, the issue of costs needs to be addressed. Chapter 23: Managing, Costs, Benefits and Your Health Care With Insurance explores more details about your health care finances and how to get coverage for your treatments and follow-up. (See also next section on Health Insurance.)

Table 21-8 Newer Approaches to Brain Tumor Therapy – 2005	
Mechanism & Key Words	Method or Drug Names
Anti-angiogenesis Prevention of new blood vessel formation, thereby preventing tumor growth.	Mostly Phase 1 • Avastin • TNP-470, SU-5416 • Angiostatin, endostatin • Pentosan polysulfate, • Platelet factor 4 • Thalidomide
Chemotherapy + anti-angiogenesis agents	Phase 1, 2 Chemotherapy+COX-2 inhibitors Celebrex
Chemotherapy – novel routes • Disruption of the blood-brain barrier • Continuous infusion (enhanced convection) • Direct instillation of chemotherapy into tumor	Phases 1, 2, and 3 Convection-enhanced delivery of drug Blood-brain barrier disruption for drug entry

Gene Therapy Injection of genes intravenously or directly into the tumor. This stimulates *programmed cell death* or other killing mechanisms.	Phase 1 Herpes and other custom-designer viruses
<u>Immunotherapy</u> Energizing and re-educating of the immune system to recognize and destroy the tumor.	Phases 1 and 2 • <u>Dendritic cell</u> immunization • Natural killer cell stimulation • Programmed cytotoxic T cells
Stem Cells Targeting of cells (search and destroy)	Phase 1 Stem cells carry pro-drugs or genes
<u>Differentiation Agents</u> Causing of tumor cells to slow their rate of growth.	Phases 1 and 2 • <u>Retinoids, Cis-retinoic acid, Fenretinide</u> • All-trans <u>retinoic acid (ATRA)</u> • Sodium <u>phenylacetate</u>, Sodium <u>phenylbutyrate</u>
<u>Radiation Sensitizers</u> Selective uptake by cancer cells.	Phase 2 and 3 • Xcytrin (<u>motexafin gadolinium</u>) • <u>RSR-13</u>
Targeting of specific "messengers" in the cancer cell's operating system.	Phases 1, 2, and 3 • <u>Signal-transduction inhibitors</u> • <u>Bryostatin, Hypericin</u> • <u>SU-101, UCN-01, Suramin</u> • <u>Matrix-metalloproteinase inhibitors</u> • <u>Bay 12-9566, Ag 3340</u> • <u>Farnesyltransferase inhibitors (FTI)</u> • <u>Tumor Necrosis-Targeting Antibodies (Cotara)</u>
Specific cell surface receptors Interference with communication or transmission of growth signals inside of a cell.	Phase 1, 2. • <u>Interferons, immunotoxin</u> delivery by antibodies (<u>IL-13-PE38QQR</u>) • <u>Tarceva, Iressa (anti-Epidermal Growth Receptor) (EGFr)</u>

WILL MY HEALTH INSURANCE PAY FOR EXPERIMENTAL THERAPY?

A *yes* answer depends upon the state or country in which you reside. California and 11 other states specifically require health insurance companies to cover "routine cancer care and support" during *all* phases of clinical cancer trials as of 8/9/2001 (see Table 21-9 for a list of the 12 states). Modeled on language approved by the Clinton administration for Medicare coverage, the laws require coverage of hospitalization, physician visits, drugs, laboratory tests, and other expenses for study participants with any type of cancer while enrolled in an approved clinical trial. (See also Table 21-10 for Internet-based insurance coverage information.)

Table 21-9 12 States with Mandatory Insurance Coverage for Clinical Trials (2005)			
California	Connecticut	Delaware	Georgia
Illinois	Louisiana	Maryland	New Hampshire
North Carolina	Rhode Island	Vermont	Virginia

Legislation has been created to encourage more cancer patients to participate in and benefit from clinical trials. Implementing this law in California alone could allow more than 3500 new people a year to be eligible, because now they could afford it. It is possible that your insurance company representative may not know this. You can refer them to the following web site, which list specific health benefits by states: http://www.insure.com/health/lawtool.cfm. Fight for your rights!

ORPHAN DRUGS AND CLINICAL TRIALS

Primary brain tumors are a relatively rare form of cancer in adults (about 30,000 new cases per year). This makes the "market" for developing specific cancer drugs a financially unrewarding proposition. Brain tumors (primary and metastatic) fit the definition of an "orphan disease":

- One that affects less than 200,000 persons in the UNITED STATES
- One that affects more than 200,000 persons in the UNITED STATES, but there is no reasonable expectation that developing and selling a drug for this disease or condition will be cost-effective.[14]

The 1983 Orphan Drug Act (P.L. 97-414) guarantees seven years of market exclusivity for the developer of an orphan product following approval by the

FDA. Thankfully, this provides an incentive for drug development companies to focus on brain tumors; Gliadel and GliaSite were developed under these terms (see descriptions of the way that Gliadel and GliaSite work in Chapters 17 and 19). Orphan status itself does not affect your conditions of participation in a clinical trial.

This chapter has described the process and content of clinical trials. Chapters 23, 24 provide additional information on insurance issues and clinical trials. Chapter 22 discusses clinical trial issues specifically for children.

Table 21-10 Web Site Resources for Clinical Trials

Subject	Web site
Acoustic neuromas	www.ANAusa.org/list.htm http://www.acousticneuroma.neurosurgery.pitt.edu www.ANAusa.org/list.htm support@anausa.org (E-mail)
Blood brain barrier disruption	http://www.ohsu.edu/bbb
Brain tumors	http://www.brainTMR@mitvma.mit.edu
Cancer and COX-2	http://www.jci.org/cgi/content/full/105/11/1511 All sites accessed and retrieved February 18, 2005.
Clinical Trial- general Finding one	www.virtualtrials.com http://cancer.gov/clinicaltrials http://www.nabtt.org http://cancer.gov/clinicaltrials/finding https://www.veritasmedicine.com https://www.veritasmedicine.com/d_index_tc.cfm?did=3&cid=0 http://www.emergingmed.com (85 listed clinical trials as of February 18, 2005)
Clinical Trial- Recruitment service by drug industry. Veritas Medicine	www.veritasmedicine.com
Clinical Trial- understanding	http://cancer.gov/clinicaltrials/understanding
Clinical Trials-search	http://cancer.gov/clinicaltrials/finding www.virtualtrials.com http://www.emergingmed.com

Germ cell tumors and clinical trials	http://www.emedicine.com/med/topic863.htm http://www.emedicine.com/med/topic759.htm http://www.centerwatch.com/patient/studies/cat564.html
Insurance coverage & clinical trials	http://cancer.gov/clinicaltrials/digestpage/private-insurers http://www.cancer.gov/clinicaltrials/understanding/insurance-coverage
Insurance coverage for clinical trials by state	http://www.insure.com/health/lawtool.cfm http://cancer.gov/clinicaltrials/digestpage/private-insurers http://www.cancer.gov/clinicaltrials/understanding/insurance-coverage
Meningioma	www.virtualtrials.com
Neurofibromatosis	http://www.nf.org/clinical_trials
Pituitary	http://www.virtualtrials.com/pitlst.cfm http://www.pituitary.org http://www.braintumors.com http://capstoneclinic-dl.slis.ua.edu/patientinfo/endocrinology/pituitary.html
Radiation sensitizer (example)	http://www.docguide.com/news/content.nsf/news/852569770057 3E1885256B22004973D C?Open&id=48DDE4A73E09A9698525688800 78C249&count=10
Tuskegee experiment	http://www.cdc.gov/nchstp/od/tuskegee/time.htm

Table 21-11 Experimental Subject's Bill of Rights

Any person who is required to consent to participate as a subject in a research study involving a medical experiment or who is requested to consent on behalf of another has the right to:

1. Be informed of the nature and purpose of the experiment.
2. Be given an explanation of the procedures to be followed in the medical experiment, and any drug or device to be utilized.
3. Be given a description of any attendant discomforts and risks reasonably to be expected from the experiment.
4. Be given an explanation of any benefits to the subject reasonably to be expected from the experiment, if applicable.
5. Be given a disclosure of any appropriate alternative procedures, drugs or devices that might be advantageous to the subject, and their relative risks and benefits.
6. Be informed of the avenues of medical treatment, if any, available to the subject after the experiment if complications should arise.
7. Be given an opportunity to ask any questions concerning the experiment or the procedure involved.
8. Be instructed that consent to participate in the medical experiment may be withdrawn at any time and the subject may discontinue participation in the medical experiment without prejudice.
9. Be given a copy of any signed and dated written consent form used in relation to the experiment.
10. Be given the opportunity to decide to consent or not to consent to a medical experiment without the intervention of any element of force, fraud, deceit, duress, coercion, or undue influence on the subject's decision.

CHAPTER 22A

Children with Brain Tumors – Special Considerations in Diagnosis and Treatment

Children are not just miniature adults. Specialist treatment can make the difference between just surviving… and quality survival.

Paul Zeltzer 2003

CHILDREN WITH BRAIN TUMORS

⚷ Key search words

- brain injury
- radiation
- late effects
- pituitary
- clinical trial

- development
- chemotherapy
- endocrine
- diabetes insipidus

- pediatric neurosurgeon
- medication
- hormone
- thyroid

CHAPTER 22A
Children with
Brain Tumor

INTRODUCTION

Previous chapters provide information about diagnosis and treatment of specific tumors and guide you on how to be the most effective advocate for your child. These techniques are the same for a spouse or a parent. This chapter provides

Children are NOT miniature adults.

important information about the unique features of the tumors and their treatment in the child. It includes information and guidelines that many families have learned and used to attain the best possible outcome. Helpful pamphlet, book,[1] equipment, and web-linked resources specifically for children, including hormonal after-effects are highlighted and referenced in Table 22A-4. Social and psychological effects of the tumor and its treatment are detailed in Chapter 22B.

Children are not miniature adults. Their bodies and brains are growing, changing and have different reactions to treatments than adults. A brain tumor in a child means that special precautions must be taken, from the dose of x-rays of a CAT scan, radiation therapy or medications, to the choice of a treatment center. As a blessing for their innocence, children with brain tumors usually respond better to our current therapies than do adults with the same tumor.

FINDING INFORMATION ABOUT CHILDHOOD BRAIN TUMORS

Cancer is the number one cause of death from disease in children,[2] and brain tumors account for 25 percent of these deaths. However, cancer is no longer a death sentence. By the year 2020, one in every 1000 United States' citizens will be a survivor of childhood cancer. In fact, more than 60 percent of children with cancer survive the disease.[3] Most child brain tumors start and grow in the lower, rear part of the brain (called posterior fossa). They differ in type and location from those in adults. (See Figures 22A-1, 2-2, 2-3.) Tumor types are listed in the glossary and in the chapters on primary tumors.

Children who are cancer survivors, however, experience a range of short and long-term effects in their medical health, psychological, cognitive

Many children will experience long-term effects: physical, psychological, cognitive & neuropsychological.

and neuropsychological functions, all of which impact re-entry to the family and classroom.[4,5] Nowhere are these effects more dramatic than with

□**Bottom Line** ➤ 60% of children with cancer will be long-term survivors.

children who have nervous system tumors, the most common of all childhood cancers. Thus you must be aggressive in seeking resources and information to make the best choices. This is how Carol deals with her doubts about being "aggressive."

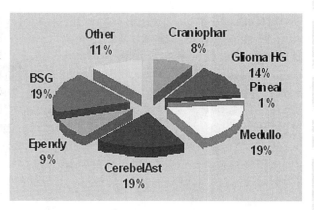

Figure 22A-1 Common Brain Tumors in Children

If you think there's something wrong with your kid...there probably is...if you request a test or something be checked out, don't fear being proved wrong. If the test comes out negative, you win, as then you know that is NOT the problem (yea. If it turns out positive then you can start treatment and your child should start feeling better.

Don't worry about hurting a doc's feelings or wounding their ego. This is about YOUR child and getting the right thing done to insure proper treatment, NOT about them. This is their job; sometimes we just have to show, push or shove them in the right direction though.

Get used to it...it will be like this for as long as you parent this child.

Carol, mom to Mandy. Norman, OK

There are many sources for additional information. Brain tumor foundations have been started by parents, like yourself, whose children were diagnosed with a brain tumor. They have priceless knowledge from direct experience including materials and support which can help you: access to state-of-the-art treatment centers (see Chapter 7 [6]); and locate important web sites, chat rooms, list-servers; and opportunities for support and advocacy (see Chapter 4 and Table 22A-4). Books devoted to children with brain tumors[1] can be found on booklists or by searching "brain tumor" or the search words on the first page of this chapter on any of the online bookstore web sites, or by doing a "Google" search (see Chapter 4).

Bottom Line ▸ Treatment at a Center specializing in children's cancer that uses the most advanced therapies & clinical trials will increase your child's chances for survival and quality of life.

Lenore and Murray, grandparents to Sophie, who has a newly diagnosed thalamic tumor, told me of a web site called "Caring Bridge." It guides you step-by-step through the process of making a personal web site for your child and family. It

> Most children's brain tumors grow in the rear part of the brain – posterior fossa.

allows you to post the latest news, findings and progress of your child as well as to upload links and photos. It's an efficient and less time-consuming way of keeping your support circle of family and friends informed, so you don't devote your limited energies to repeating the same routine on the phone 20 times a day. As a physician I had no idea how important this could be (see Table 22A-4).

COMMON QUESTIONS ABOUT BRAIN TUMORS IN CHILDREN

WHY DID MY CHILD GET A BRAIN TUMOR?

You will hear from well-meaning friends, television news programs, and magazines that fast foods, too many diet soft drinks, cell phones, and marijuana are the causes (see Chapter 24: Heredity and Other Causes of Brain Tumors). Forget it! You did not do anything wrong. About 5 percent of people with brain tumors have an inherited tendency to get one. If by chance there is a gene(s) that the family inherited, you received it from someone else, and it is only one of 15,000 other genes you have passed on to your family. You are no more responsible for that than your children's eye color or height.

WHY DO I FEEL ASHAMED OR GUILTY WHEN I KNOW I SHOULD NOT?

You teach your child not to stick his or her hand on a hot stove, to cross the street after looking both ways, and to wear seat belts in the car. These are your responsibilities to make them safe. Then below your radar screen, a tumor comes in… and your lives seem irreversibly changed.

It is normal to feel guilty, hopeless, and worried. Nevertheless, you will move forward through that and do whatever is necessary to help your child. As a children's oncologist and brain tumor specialist, I have never met a parent who did not suffer from guilt. It happens and you cannot prevent it.

▭**Bottom Line**➝ I have never met a parent who did not suffer from guilt. You could not prevent this brain tumor!

Many parents may go through one or more of five stages in coming to terms with their child's illness:

1. Denial: "I don't believe it. The diagnosis must be wrong."
2. Anger/rage: "Why us?" "What did I or someone else do wrong?"
3. Bargaining: "Please let her live until she can go to school… or until she is married."
4. Depression: "I cannot bear this!"
5. Acceptance: "Okay. What can we do to beat this thing?"

Not every one follows the same pattern, so don't be distressed if you do not experience this sequence. But it is normal to have one or more of these reactions.

What Do I Tell People?

Hearing this kind of news can cause a range of reactions. Some friends or family might venture a question. Others may not ever want to know the details. But when someone does say, "If there's ever anything we can do…?" Do not hesitate to reply, "We could use help with carpools, feeding the pets, taking our other children out or to school, preparing, meals," and so on. Share as much as you are comfortable with, including your personal needs. Know that while some may be willing to assist, others may withdraw.

> If friends offer help, say, "Yes!"

What Do I Tell My Child?

You know your child better than any one else. In my experience, parents should tell their child in their own special way about the *here and now*, exactly which event or procedure is going to happen each day in the hospital or clinic. If there will be an uncomfortable procedure (blood drawing, spinal tap etc) then tell them what will occur … and what you are doing to alleviate any discomfort that may occur. This then becomes your responsibility to discuss with the doctors which symptomatic treatments and precautions will eliminate the discomfort (anesthetic cream on skin, conscious sedation for spinal tap or bone marrow exam, music, hypnosis etc.). Likewise, for the MRI scans. Talk with the nurses about the procedures they use with the MRI scanner.

> Talk with your child about here and now: This…will happen today. I am going to be with you… always.

If you lie and the child finds out the truth, then he or she cannot rely on you as much for support. Few children ask initially, "Am I going to die?" The frank answer is that we will all die someday, and the truth is that they are sick. Clarify that you are going to stand by them every step of the way. Unlike adults, the child fears losing contact with his parents or separation (abandonment) more than any threat of dying.

Should We Look Into Controversial Treatments?

Parents faced with a diagnosis of brain tumor in their child are often bombarded with suggestions from well-meaning friends and family. There are many questionable and controversial treatments using diet, "natural products" that promise cures (see Chapter 18: Complementary, Alternative, and other therapies). Most do not meet the test of validity; they only give testimonials. I suggest contacting any of the major brain tumor organizations (ABTA, NBTF, BTS) with links in Chapter 4: Searching the WEB and Internet, or www.virtualtrials.com for more information on specific treatments.

What Is the Controversy about Radiation Dose and Diagnostic CAT Scans?

A computerized axial tomograph (CAT), also called a computerized tomographic (CT) scan, is a 3-dimensional x-ray picture of the brain used for diagnosis and follow-up. The machine emits a lot of radiation (four to 30 times that of a chest x-ray) to get the many images needed to reconstruct a 3-D picture of the brain. For many years, children were receiving adult doses of radiation with each scan.[7] Now children receive lower doses. Ask the radiologist if the CT machine has been recalibrated for a child's dosage. If not, go somewhere else. Unless it is an emergency, it adds to the lifetime risk of getting a secondary cancer (either a brain tumor or leukemia.). This does not apply to MRI machines as they use magnetic energy, not x-rays.

> Doses of X-rays for CAT scans and medications must be adjusted for the age & weight of the child.

How Do Doctors Calculate Medication Dosages for Growing Children?

It seems obvious that a six-month infant should receive a smaller dosage of dexamethasone or chemotherapy than a five-year old child should. A five-year-old's dose could be fatal for an infant. But how do the professionals calculate each

□ **Bottom Line** Every child should have a treatment plan directed by a Team at a major center for childhood brain tumors.

dose? Various parts of an infant grow and use chemotherapy at different rates. Dr. Archie Bleyer, when working at the National Institutes of Health, found that when dosing infants with methotrexate to treat the nervous system, the young child's head and its total spinal fluid volume increased rapidly after birth and reached near adult levels at about three years of age.[8] The recommended doses are adjusted according to this model.

In contrast to the nervous system, when calculating doses of medicine for the rest of the body, the *correct* dose is most closely related to a combination of the weight and the body's skin surface area (BSA). BSA is a calculation of how much skin is exposed to the air. There are now pocket diagrams, formulas, and even on-line web sites to arrive at the correct dose.[9]

Why is this important? A six-month, twelve-month or three-year old grows during therapy and the correct dose three, six, and 12 months later will be too low, if only their starting dose are used. Pediatric oncologists are very familiar with making these changes. More information on chemotherapy is in Chapter 17: Treatment, and Chapter 19: Medications.

REASONS TO CONSULT A PEDIATRIC NEUROSURGEON FOR YOUR CHILD'S TUMOR

The reasons are simple and clear: survival and quality of life. I am asked frequently why a specialist surgeon is needed and I answer, "Children are not miniature adults!" The accompanying chart shows the death (mortality) rates within two to four weeks of brain surgery for children over the past 70 years (see Table 22A-1).

TABLE 22A-1 Reduction in Neurosurgical Deaths: 1930-1999		
Author	Year	Deaths %
Cushing	1930	20/61 (32)
Spitz	1947	16/67 (24)
Newton	1968	11/35 (31)
Aron	1971	3/20 (15)
Mealy & Hall	1977	4/37 (11)
McIntosh	1979	11/85 (13)
Mazza, et al	1981	4/36 (11)
Zeltzer, et al	1999	-/400 (< 1)

The most famous North American neurosurgeon, Harvey Cushing (circa 1930), watched 32 percent of his child patients die during or just after surgery! Surgical death rates have dropped steadily over the last 20 years due to both better anesthesia and neurosurgical techniques. These have been developed by *pediatric* neurosurgeons who work closely with teams of other children's medical specialists.

In North America, about 50 percent of children with brain tumors are operated on by general neurosurgeons and the other 50 percent by pediatric neurosurgeons. A study by Dr. Leland Albright and myself found that pediatric neurosurgeons performed more complete tumor removals than general neurosurgeons, with no increase in brain damage or death rates.[10] We do not know if the same is true for patients in other countries.

THE CHOICE OF NEUROSURGEON CAN AFFECT YOUR SURVIVAL

The choice of neurosurgeon can have a major impact on your child's chance of survival. The accompanying chart shows survival rates of children with three major types of brain tumors. The data shows what happens if more or less than 90 percent of tumor is removed (see Table 22A-2). (This is similar to the results analyzing more or less than 1.5 cm^2 [less than a square inch] of remaining tumor on the postoperative MRI.) There is a striking *survival advantage* when more tumor is removed. For children with medulloblastomas, a 25 percent difference in survival rate (75 percent vs. 50 percent) exists five years later, depending on the skill of the neurosurgeon in removing those last bits of tumor. So, if the surgeon did not completely remove the tumor the first time, this means that the possibility exists to remove more in a second operation and increase the chances for survival.

> You could benefit from a 2nd opinion and 2nd surgery for an incompletely resected tumor.

Table 22A-2 Average Five Year Survival for Children with Brain Tumors by Amount of Tumor Removed		
	More than 90% resection	Less than 90% resection
Medulloblastoma	75 %	50 %
Anaplastic Astrocytoma	42 %	14 %
Glioblastoma	27 %	4 %

Bottom Line → Children should be cared for by Pediatric neurosurgeons & Pediatric oncologists for best quality of life and survival.

Is a Second Opinion or Surgery Needed?

To see if additional surgery would have benefited the children with medulloblastoma above, Drs. Albright, Wisoff, and I reviewed the MRI scans of 80 medulloblastoma patients who had subtotal or incomplete resection and who had no tumor spread elsewhere (stage M-0). We concluded that in 66 percent of those patients, a complete resection *could have* been performed...if the surgeons had seen the child after the first operation. Why? Experience and training are the likely answers. Pediatric neurosurgeons work very closely with pediatric oncologists, operate more frequently and have better technical expertise with these tumors in infants and older children. Thus, they know the importance of complete resection and understand it makes a difference.

I have seen many child patients in whom the operating general neurosurgeon did *not* take an MRI after surgery to see how much tumor remained; and the oncologists based their therapy solely on his operative report. I never saw this happen with a pediatric neurosurgeon.

The message is clear: Ask the neurosurgeon if he will order a postoperative MRI scan. If not, request one to determine how much tumor remains.

Tumor Staging: Why Is It Important Before or After Surgery?

Staging is an assessment and measurement of how far the tumor has spread. Has it traveled to other parts of the brain or spinal cord, or even to the bone marrow or lymph glands? The amount of tumor and *its spread* determine the treatment choices – directed and stronger therapy for remaining tumor; or less therapy if no residual tumor.

> Staging is important before any therapy starts.

Staging is commonly performed with the PNET group of tumors such as medulloblastoma, pineoblastoma, ependymoblastoma, etc., which account for more than 25 percent of all childhood brain tumors. Gliomas may metastasize, but rarely at diagnosis (studies say in about 15 percent of cases at some time in the course of the illness). The current staging system was developed by Dr. C. Chang[11] (see Table 22A-5 at end of this chapter). Our group showed that it was the "M" stage part, not the "T," that was important in assigning therapy and later survival for PNETs.[12]

Bottom Line ➡ Each child needs to have their treatment care plan directed by a specialist team at a major center for childhood brain tumors.

WHAT IF THE NEUROSURGEON CANNOT REMOVE THE ENTIRE TUMOR?

It does not mean the neurosurgeon is incompetent! Excellent neurosurgeons do not always get a complete removal of medulloblastomas or gliomas. These tumors are challenging and can look the same as normal brain, especially inside the fourth ventricle near the brain stem, or if wrapped around the brain stem or hiding in a crevice.

An excellent neurosurgeon will review the postoperative MRI films and consider if a *second* surgery offers the child a better chance of survival. Thus, a parent should feel reassured if the neurosurgeon considers and recommends a second surgery.

What are the options, if your child had a less-than-complete tumor resection? Ask for a consultation by a pediatric neurosurgeon at another center to evaluate whether additional surgery might make a difference. For example, if the tumor is staged (see Table 22A-5) and there is tumor in other parts of the brain or spinal cord (stages M-2 or M-3), then additional removal of the main tumor may not affect outcome.

> Survival is dependent on skill of your neurosurgeon & amount of tumor remaining.

CAN YOU OPERATE TWICE ON THE SAME TUMOR?

There is no limit to the number of operations on the same tumor for the same patient. The consideration must always be "Will the child have a greater chance of benefit than harm from re-operation?" I had a patient for example like Carrie, who had her first operation at 15 months of age for an "atypical" brain stem glioma. She required surgery 2 ½ years later for regrowth after chemotherapy as well as three shunt revision surgeries, and partial surgical resections at ages eight, 13 and 20. This is not uncommon.

WHAT ABOUT PAIN CONTROL FOR CHILDREN?

Treatment of pain in children is sometimes like the weather: "Everyone talks about it," but nothing is done about it.. There are initiatives, hallway signs and badges, talk of pain being the 5th vital sign along with a pulse, breathing, blood pressure and temperature. Pain can occur after surgery or for other reasons My experience is that children, in and out of hospital, still experience untreated or under-treated

Bottom Line Pain is another responsibility for parents to monitor. Insist on appropriate pain management.

pain; and often, they learn to live unnecessarily with pain. Ineffective pain treatment is more prevalent in places less familiar with children's cancer.

WHAT CAN YOU, AS THE PARENT, DO ABOUT IT? THERE ARE THREE POSITIVE ACTIONS:

- You must be vigilant.
  If you think your child is in pain, you must directly and aggressively mention this to the nurse or doctor caring for your child. Unfortunately, many professionals believe that because the brain itself has no pain sensation, then children should not have pain after surgery. Baloney! They have injured muscle tissue, cut bone and bone coverings (periosteum, scalp), meninges (coverings of the brain), all of which have pain fibers.

- You must ensure that the medication is given.
  It must be given regularly around the clock, not just when your child feels the pain or it becomes unbearable. It should never be given as an intramuscular shot (ouch!); rather pain medication should be administered as a pill or through the intravenous line.

- Be assured your child will not become a drug addict.
  Many physicians are fearful that children will become addicts if they receive morphine, codeine or other narcotic drugs. Baloney again! Studies show the opposite: Untreated pain prolongs hospitalization and slows recovery. Fear of stopping respiration as a potential side effect is also overrated.

CLINICAL TRIALS

SHOULD YOU PERMIT YOUR CHILD TO PARTICIPATE?

For most cancers, children on clinical trials live longer than those who do not participate in an experimental study.[13] The national clinical trials program for children has been responsible for lowering the death rate from all cancer by 50 percent over the past 30 years. It has led to the cure for most childhood cancers: Wilms' tumor, sarcomas, lymphoma, and leukemia. Now these same national and international programs are focused on improvements for childhood brain tumors.[14]

As explained in Chapter 21, I am emphatically pro-trial and I make no apologies! Trials are the best way to get the most advanced, state-of-the-art therapy when your doctors do not know which of two or three therapies is best. As a bonus, the average person treated on Phase 1 and 2 clinical trials has improved survival compared with those on "best available" conventional treatments. That is even more remarkable considering most Phase 1 studies test for drug toxicity rather than for effectiveness. Chances are that anyone in a trial receives more careful monitoring and prevention of complications.

Unfortunately, we do not have the cure for all brain tumors. We can, however, provide care that will give children a better chance of survival than what existed five or 10 years ago. Clinical trials are one way to achieve this objective. Only about 3 percent of all adult cancer patients participate in clinical trials, compared with more than 75 percent of children. Government has recognized that it is less

> Clinical trials are tightly monitored – many safeguards are in place to protect children from errors and inappropriate treatment.

expensive to cure a child than give sub-optimal treatment. To this end, legislation has passed in at least 12 states (see Chapter 21: Clinical trials, Table 21-7; and Chapter 23B: Receiving Health Care Benefits from Your HMO or Insurance Company: challenges a brain tumor patient must face) to encourage more child and adult cancer patients to participate in clinical trials. Implementing this law in California alone will allow more than 3500 new adults and children per year to be eligible.

> *The law requires that an insurance company or HMO must pay for care administered in conjunction with an approved (major Group sponsorship) clinical trial.*

An advocacy group will help you battle the insurance company or HMO, if they refuse to pay. (See http://www.childhoodbraintumor.org/ombuds.html and Tables 23B-2, 23B-3.)

Repeating the lessons of Eve and Adam in the Garden of Eden, the clinical trial is seeking knowledge, and you and your child are part of that search. I do not believe for a moment that your child will suffer or be punished; rather, the trial can lead you to the chance for an improved outcome, rather than fear of the unknown. Chapter 21: Clinical Trials has the answers to the most frequently asked questions (FAQs) like: What is a trial? How do I choose a trial? Who develops the trial?

Bottom Line The law requires an insurance company or HMO to pay for care in an approved clinical trial.

Will My Child Be a "Guinea Pig" in a Clinical Trial?

Do you remain vigilant in understanding the details of the trial, its implications, and protect your child? Yes. But many safeguards are in place to protect children who participate in clinical trials from errors and inappropriate treatment. Most pediatric oncologists and neuro-oncologists caring for children are part of one or more clinical trial groups that develop their own trials, as well as participate with others. They know the legal and ethical requirements of informed consent. More importantly, the standard of therapy in the textbooks is five to 10 years old. The clinical trial tests the best-known, most advanced concepts in therapy for children in your own community and worldwide.

> Clinical trials provide treatments that give children a better chance of survival than 5 or 10 years ago.

An example: In 1983, most clinicians were aware that radiation therapy to the brain tumor of an infant or young child was associated with significant brain damage and later mental retardation. It was especially devastating to children three years of age or less. In 1984, Drs. Jon Finlay (now in Los Angeles), Russ Geyer (Seattle), Jeffrey Allen (New York) and I worked together to develop a clinical trial to delay or omit radiation and substitute an initial chemotherapy-only approach to avoid the irreversible brain toxicity from radiation. This had never been attempted before on a national basis. We found that the survival results were no worse than with historical controls[15] (20 percent at five years). However, the surviving infants were more mentally intact. A chemotherapy-only approach for initial therapy is now considered the "gold standard" for infants with or without residual tumor.

> Seek a Radiation Center having experience with children.

What If You Do Not Want "Standard" Therapy in a Clinical Trial?

For trials that compare two or more different treatments, some parents are concerned that their child will receive the older, standard therapy and not the new one; others do not want to take the risk of a (less reliable) new treatment. This is a major dilemma. I counsel families that if the doctors, based on knowledge, cannot decide which is *the best* treatment, how can the parent be responsible for deciding a best therapy? I think that having the computer decide is a better approach. Besides, I know that just being on the study will improve the child's chances for survival. A parent need only be responsible for understanding the potential risks and deciding if they are tolerable.

RADIATION THERAPY

ARE THERE CHILDREN'S RADIATION ONCOLOGY SPECIALISTS?

The answer is yes... and no. There are no formal Board certification examinations for child radiation specialists. Again, experience counts for a lot. Radiation therapy is both an art and a science. Techniques like shaping the radiation fields, strength and timing of the beams, having a friendly, non-threatening environment, and having available pediatric anesthesia specialists, if needed, are only available in large centers that can support a relatively small child population. In addition, there are new treatments that have been used in adults that might find their way into child clinical trials: radiation sensitizers, GliaSite tumor implant of radioactive therapy, Radiosurgery, and radioactive antibody treatments, to name a few. Larger centers most likely are in a position to offer these.

I strongly suggest that parents "shop around" for the radiation therapist who sees at least 25 child patients per year. Currently, there are one or two radiation centers in most states that have such a program. These can be found on www.virtualtrials.com or through any pediatric oncology center associated with a university program (see Chapter 7 [6] and Tables 7-7, 7-9).

WHAT ARE THE ISSUES OF LOWERED RADIATION DOSAGE ON YOUNGER CHILDREN?

In an attempt to lessen the toxic effect of radiation on the young and developing brain, several studies attempted to lower the radiation dose to the *tumor sites* in the head and spine of infants; the survival outcome was worse in almost all these studies. The tumor is not nice or forgiving because it is growing in a young child. The tumor grew when less radiation was used. These are choices that no parent would ever *want* to make:

- Therapy to hopefully cure the tumor, but that likely delays a child's neurological development.
- No or inadequate treatment.

The preventative ("prophylactic") radiation dose to the brain and spine in PNETs is less (2400-3600 cGy) than the usual tumor dose (5500 cGy). Many studies have incorporated even lower doses to minimize brain damage, but the benefit of this approach has not yet been established. The best advice that I can give at this time is that the parent should know all likely risks and how they might be evaluated and possibly alleviated. Clinical trials also are studying this question and may be advantageous for your child. (Refer to important questions to ask your Radiation Oncologist before any treatment starts in Chapter 5: The Team[6]; also Chapter 17: Treatments; and Chapter 21, Clinical Trials.)

> Tumor-directed radiation (higher dose) is at the tumor site; Prophylactic radiation (lower dose) is to unaffected areas.

RADIATION THERAPY AND MY CHILD'S BRAIN FUNCTION

Should I be concerned? Yes, absolutely. Two points to make:

1. Following surgery, radiation therapy is the most effective treatment against brain tumors.
2. Radiation to major portions of a young child's upper brain can potentially lead to major brain injury and affect his or her later intellectual development. The above statements are true and therein lay the dilemma: parents and doctors

> Ask about pros & cons of different radiation techniques and dosages.

share very different perspectives. Radiation oncologists typically focus on #1 rather than #2. Logically the doctors view radiation as a life saving therapy that is painless to administer. However, as a group, radiation oncologists tend to downplay the long-term effects of their treatment. Like many physicians, they take a short-term view and thus do not deal with some tough questions you might have, such as:

a. How will the treatment affect my child in the long-term?
b. What are the chances my child will be graduated from high school?
c. What activities of daily living will he or she become incapable of doing?
d. Will my child be able to care for himself/herself as an adult?

While no one can predict for an individual, information shows that children may have significant problems depending on the child's age and the brain location where he/she received the radiation: the younger the child, the more severe the consequences. Understanding these possibilities allows for early recognition of problems and appropriate specialist care. For example, undiagnosed hypothyroidism can affect normal development and quality of life. This is preventable.

SPECIFIC LATE EFFECTS OF TREATMENT OR THE TUMOR

RADIATION-RELATED

Head (cranial) radiation can produce pronounced effects on the child's brain function. Also certain parts of the brain, like the pituitary gland and frontal lobes, are more sensitive and vulnerable, with glandular problems and decreases in intelligent quotient (IQ) over time.[16] Radiation can affect concentration, memory, organization, planning, eye-limb coordination, writing and drawing and other fine motor skills.[16] These problems are sometimes diagnosed as attention deficit hyperactivity disorder (ADHD) because of the child's distractibility, impulsivity, and concentration difficulties. It is, however, usually more complicated than this.[17] Dr. Sam LeBaron and I found, to our surprise, that even radiation to the lower part of the brain, the cerebellum (considered then not to affect memory and thought processes), produced cognitive deficits over time.[18] The effects were more pronounced in the youngest children.

CHEMOTHERAPY-RELATED

Chemotherapy also can cause side effects that affect learning. Children with brain tumors who received chemotherapy reported fatigue, decreased energy, weakness, hearing impairment, and irritability.[19] Cisplatin can affect hearing (auditory processing). However, other chemotherapies can affect cognitive abilities. Children with leukemia who received intrathecal (injected into the spine) chemotherapy had poorer academic achievement, as measured by tests in reading, spelling, and arithmetic.[20] This may be less relevant as most children with brain tumors do not receive intrathecal therapy.

Many hormonal imbalances can be treated: hypothyroidism, premature puberty, short stature.

SURGERY-RELATED

Cerebellar mutism is a condition in which the child stops talking within a few days after surgery and may develop profound swallowing and movement difficulties. It is now increasingly recognized as a complication of posterior fossa surgery.[21,22] Recovery can be complete or partial or with permanent disability.

Hormonal Problems Associated with the Tumor or Its Treatment

One or more endocrine conditions are present in 43 percent of childhood brain tumor survivors.[23] Five years after diagnosis, there is a significantly increased risk of hypothyroidism, growth hormone deficiency, and the need for medications to induce puberty or to treat osteoporosis (see Table 22A-3). Hormonal imbalances could contribute to the one or more cardiovascular conditions that were found in 18 percent of survivors, with an elevated later risk for stroke, blood clots, and angina-like symptoms.

Hormone excess can occur when a tumor is in or near the pituitary gland. More problems in children arise, however, from deficiencies caused by the tumor, surgical removal, chemotherapy, or radiation to the involved area. Common hormonal problems are listed in Table 22A-3, along with frequent symptoms, tumor types and locations, and causes. Many are reversible with correct treatment. See also Chapter 20: Side Effects and Later Effects of the Tumor or Treatment.

Craniopharyngiomas, for example, are found mainly in children (four to 14 years) and are commonly associated with abnormal function of the pituitary gland. These *benign* tumors grow out from the pituitary gland stalk and are not, strictly speaking, a cancer. Their symptoms depend on the speed, size and direction of the tumor growth. Eyesight difficulties, headaches, and frequent urination can occur months or years before the diagnosis. Excess prolactin secretion causes breast milk production in both sexes. These deficiencies also can emerge months or years following therapy.

Table 22A-3 Effects on Hormones in Children with Brain Tumors

Symptoms	Tumor types	Affected Hormones	Location/ causes of damage
Short stature, slow growth, low blood sugar	Craniopharyngioma (CP). Hypothalamic gliomas	Growth and sex hormones, others	Pituitary gland. Surgery, radiation
Weakness, pale skin, feeling cold, constipation, slow growth, hair loss	Hypothalamic gliomas, CP, brain stem glioma, posterior fossa tumors, PNET) i.e. medulloblastoma,	Thyroid hormone	Surgery, radiation to pituitary gland; Radiation to spine or cerebellum, brain stem
Weakness, vomiting, fainting, low sodium in blood	Pituitary or adrenal gland tumors, hypothalamic gliomas	ACTH, cortisone, mineralocorticoid	Pituitary gland or hypothalamus. Surgery, radiation
Inadequate progress thru puberty, lack of breast and pubic hair development, no menses	Craniopharyngioma, hypothalamic gliomas, Pituitary or adrenal gland areas;	FSH, LH (Gonadotropins) e.g., sex hormones	Surgery, radiation to pituitary gland or hypothalamus; radiation to spine, ovaries, testicles
Excess urination	Posterior pituitary tumors, germinomas, histiocytosis, cranio-pharyngiomas	Anti-diuretic hormone (ADH) deficiency	Surgery, radiation to posterior pituitary gland
Early puberty & menses	Craniopharyngioma, optic pathway-hypothalamic gliomas, PNETs	Excess or early secretion of sex hormones	Surgery, radiation, tumor of optic nerve, other brain locations

SUMMARY

A child with a brain tumor, or who has been treated for a brain tumor, must be evaluated and followed for any possible deficiency of the hypothalamic-pituitary axis. Specifically, this means evaluation for deficiencies of growth hormone, thyroid hormone, cortisol, vasopressin (the hormone that allows the kidney to concentrate urine) and the hormones that control puberty, LH and FSH. Type and location of tumor and the course of treatment influence the possibility of finding any of the above.

In spite of these findings, some long-term survivors of brain tumors are able to conceive and have normal children.[23,] All this means that you should not "just be glad he/ she is alive," but rather know that long-term medical follow-up is important to treat conditions and prevent problems.

FURTHER READING

Chapter 20 also includes detailed discussions of possible late effects of the tumor or specific treatments. The sense I want to give in this chapter has been that children are not miniature adults. There are specific aspects to diagnosis and treatment that deserve careful consideration and expertise.

The next chapter, 22B covers another, different aspect of late effects; rehabilitation, psychological issues and re-entry to school, and the family unit, after successful therapy.

CHAPTER 22A
Children with
Brain Tumor

Table 22A-4 Internet Resources for Childhood Brain Tumors

Organization/ Resource	Web site
Basic information about the brain for kids	http://faculty.washington.edu/chudler/introb.html#bb
Caring Bridge- posting your child's progress on the web	http://www.pilink.com
Cerebellar Mutism	http://health.groups.yahoo.com/group/cerebellarmutism
Chat group- to get started	http://health.groups.yahoo.com/group/Pediatricbraintumors/
Clinical trials	www.virtualtrials.com http://acor.org http://clinicaltrials.gov/ct/search?term=brain+cancer&submit=Search http:/cancer.duke.edu/btc/Treatment/ClinicalTrials.asp http://www.nccf.org/childhoodcancer/clinicaltrial.asp http://www.pbtc.org/public/BTlinks.htm
Endocrine (Thyroid) information	http://www.healthy.net/asp/templates/article.asp?id=528 http://www.thyroid.org/patients/brochures/Hypothyroidism%20_web_booklet.pdf http://www.thyroid.org/patients/brochures/HypothyroidismFAQ.pdf (See Chapter 20, Side effects and late effects of treatment)
Every organization from "ABTA" to "Zink the Zebra"	http://www.acor.org/ped-onc/ccorg.html http://www.acor.org/ped-onc/links/sitelinks.html
General information about tumors in children	www.virtualtrials.com http://www.cancer.med.umich.edu/learn/pwccbraintumors.htm http://www.btfcgainc.org/index.asp http://www.acor.org/ped-onc/resources/supportorg.html

Helpful services	http://cancer.duke.edu/btc/resources/btfsc.asp http://www.pbtfus.org/PatientResources/Questions/page1.htm http://www.cancercare.org/CancerCareServices http://www2.edc.org/lastacts/archives/archivesMarch00/featureinn.asp www.childhoodbraintumor.org
Late Effects and Guidelines for Children (Childrens' Oncology Group-COG)	http://www.candlelighters.org/treatmentcoglateeffects2.stm http://www.childrensoncologygroup.org/disc/LE/default.htm
Ombudsman Program for HMO, Insurance/ advocacy	www.childhoodbraintumor.org/ombuds.html
Support, hope, financial aid and great links	http://www.braintumor.org/patient_info/surviving/pediatric_info http://www.btfcgainc.org/index.asp http://www.cbtf.org http://www.acor.org/ped-onc/cfissues/financehelp/finhelp.html
Online Support Groups by Email	
Books	Shiminski-Maher, Tania. Childhood Brain & Spinal Cord Tumors: a Guide for Families, Friends & Caregivers. O'Reilly & Associates, Inc, 2002, Sebastopol, CA: Hamaguchi, Patricia. Childhood Speech, Language, and Listening Problems: What Every Parent Should Know. Publisher: John Wiley & Sons Inc, Aug 2001, , NY. ISBN: 0471387533 Field M. J. Behrman RE, Editors, When Children Die: Improving Palliative and End-of-Life Care for Children and Their Families. Committee on Palliative and End-of-Life Care for Children and Their Families. ISBN 0-309-08437-7
Hypothalamic Hamartoma Online Support	http://www.hhugs.com E-mail: rwdavis@logan.net E-mail: medulloblastoma-owner@yahoogroups.com
Medulloblastoma Online Support	
Optic-Glioma Online Support	E-mail: optic-glioma-subscribe@yahoogroups.com

| Parents of Children with ependymoma | Email: Ependyparents@braintrust.org. List Captain: J Dombrowski ependyparents-captain@braintrust.org |
| Pediatric Brain Tumor Online Support Group | E-mail: pediatricbraintumors-subscribe@yahoogroups.com http://health.groups.yahoo.com/group/Pediatricbraintumors http://groups.yahoo.com/group/Pediatricbraintumors |

Table 22A-5 Chang Stages Of Tumor (T) And Metastasis (M) for PNETs [10]

	T stage
T-1	Tumor < 3 cm in diameter and limited to the classic midline position in the vermis, the roof of the 4th ventricle, and less frequently to the cerebellar hemispheres.
T-2	Tumor > 3 cm and invading one adjacent structure or partially filling 4th ventricle.
T-3a	Tumor further invading two adjacent structures or completely filling the 4th ventricle with extension into the aqueduct of Sylvius, foramen of Magendie, or foramen of Luschka, thus producing marked internal hydrocephalus.
T3b	Tumor arising from floor of 4th ventricle and filling 4th ventricle.
T-4	Tumor spread through Aqueduct of Sylvius to involve 3rd ventricle , midbrain, or down into upper cervical cord.
	M stage
M-0	No gross subarachnoid or blood-borne metastasis
M-I	Microscopic tumor cells found in cerebrospinal fluid
M-2	Gross nodular seeding in cerebellum, cerebral subarachnoid space or in 3rd or 4th ventricles
M-3	Gross nodular seeding in spinal subarachnoid space
M-4	Outside the nervous system (Extra-neuraxial metastasis)

CHAPTER 22B

Children and Brain Tumors – Longer Term Psychological and Social Issues

For most children with a brain tumor, "normal" is relative. Often there is a new normal that is not the same as the one before the illness. Perhaps this is the most difficult challenge for child and parent alike.

Paul Zeltzer 2003

Life is sometimes good. It is not always fair.

Anonymous

⚷ **Key search words**

• brain injury	• child	• development
• pediatric	• late effect	• side effect
• neuropsychology	• school	• Individual Education Plan
• IEP	• 504	• camp
• hospice	• QOL	

You might hear from friends and the school that cancer survivors in general have few psychological problems.[1,2] This is not so for many children with brain tumors. Changes in the child's physical appearance from dexamethasone, or hormonal imbalance such as early puberty affect the child's body image; this can cause depression or social anxiety.[3,4,5] Long-term problems also have been called the "silent illness" by Sheryl Shetsky, an adult brain tumor survivor.[6] She observes that many children (and adults) *appear* alright, but it is the speed of information processing by their brain which suffers. The deficits are not appreciated until a conversation or competition in the school uncovers the problem.

To further complicate matters, a recent study showed that brain tumor survivors know little about their illness, including their diagnosis.[7] Such deficits could impair survivors' future ability to seek and receive appropriate long-term follow-up care. Hence your attention to record keeping and organization will pay dividends for your child (see Chapter 3).

PSYCHOLOGICAL AND SOCIAL LATE EFFECTS

Children with brain tumors and their parents suffer a "double whammy" that survivors of other cancers do not share. They experience the trauma of the disease (intravenous injections, feeling unwell, facing mortality, nausea, vomiting, school and home absences, and changed body image). In addition, they live with long-term effects produced by the tumor, surgery, radiation, and chemotherapy on the brain; these can be pronounced and permanent. Many clinical trials for brain tumor treatment now have "Quality of Life" (QOL) outcome measures that let the investigators and parents know the psychological

> Brain Tumor Double Whammy: Difficult Treatment of the disease & long-term effects.

and functional capacities of these children after completion of therapy. The actual long-term effects are now better appreciated than in previous decades (see Table 22B-1).[8] In terms of prevalence, clinically significant psychological distress was found in 11 percent of adult survivors of childhood brain tumors.[9]

Table 22B-1 Long-term Psychological & Physical Problems in Survivors of Chilhood Brain Tumors

Problem (Reference #)	
• Post-traumatic stress disorder (PTSD) [10]	• Thyroid, growth & sexual maturation
• Inhibition and withdrawal [13]	• Unfounded body complaints[18,19]
• Discouragement related to school difficulties[18, 23]	• Complaints of intense stress[19]
• Peer relationship difficulties [39]	• Anxiety and panic,
• Loss of independence in adolescence [11]	• Behavior problems [12]
• Job seeking/ retention [13]	• Infertility [14,15]
• Concern about attracting the opposite sex and about career/ relationships	• Cerebellar mutism/ posterior fossa syndrome[16]

LATE EFFECTS GUIDELINES FOR SPECIFIC TREATMENTS

How do parents know if their child has a "late effect?" First, ask your health care professionals at the center you receive treatment. Second, use all the references in the last table in this and the previous chapter. You also can contact the Children's Oncology Group for many useful resources including this guide, Children's Oncology Group Childhood Cancer Survivor Long-Term Follow-Up Guidelines.[17]

> *Children's Oncology Group Childhood Cancer Survivor Long-Term Follow-Up Guidelines … provides recommendations for screening and management of late effects that may potentially arise as a result of therapeutic exposures used during treatment for childhood cancer. These guidelines represent a statement of consensus from a panel of experts in late effects of treatment for pediatric malignancies. The recommendations are based on a thorough review of the literature as well as the collective clinical experience of the task force members, panel of experts, and multidisciplinary review panel (including nurses, physicians, behavioral specialists and patient/ parent advocates).*

> *Implementation of these guidelines is intended to increase awareness of potential late effects and to standardize and enhance follow-up care provided to childhood cancer survivors throughout the lifespan.*

> *(See http://www.childrensoncologygroup.org/disc/LE/default.htm)*

The facts that you need to know can be found by asking the right questions (see Chapter 5: The Team). The e-mail below is from the mother of Jordan who has cerebellar mutism. She stopped talking, had difficulty in swallowing and maintaining balance shortly after surgery (see Chapter 20: Side Effects and Later Effects).

I guess what this all boils down to is this...don't give up. Give yourself credit for getting through the last 10 months. Everyone has times that they feel worn out. Encouragement and love go a long way in helping a child. I tell Jordan she can do anything. She's only limited by what she thinks she can't do. ...We try everything and do things we never would have done before. We try to live each day enjoying our time together.

My advice: watch what the therapists do during their sessions and look for things you can incorporate into your home routine. Read to him and have him try all kinds of food. Try a small cocktail straw if he has trouble swallowing. Take him places he used to like to go to. Hang things on the ceiling to look at; suspend balloons from the ceiling to encourage him to move his arm up to them to push them around. Educate yourself. Most of all just be his cheerleader. Ruth, mom to Jordan, medulloblastoma.

Parental Role in the Child's Adjustment

It now becomes part of the parents' responsibility and burden to ensure that their child receives appropriate assessment and rehabilitation for the child's deficits. This is not an easy task in an era of shrinking health benefits, school budgets, and with little available guidance.

> Your child's school success may be dependent on your taking charge and working the system.

Some factors that help in positive adjustment are not under the child's or parent's control. These include absence of learning difficulties, functional and physical limitations.[1,18,19] On a positive note, there are factors that are more under your control and that predict better psychological adjustment:

- The less the children believe their physical appearance is affected by cancer.[20]
- High levels of support from the family, classmates, the school and the hospital.[5]
- Social skills training targeted to the child's problems (understanding slang, body language, etc.).[21]

Read how Martha sees her son and how this might affect the positive vision for his future:

At age 3, Michael's 5.5 cm tumor was in his midbrain, hypothalamus, and optic tract. The first resection got about 60 per cent; then the chemo kept it stable for 18 months. The second surgery got another 70 percent of what was left. He went on Temodar Sept. 2002 and the last MRI showed that the tumor actually shrank about 20 per cent. Michael is now 6 years old, has left-side weakness, no left peripheral vision and some learning issues. He gets therapy both from school and outside (PT/OT, traumatic brain injury therapist/ teacher for the visually impaired/ and speech). He compensates very well for the weakness and vision; he also has a very bad stutter.

On paper it sounds very pitiful, but you wouldn't know all of his issues by looking at and playing with him. He is also the most outgoing boy and very active. He amazes me on a daily basis.

Martha, mom to Michael, Newhaven, CT.

TRANSITION BACK TO SCHOOL

LEGAL RIGHTS OF EVERY CHILD WITH A BRAIN TUMOR

Under Federal Law, P.L. 94-142 (1975), children with identified disabilities are entitled to a free and appropriate public education.[22,27]

The passage of P.L. 94-142 and Section 504 of the Rehabilitation Act and the more recent passage of P.L. 99-457 and P.L. 101-476, the Individuals with Disabilities Education Act (IDEA) 1990, guarantee access to school for children with chronic and handicapping conditions. Children with special healthcare needs must be integrated into the regular school setting, and schools must modify and adapt their environment and programs to accommodate these children. Section 504 prohibits discrimination based on disability in programs and activities, public or private that receive federal financial assistance.[22]

Children with brain tumors usually fall under the category of "orthopedically impaired" or "other health impaired". "Federalese" language reads that children with cancer may have "limited strength, vitality, or alertness due to chronic or acute health problems which adversely affect educational performance."

The Individual Educational Plan (IEP)

More than 35 per cent of survivors report significant school difficulties. This means that objective assessment of your child's strengths and weaknesses is a must.[23] This process usually starts with the following tests and evaluations and concludes with a plan of action – the Individual Educational Plan (IEP). The following studies will serve as the basis for developing the IEP that is specific to your child:

- Medical history and physical examination by a primary care provider;
- Neurological examination; and
- Neuropsychological assessment.

IEP students usually have serious *academic,* or *learning,* problems that prevent them from meeting the standards of the class. Therefore, an IEP includes the availability of instruction from resource teachers in the Special Education Department, as well as program modifications and accommodations. The testing and steps in gathering this information are outlined in Table 22B-2.

In the public school system, the parent of a student with physical, emotional, or learning disabilities must submit a "Request for Special Education Assessment." Within 15 days, he/ she should

> IEP students require Resource Specialty teachers and accommodation for their unique challenges.

receive a written response. An evaluation determines if the student qualifies for *special accommodations* and *modifications* under an IEP. The Special Education Department of the school (District) is responsible for seeing that an IEP is followed and that the student's needs are met.

The 504 Plan

If a student does not need or meet the criteria for an IEP, the student might qualify for a *504 Plan*. A 504 Plan involves only modifications and accommodations in the student's program (no resource teachers).[22] An administrator or counselor and the classroom teacher, rather than the resource teachers in the Special Education Department, are responsible for carrying out the modifications and accommodations stated in the student's 504 Plan. The ultimate responsibility for implementation of either plan rests with the school principal.

Table 22B-2 Roadmap of Preparations for Return to School	
Evaluation/ Follow-up	Result
1. Medical (physical) and Neurological examinations	Treatment Plan for physical therapy, speech and occupational therapies, and total rehabilitation.
2. Neuropsychological assessment	Areas of strength, weakness → Individual Educational Plan (IEP) – his/ her best chances for recovery and adjustment.
3. School/ Teacher receives IEP or 504	Implementation in classrooms to benefit child.
4. Parents seek continuing retraining for short- & long-term memory, organization, attention and processing skills	Periodic evaluations of progress, assessment of learning and improvement.

NEUROPSYCHOLOGICAL TESTING: WHAT IS IT?

Neuropsychological testing does *not* aim to mark you or your child as "crazy" or "retarded." It is a method to find out what portions of the brain and its circuits are working well and which ones are affected by the illness or treatment (see Table 22B-3). This will ultimately help you understand and develop a logical, coordinated rehabilitation program and educational plan.

Parents must talk to the Principal if they are unhappy with implementation of 504 or IEP plans.

Table 22B-3 Major Brain Areas & Functions Assessed by Neuropsychological Testing	
Domain-anatomic area	Function
Frontal lobes	Executive function: decisions, initiating activities
Occipital and parietal lobes	Visual-spatial coordination
Occipital-frontal lobes & motor strip	Eye-hand coordination
Temporal lobes and hippocampus	Visual and hearing memory
Third ventricle	Emotional regulation, initiation of behavior
Cerebellum	Motor coordination, attention

After neuropsychological testing, many parents tell me the importance of pursuing cognitive remediation or brain injury retraining. This helps "beef up" mental skills such as short- and long-term memory, organization, attention, and processing skills. With this information, you will be able to help your child attain his or her best chances of recovery and adjustment.

For example, if there is a subtle hearing-processing deficit, then school work could be better presented in written form for *visual* processing. If concentration is affected, then *timed tests* may need to be adjusted. Some school districts will perform neuropsychological testing, but the wait can be one to two years! If possible, have the testing performed privately to speed up the process.

POSITIVE *ATTITUDES* THAT AFFECT SUCCESSFUL SCHOOL REENTRY

Returning to a normal routine soon after diagnosis is essential for the child with cancer, as "normality" has a significant effect on a child's general adjustment and self-esteem. School to a child is like work to an adult. When a child is out of school for a long period of time, he or she is "unemployed" and may experience depression, apathy, and poor self-concept.[24]

The following parental concerns and actions can affect the quality of the child's adjustment:

- Feelings and actions of uncertainty about the child's future.
- Expectations that emotional and physical efforts of returning to school will be "too much" for the child.[25]
- Allowing him/ her to stay home. The pattern of absenteeism becomes a cycle and the child ultimately refuses to attend school.[26]
- Separation anxiety by both parent and child can manifest as school phobia.
- The school may not be responsive to the child's needs.
- The school may not respond appropriately to parents' concerns or requests (IEP).

POSITIVE *ACTIONS* FOR A SUCCESSFUL SCHOOL RE-ENTRY

Both parent and child have been through a major trauma and their reactions of uneasiness are understandable. Successful school re-entry depends on cooperation between the family and the school. Seven factors become action items for the parent or child's advocate to resolve (see Tables 22B-4, 22B-5). Is it a smooth process? Not always. Read what one parent experienced:

□ **Bottom Line** ➤ School to a child is like work to an adult.

The most important point for all of you is to not give up. This has been a harder fight than fighting the tumor. After five years of fighting the school district, I am finally on the right track. At yesterday's IEP day 2, we finally got Speech, PT, Behavioral Planning and Vision Evaluation to get on board and recheck her status in three months.

I highly recommend checking into an attorney because in my case the attorney cost the same as the advocate who was going to charge me. The district ended up having to pay some of the attorney's fees; they don't have to pay the advocate, ever.

I have had as many as 25 people in my IEP meeting, OT-3 , PT-2, speech-3, Regional Center, Director of special Education, Pychologist-2, CCS supervisor, District behavior specialist, Vision specialist, School of the Blind representative, NJ Deaf Blind representatives, teachers, School director at the private school the district placed her, myself and my attorney.

I had reports contradicting just about everything that the district said. I let it be known that I was planning to report the district personnel to their licensing boards for failure to do their jobs. For every report that they gave denying her needs, I had two or more saying that she needed the help. They were more afraid of me than their boss. One therapist stated she had to ask permission to recommend service, since it would cost the district so much money to give it. This is against the law, and if I reported this she could lose her license to practice.

Lucy, mom to Hayley. Morristown, NJ

Table 22B-4 Seven Parental Steps to Promote Successful School Reintegration[27]
1. Request in writing a meeting to formulate & update your child's IEP. Insist that the IEP details the specific goals that meet his/her needs.
2. Provide the school with accurate and up-to-date medical information.
3. Communicate regularly with school personnel regarding the child's condition.
4. Encourage and facilitate continued interactions with classmates and peers.
5. Ensure that the child keeps up with his or her school assignments.
6. Encourage participation in ordinary tasks, responsibilities, school activities[28,29]
7. Follow-up progress with the school. Show appreciation for teacher/ school efforts.

By following these guidelines (see Tables 22B-4, 22B-5), parents demonstrate to their child an optimistic expectation that the child will indeed survive.[30] Hiding the facts of the illness or not dealing with it directly does not help in this adjustment.

Note: Even if your insurance does not list neuropsychological testing, you can request or appeal for insurance coverage based on medical diagnosis. (See ombudsman, Table 22B-7 and Chapters 23A, 23B: section appealing denials.)

Table 22B-5 Checklist of Major Components of School Reintegration	
Component	Comments
1. Individual Education Plan	IEP is every child's legal right in the USA
2. Neuropsychological Testing Neuropsychologist School Psychologist	Schools can have 1-2 year wait to test child. Private testing speeds up process. It can be expensive ($1200-$2500). The Neuropsychologist, Social Worker, Speech Therapist, etc. are links to school for IEP implementation/peer education.
3. Physical Therapy/ Speech and Occupational Therapy	As indicated by testing, assessment
4. (IEP) Teacher / School Counselor/ Child Life Specialist, Social Worker	Coordinate classroom/ teacher/ student education. Ask your Pediatric Cancer Center for help.
5. Family	Home and friends play a large role
6. Peers	Peers need information about the illness & effects
7. Parent Advisory Council (PAC) Call district Special Education Director, for contact.	School districts are mandated by law to fund PAC advisor for special needs students (informs you of your rights regarding IEPs and IDEA (Individuals with Disabilities Education Act).

PREPARATION AND SUPPORT OF THE CLASSROOM TEACHER

There are several components here, including knowledge of all relevant information about the child and his or her illness.[31] In my opinion, the recent privacy legislation (HIPAA) may, in fact, impede important communication of key facts needed for teacher preparation. The teacher should be aware of the following:

> Regular contact with teachers and positive support will help.

1. Type of cancer that the child has, its symptoms, and general prognosis.
2. Treatments and their side effects.
3. Awareness of parents' wishes for what classmates and school personnel should know about their child's illness.
4. How effects of the disease and treatments can affect skills needed for learning, such as attention, memory, language, nonverbal and motor skills (IEP review).
5. Psychological effects of cancer and issues such as anxiety, behavior problems, emotional difficulties, peer relationships and frustration related to school difficulties.
6. Teachers should receive a schedule of upcoming medical appointments to help the child prepare and anticipate absences.
7. Assistance from the treating Pediatric Oncology Center to educate and dispel myths (Child Life professional).

PREPARING THE CLASS FOR THE CHILD'S RETURN

The teacher should have a classroom presentation given by the hospital or school liaison regarding the child's disease. Most children's oncology programs have "Child Life" specialists or nurses who are experts in providing this information. They can explain from the child's perspective, answer questions, and clarify cancer stereotypes.[32,33]

The teacher should use the knowledge that he or she has gained in modifying goals, teaching methods and disciplinary practices. This is part of the specific IEP. The child may show academic and behavioral problems as a result of treatment for which the teacher may need to adjust. Appropriate expectations, however, should be maintained regarding the child's schoolwork.[34] If the child is unable to attend school, the teacher can facilitate classmate support by encouraging contact with the child, such as writing letters or cards.[35]

In preparing the class for the child's re-entry, the designated individual (psychologist, school nurse, child life, social worker) might describe the patient's hospital experiences, provide information about the child's specific illness in an age-sensitive manner and discuss social support and teasing. Importantly, this is the time to establish the patient as the expert on his or her disease.[36] The school psychologist may offer support to school personnel or refer child and family to support groups, individual counseling, or for social skills training.[26]

POTENTIAL PROBLEMS: FINDING AND USING SCHOOL RESOURCES

Many teachers express feelings of shock, worry, uncertainty and frustration by having a child with cancer in their classroom.[37] Some teachers seek support and information from the school nurse. However, teachers report that a lack of visibility, accessibility, and rapport prevent them from receiving support from the school nurse. Thus, the school psychologist, child life, or social worker may be an alternative to establish a source of support and information for teachers.[38]

> Many children are anxious about cancer in a classmate. Establish your child as the expert on his/her disease.

IMPORTANCE OF PEER SUPPORT

Peer contact is important. Fear and lack of information can affect actual contact time of peers with the child. Research has shown the following:

1. Better social support from classmates is correlated with higher psychosocial adjustment for children with cancer.[39]
2. Peers who are knowledgeable and informed about the disease are more likely to accept and interact with children who have cancer.[40]
3. Peers influence treatment and medication compliance; that is, the child is more likely to ignore treatment and medication rules, if they interfere with social situations.[18,32,41]
4. Children often have misconceptions about the disease. Preparatory conversations can dispel myths that may affect the way in which peers treat the child.
5. Children's knowledge about the disease varies according to their developmental level.
   a. Elementary school students ask questions such as "What is cancer?" "Can he die from it?" "Can I catch cancer?" "Can she still play?"
   b. Middle school and high school students ask harder, more theoretical questions.[42] "What will dating be like?" "Will she be able to work or have a career?"

REINTEGRATION RESOURCES FOR PARENTS AND SCHOOL

Twenty five per cent of all long-term cancer survivors received special school services related to learning problems.[43] The needs for children with brain tumors must be much higher, but no similar needs-data are yet available for brain tumor survivors. Their learning problems are aggravated by the high rate of absenteeism that results from hospitalizations, treatments and treatment side effects.[44] Children with brain tumors may be eligible to receive services below, as part of their IEP plan, to benefit from their educational experience:

> Parents can help socialization with invitation to after school 'play dates,' games, outings.

- Hearing and speech pathology;
- Counseling and psychological services;
- Medical services;
- Occupational and physical therapy; and
- School health services (e.g., services provided by the school nurse).

Dr. Ernie Katz developed *The Cancervive Teacher's Guide for Kids with Cancer, and the School Reintegration Program.*[31] This program uses the school psychologist, for example, in the roles outlined above. In addition, it provides a sample classroom presentation and a list of resources for information on cancer. It has been evaluated positively by teachers, parents, and children.[45]

The solutions discussed in this section require a tremendous effort and cooperation with school personnel. Even if a student has an IEP or 504 Plan, the plan is only as good as the people who implement it. Caring school administrators, nurses, and teachers are often willing to accommodate students even without an IEP or 504 Plan. We need to continually acknowledge the individuals who are helping us every day. It is important to express appreciation periodically to those who are helping your child succeed in school.[46]

SUMMER CAMPS

Camping as a "Rite of Summer" is a uniquely North American experience from which many children have benefited. More than 20 years ago, a boy named David (a leukemia survivor) was denied admission to summer camp only because he was receiving chemotherapy. As a result, his mom founded a camp in Los Angeles for David and others like him and helped promote the creation of similar camps that are now thriving across the USA,[47] in Canada, Europe, the Middle East and Africa.

Paul Newman, actor and chef, along with his partner AE Hotchner, have been heroes in the expansion of camps for seriously ill children. The Association of Hole in the Wall Gang Camps supports programs around the world, including the namesake facility in Ashford, CT and Barretstown Gang Camp in Ireland, and several other across the US.[48] Additionally, many pediatric oncology divisions in the

Summer camp experience is available & free of charge for most children with brain tumors.

USA and Canada host camp sessions using their own medical staff. Most are offered at no cost (see Table 22B-6).

SEND MY CHILD TO CAMP?

Sending your sick child away to camp may seem like the very last thing a sane parent would do. But it may be the best thing you could do, both for you and your son or daughter. Even for the healthiest child, camp is magical. The freedom and adventure, the friendships made, the secrets shared, the songs sung, the accomplishments attained – all contribute to a sense of independence and pride. Most importantly, camp is what normal, healthy children do.

Isn't that precisely what a child with cancer needs to do as well? Add to the basic fun of camp, the common element of cancer – "Oh, do you take dexamethasone, too?" and the inspiration of older campers and counselors – "I had a brain tumor about 14 years ago. I know what you're going through." All that and the relief of being away from the hospital, and you have just what the doctor ordered: sleep away camp!

What this means for you and your child is that a summer camp experience is within reach. There will be experienced counselors and oncology-trained physicians to care for your child while he or she does things never felt possible before. To enroll, parents should contact the social worker at their local pediatric oncology program to learn about necessary preparations to have this experience (see Table 22B-6).

CHAPTER 22B
Children's
Longer-term
Issues

Table 22B-6 Camps for Children with Brain Tumors in the United States, Europe, & Middle East		
Camp	Website / E-mail	Telephone
The Association of Hole in the Wall Camps Camp Sunshine, Maine	www.holeinthewallcamps.org http://www.campsunshine.org http://www.hitwgcamps.org e-mai: info@holeinthewallcamps.org	One Century Tower 265 Church St, #503 New Haven, Connecticut 06510 Ph. 203-562-1203 Fax 203-562-1207 207-655-3800
Ronald McDonald Camp Programs	http://www.campronaldmcdona ld.org/goodtimes/index2.htm California http://www.coca-intl.org e-mail: rjhamdg@juno.com	COCA, International Ph. 856-756-7900 ext 5261 Fax 856-966-5957
USA, Australia Camps	http://www.acor.org/ped-onc/ cfissues/ckcamps.html http://www.acor.org/ped-onc/ cfissues/camps.html	
Candlelighters All Camp contacts	www.candlelighters.org e-mail: info@candlelighters.org	3910 Warner Street Kensington, MD 20895 Ph. 800-366-2223 / 301-962-3520

EFFECTS ON THE FAMILY

FINANCIAL COSTS

Cancer in a child is the most difficult challenge most parents will experience. The effect on the family finances is also significant – the average family spends 25 per cent of their income, over and above what insurance covers, when cancer strikes a child. Thirty-seven per cent of families needed to borrow money because of the financial effects of the child's illness.[49] Those with severe physical effects from the tumor clearly face even greater costs – physically, financially, and emotionally. Many families also care for their child at home, rather than in a hospital, and use family resources to manage these mammoth challenges.

SIBLINGS AND EXTENDED FAMILY

The whole family may feel distress. There might be uncertainty, loneliness, low self-esteem, symptoms of post traumatic stress disorder (PTSD) for the child, as well as distress related to adjustment for siblings.[50,51] These problems seem to be worse in poorer families (if income is affected), in families that lack religious affiliation for support, or where chronic illness affects another family member.[9]

For these reasons, it is very important to get the most support possible from family, friends, and community resources (See also Chapter 3: Getting Organized and Chapter 5: The Team). A mother echoes her feelings below:

> 37% of families borrow money due to financial effects of their child's illness.

Sometimes I want to scream and say "I want the world to stop cause I can't deal with it anymore. Don't you know my son has a brain tumor? How can you expect me to carry on any normalcy when all I want to do is find a way to get him back?" ...But I don't do that. I get up, get dressed and go out in the world and try to blend in to everyday living. I listen to other people talk about their lives and make idle comments and laugh at their anecdotes, but on the inside I am crying 'cause it's so hard.

A mom who is there. Bakersfield, CA

The divorce rate for parents of children with a serious illness is at least 50 percent. There are very helpful organizations that understand this problem and can offer specific help. Contact the major brain tumor organizations for children. WE CAN at http://www.wecan.cc/mission.html is such an example in California (see Table 22B-7).

As I mentioned, siblings at home can suffer, no matter how well the parents prepare for being absent; it is unavoidable I found out about these effects in an unusual way. Each year I volunteer as a summer camp physician at the Barretstown Gang Camp in Ireland for children with cancer. This camp accepts children from all over Europe. Of the eight sessions, we always have at least one 10-day camp session devoted only for the siblings. Each year we record the number and types of visits to the camp medical facility. The siblings have *more* visits during the 10 days than any sessions of children with AIDS or cancer, 50 per cent of whom were actively receiving their chemotherapy! We interpreted this to mean these children needed as much attention as their sibling with cancer. *Normal* siblings may have medical and other needs that are not being met.[52]

> Divorce rate for parents of children with a serious illness is 50%.

THE NEW NORMAL

Getting back to school and reintegrating with the family is one way of getting back to normal. For most children, the term *normal* is relative, and there often is a new normal unlike the one before the illness. Perhaps this is the most difficult challenge for a child and parent alike.

Is this easy? No. The challenges usually begin after surgery, rather than ending there. So many areas of your child's development must be cared for. My hope is that finding, learning and using the available information will make your journey a little smoother. I've had many patients with medulloblastoma, cerebellar mutism and paralyses or weakness who entered University, attained work and became productive citizens. There is hope. The most recent study of more than 1000 brain tumor survivors receiving no or many types of therapy reported that only 11 per cent had an overall prevalence of significant psychological distress.[9] Always remember, your participation and championing will help your child attain the maximum benefit possible.

> There is often is a new normal unlike the one before the illness.

One adult survivor of childhood cancer shares what he wanted from his physicians:

> ... *to be understanding of the very deep needs...and to the authentic but often unspoken, expressions of ... anxieties about physical and emotional pain, loss of control over personal destiny, and plain dread of dying and of the end of cherished relationships.*[53]

> Brad Zebrack

Physicians need to be sensitive to these words.

WHEN IS IT TIME TO SAY, ENOUGH?

This is the decision that every parent I have ever met dreads. And yet some will have to grapple with it. The most profound answer I have heard was spoken in the words of a mother who traveled that path and was advising another parent.

> *Hope should be with you forever, despite the outcome. If you have a good relationship with God, you will not give up hope, hope that your child will be*

miraculously healed, or hope you will see him again. Do you know I don't think I ever asked Gary's doctors what his odds were? Why? Because I already knew what they were: 100 per cent if it was God's will, and 0 per cent if it wasn't.

Now, when do you know when enough is enough? You will know, Denise. I asked my neuro-oncologist the same question when Gary relapsed the second (last) time. She told me the same thing, you will know. She also told me that they would support us whatever we chose to do. I told her we would never stop trying something else... but you know what, we did.

It is so easy to make these decisions when your child still feels good and is still so much himself. Our decision came the day of Gary's last doctors appointment in Birmingham. Of course, we didn't know it was going to be his last appointment. He walked to the car that morning and it was the last time he ever walked again unassisted; and of course he eventually couldn't walk at all. There was never any question what we should do. We just knew. However, if you have to ask when enough is enough, this is not the time.

I put this section last, not because it is unimportant. Rather, it is secondary in the order of how we approach the issue of our mortality and the need for hope to carry on. Melanie spoke about her changed perspective this way:

We all have a new way of looking at things. We all have a "new normal." We have an adjusted level of what sick means... a new definition of stress. We tend to see things in a different way than our friends and family. We value things on a different scale. I liken it to becoming a parent. My single childless friends cannot fathom the love that I have for my children. They have had a glimpse of what it is like to love someone in relationships that they have had over their lives (i.e. family , friends and lovers); but none can compare to that of having a child. This is how I describe the feeling of having a terminally ill child. It is something that cannot be explained or put into words or fully understood until you are in that situation.

Do I Talk with My Child About Dying?

Often a parent will think that talking about the seriousness of the illness is taboo or incorrect. Fortunately, there is helpful information about how to handle such a sensitive subject.[54] But the study to answer this question almost was not performed! A proposed nationwide postal questionnaire to Swedish parents who had lost a child due to cancer between 1992 and 1997 was *denied* approval by the local ethics committee. However, the pilot study to assess the harm and benefit of the questionnaire was approved and 95 per cent of parents found the pilot study valuable. The results showed that 423 (99 per cent) of parents found the investigation valuable, 285 (68 per cent) were positively affected, while 123 (28 per cent) were negatively affected by the study questionnaire.[55]

None of 147 parents who talked with their child about death regretted it.[45,55] In contrast, 69 of 258 parents (27 percent) who did *not* talk with their child about death regretted not having done so. Parents who sensed that their child was aware of his or her imminent death were more likely to regret not having talked about it. The child's age was related to both having talked about death and the parents' regretting not having talked about it. The conclusion was that parents who sense that their child is aware of his or her imminent death more often later regretted *not* having talked with their child than do parents who do not sense this awareness in their child. No parent later regretted having talked with his or her child about death.

WHAT IS A HOSPICE?

End of life care is discussed in detail in Chapter 25: Your legacy. A helpful and informative reference for understanding the unique aspects of hospice services for children also can be found at http://www2.edc.org/lastacts/archives/archivesMarch00/featureinn.asp.

Table 22B-7 Internet Resources for Childhood Brain Tumors

Organization/ Resource	Website
Basic information about the brain for kids	http://faculty.washington.edu/chudler/introb.html#bb
Caring Bridge- posting your child's progress on the web	http://www.pilink.com
Chat group- to get started	http://health.groups.yahoo.com/group/Pediatricbraintumors/
Every organization from "ABTA" to "Zink the Zebra"	http://www.acor.org/ped-onc/ccorg.html http://www.acor.org/ped-onc/links/sitelinks.html
Helpful services	http://cancer.duke.edu/btc/resources/btfsc.asp www.childhoodbraintumor.org Email- cbtf@childhoodbraintumor.org http://www.pbtfus.org/PatientResources/Questions/page1.htm http://www.cancercare.org/CancerCareServices http://www2.edc.org/lastacts/archives/archivesMarch00/featureinn.asp
Late effects	http://www.candlelighters.org/treatmentcoglateeffects2.stm http://www.leukemia-lymphoma.org/all_page?item_id=104428
Late Effects Guidelines for Children (Childrens' Oncology Group-COG)	http://www.childrensoncologygroup.org/disc/LE/default.htm
Returning to school Children's Brain Tumor Foundation. Candlelighter's Foundation. Educating the Child with Cancer IEP and "504" provisions	http://www.cbtf.org/school.html http://www.acor.org/ped-onc/cfissues/backtoschool/cwc.html http://www.candlelighters.org/bookeducating.stm http://www.squirreltales.com/articles/school_letter.html http://www.wrightslaw.com/info/section504.ada.peer.htm
Speech and Language resource:	20312 Watkins Meadow Drive Germantown, MD 20876 (301) 515-2900 Toll-free: (877) 217-4166

Table 22B-7 Internet Resources for Childhood Brain Tumors (continued)

Support for Parents of Children with Cancer	http://www.wecan.cc/mission.html
Support, hope, financial aid and great links	http://www.braintumor.org/patient_info/surviving/pediatric_info http://www.btfcgainc.org/index.asp http://www.cbtf.org http://www.acor.org/ped-onc/cfissues/financehelp/finhelp.html
Wish Fulfillment	http://personal.nbnet.nb.ca/normap/wish.htm
Books	Hamaguchi, Patricia. Childhood Speech, Language, and Listening Problems: What Every Parent Should Know. Publisher: John Wiley & Sons Inc, Aug 2001, , NY. ISBN: 0471387533
	Field M. J. Behrman RE, Editors, When Children Die: Improving Palliative and End-of-Life Care for Children and Their Families. Committee on Palliative and End-of-Life Care for Children and Their Families. ISBN 0-309-08437-7
Online Support Groups by E-mail	
Hypothalamic Hamartoma Online Support	http://www.hhugs.com E-mail: rwdavis@logan.net
Medulloblastoma Online Support	E-mail: medulloblastoma-owner@yahoogroups.com
Optic-Glioma Online Support	E-mail: optic-glioma-subscribe@yahoogroups.com
Parents of Children with ependymoma	Email: Ependyparents@braintrust.org . List Captain: J Dombrowski ependyparents-captain@braintrust.org
Pediatric Brain Tumor Online Support Group	E-mail: pediatricbraintumors-subscribe@yahoogroups.com http://health.groups.yahoo.com/group/Pediatricbraintumors http://groups.yahoo.com/group/Pediatricbraintumors

CHAPTER 23A

Health Care Coverage Systems at-a-Glance – What a Brain Tumor Patient Must Know

It is not fair! You may not feel great after surgery or during radiation and chemotherapy. Few healthy people can decipher the modern insurance claim form. How about some distraught person with a brain tumor or their worried family? My advice: while you are feeling good, get a lawyer on retainer and find out the telephone number of the state insurance board. You may need both.[1]

Key search words

• health insurance	• HMO	• PPO
• federal program	• state insurance	• medicare
• medicaid	• SSI	• SSDI
• social security	• family medical leave act	• FMLA
• HIPAA	• medications	• private insurance

This chapter describes the different health care coverage systems and explains the ground rules that you must know to receive the care you need and deserve. There is a natural overlap between this and Chapter 23B. In both chapters, I give many examples of how you can: challenge denials of care; receive benefits that at first are denied; and take maximum advantage of your healthcare system. Included are many scenarios that people, like you, have used successfully. This chapter builds upon Chapter 3, Get Organized.[2] In that chapter I recommended setting up a file for financial and insurance communications. In this and Chapter 23B, you will learn how to understand and use this information to your benefit. I have marked insurance-related terms with this symbol.* The definitions can be found in the special section at the end of this Chapter, so you won't have to thumb through the larger, more general Glossary.

Many people do not realize that their own physician may not be the final decision-maker regarding treatment they must receive. A high school educated clerk hired by the insurance company may be the first to make decisions of whether to pay for medications, tests, or surgery, based on a checklist. To turn things in your favor you need to know more about how insurance companies work. Read on!

HEALTH CARE COVERAGE SYSTEMS: WHICH ONE DO YOU HAVE?

First, here is a brief look at how the health care works in the United States. There are at least five parallel systems:

1. Privately- or employer-paid managed health care programs with a variety of flexible options. The majority of "insured" people have these types of coverage today: HMO, PPO, POS plans. (See Glossary at end of chapter for definitions.)
2. Private indemnity insurance: fee-for-service with complete freedom to pick and choose doctors, hospitals etc.
3. Federal Medicare coverage: for everyone 65 years of age and older.
4. State/ Federal basic coverage for the disabled or poor who lack private insurance: Medicaid, SSI are examples of these.
5. Federal government-sponsored Veterans Hospitals and clinics and hospitals (Walter Reed) for federal employees (Congresspersons, Military, etc)

Each system has unique features you must understand to derive maximum benefit. Some may allow overlap or provide additional coverage. For example, Medicare

▭**Bottom Line** ➡ The insurance companies or HMOs want to pay out as little as possible in money or services.

enrollees can buy (only one) supplemental coverage (Medi-Gap) for non-covered Part B, outpatient expenses that are not covered under their Part A plan. The first half of this chapter explains the components of these systems and how you can use them.

MANAGED CARE ORGANIZATIONS

WHAT IS A HEALTH MAINTENANCE ORGANIZATION (HMO)?

These are prepaid health plans. As an HMO* member, you have paid a monthly *premium**. In exchange, the HMO has agreed to provide comprehensive care for you and your family, including doctor visits, hospital stays, emergency care, surgery, lab tests, x-rays, and therapy. The HMO arranges for care either directly in its own group practice or through doctors and other health care professionals under contract. Your choices of doctors and hospitals are limited to those having agreements with the HMO. Exceptions can be made in emergencies or when medically necessary. You are assigned a *primary care doctor** who coordinates all your needs and referrals.

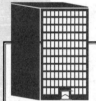

Many people like HMOs because they do not require claim forms for office visits or hospital stays. Instead, members present a card, like a credit card, at

An insurance company clerk can decide whether to allow medications, tests, or surgery.

the doctor's office or hospital. There may be a small *co-payment** for each office visit, such as $5 for an appointment with your doctor or $25 for an emergency room treatment.

HOW DOES AN HMO WORK?

It is best for the HMO to invest in preventive services for common diseases, immunizations, well-baby checkups, mammograms, and so forth. Once you are labeled a high financial risk, they want to care for you as economically as possible, within the written contract agreement. Remember, HMOs receive a fixed fee for your covered medical care. They will usually provide you with *a* specialist, rather than *the* specialist. They know that most people never read the details of their health plan unless they need to use it; they rely on that tendency.

If you don't know insurance lingo, review the glossary at end of chapter 23A.

In some HMOs, doctors are salaried, and they might be rewarded by limiting referrals. Other HMOs use independent groups of private physicians, known as individual practice associations (IPAs),* which contract with the HMO. You select a doctor from a list of participating physicians that make up the IPA network. If you are thinking of switching into an IPA, ask your current doctor if he or she participates in the plan.

You are either assigned a physician or asked to choose one to serve as your primary care doctor. This physician monitors your health and provides (or limits) treatment options, and refers you to specialists and other health care professionals. Usually, you cannot see a specialist without a referral from your primary care doctor. This is the major way in which HMOs limit your choice.

> In an HMO, you select a doctor from a list of participating physicians.

The relationship with your primary physician is essential to getting the level of services that you need. Your primary doctor has discretion in recommending referral physicians; therefore, you must be prepared to make your best and most well-founded arguments to this person (see Table 23A-1).

Table 23A-1 Seven Steps for the Best Possible Care within an HMO
1. Collect and organize your medical information, described in Chapter 3: Getting Organized.[2]
2. Ask your primary physician if he or she will serve as the team leader to consolidate your treatment and interpret what the specialists are saying.
3. Ask your primary physician which specialists have the most experience with brain tumors. Obtain a referral to these professionals. Tell them why you chose them after you meet them.
4. Use the *Eight-Point Preparations for the Second Opinion* checklist in Table 6-2, Chapter 6: Experts and Second Opinions, when you actually visit the specialist.[2]
5. Share the results of your research from all sources with the specialists and ask them to comment on whether these apply to you.
6. If a particular treatment is not available to you through your HMO, ask whether it is unavailable in your Plan, unproven or if cost is the reason that you cannot receive it. If it is the latter, then petition the Ombudsman for an outside referral, as the service is not provided.
7. In California a 1998 law entitles you to an independent review, if your HMO refuses service.

Can an individual convince a system to help? He or she can, according to Sheryl, brain tumor advocate and President of the Florida Brain Tumor Association:

What they do is take advantage of people who aren't well enough to fight. It's all about the numbers for them, not about the person. So, if you don't have the energy to fight, they are the winners. You need to have an advocate who can fight for you, take on the insurance companies, and beat them down to the mat. I've been doing that for 12 years and been successful at it.

I am the 1percent ...the nightmare they can only imagine. But they turned me into someone I don't like; it's a matter of survival. Once they denied a routine MRI. My oncologist had ordered it; I take one every four months and have for years, especially since I had my last tumor recurrence. My primary care doctor's office called to tell me that the insurance company denied the MRI. (It is very important to have a primary care doctor who supports you and understands the seriousness of the problem).

I called the insurance company myself and spoke to the Medical Director. I told him that if he were a real doctor, he would know that prevention is good business for his company – think what it will cost them if we catch the tumor on the move later? And if anything happens to me while fighting this garbage, they would regret ever hearing from me. I asked him if he graduated from Harvard Medical School? He was clueless about brain tumors. Then, I submitted a couple of letters, sent all my latest records, and appealed the decision to try to ruin my life.

> Managed care requires you obtain written insurance company approval *before* admission to a hospital.

I beat them up...and I won. They make this system discouraging, purposely. It works in their favor in most cases. For me, I've always enjoyed a challenge... and I am really sore loser.

Sheryl, Boca Raton, FL

Sheryl has made it easier for all people with brain tumors. Preparation for the challenge ahead means that you can and will survive the system.

THE PREFERRED PROVIDER ORGANIZATION (PPO)

The *preferred provider organization** (PPO) is a combination of a traditional fee-for-service medical plan and an HMO. Like an HMO, there are a limited number of

Bottom Line The primary care doctor should coordinate all recommendations and medications prescribed by specialists.

doctors and hospitals from which to choose. When you go to doctors in the PPO, you present a card and do not have to fill out forms. Usually, there is a small co-payment for each visit. For some services, you may have to pay a *deductible**♣* and *coinsurance♣*.

As with an HMO, a PPO requires that you choose a primary care doctor to monitor your health care. Most PPOs cover preventive care. This usually includes visits to the primary doctor, well-baby care, immunizations, and mammograms. The primary care doctor should be in charge of coordinating all recommendations and medications prescribed by specialists.

> Your primary doctor has discretion in recommending referral physicians.

If you see a doctor that is in the network, the PPO will generally pay 80 to 100 percent of the medical bills, after you pay the deductible and fill out claim forms. If you see a doctor out of the network, the PPO will pay a lower percentage of the bill (such as 60 per cent), and you pay more out of pocket. Some people like this option because it means they won't have to change doctors to join a PPO, even if their doctor is not a part of the network.

> PPO is a combination of a traditional fee-for-service medical plan and an HMO.

Although many plans require payment of co-insurance that counts toward an annual out-of-pocket maximum, you only have to pay this percentage until you reach the annual limit. Once you have paid an out-of-pocket maximum of $2,000, for example, the insurance plan will pay 100 per cent of your claims from that point on, up to the maximum of your policy.

> If you see a doctor out of the network, the PPO will pay a lower percentage of the bill (about 60%), and you pay more out of pocket.

Sheryl, the brain tumor advocate, also has had experience with networks and PPOs. She has a no-nonsense attitude toward getting her medical needs met:

> *Oh boy, are you serious? You've really struck a sour note there with me. I've been fighting them for 12 years, and I mean brutally. My needs require out-of-network care. They think they can tell me when to get a MRI? with the clowns on their list to see? I don't think so. I know all of them in the book. I wouldn't bring a parakeet to any of them!*

I promised them that if they didn't get me the referrals that both my husband and I needed, I would make them more miserable than they ever could imagine. Seems like I'm always in fight mode.

Sheryl, Boca Raton FL

THE POINT OF SERVICE (POS) PLAN

A POS* plan is the most versatile of plans, providing three types of coverage – one that functions like an HMO plan, another that functions like a PPO plan and the third that functions like an *indemnity plan.** Members of a POS plan can use all three types of coverage at any time, switching back and forth between them as needed. Each level of coverage is called a "tier."

> A POS plan is the most versatile plans, providing three types of coverage.

- Tier 1 functions just like an HMO. If you choose to receive your care through your primary care physician in your HMO, you will only be responsible for a co-payment (small) and no annual deductible. Your primary care physician refers you to other specialists within the HMO.
- Tier 2 functions like a PPO. You can self-refer to any provider in the PPO network of physicians. The insurance will pay for a certain percentage of the medical charge. You will be responsible for an annual deductible and co-payments.
- Tier 3 functions like an indemnity plan. You can self-refer to a provider of your choice outside the network. The insurance will pay for a lower percentage of the medical charge than in tier 2. You are responsible for higher annual deductible and co-payments than Tier 2.

Although many POS plans require you to make co-payments, you pay this percentage only until you reach your annual *out-of-pocket** maximum. If you have a maximum out-of-pocket of $2000, for example, the insurance plan will pay 100 per cent of your claims after you have paid this amount.

> POS plan Members can use all three types of coverage at any time. Each coverage level is called a *tier.*

THE INDEMNITY PLAN

This is the older, traditional type of policy that is rare and expensive today. Indemnity plans* allow you to choose any doctor or hospital when seeking medical care. These plans typically have a deductible, which you must pay before the plan will pay for any medical expenses. Once you have paid the deductible, the health plan will typically pay 70 to 80 percent of the medical expenses. The percentage of charges that you will pay is called co-insurance.* The remainder of the bill that needs to be paid by you is called patient liability. Indemnity plans vary greatly, and you will need to check the particulars of your plan and the lifetime maximum it will allow.

Although many plans require a patient liability of 20 per cent, you only have to pay this percentage until you reach your annual maximum out-of-pocket. If you have an out-of-pocket maximum of $2000, for example, the insurance plan will pay 100 per cent of your claims after you have paid this amount.

INFORMATION YOU NEED TO KNOW ABOUT YOUR PLAN

THE RULES OF YOUR HEALTH PLAN – 15 QUESTIONS TO ASK

You need to find out more about your provider. Look in your plan booklet or call the service administrator for explanations. Be prepared to wait on the phone a long time after you have navigated the automated voice tree ("press #1 if you want...") answering system.

Here are 15 questions to get started:

1. In the HMO or PPO network, are there neurosurgeons, radiation therapists, neurooncologists and so forth with expertise in brain tumors? Do they each see more than 25 brain tumor patients per year?

A growing body of evidence shows that the patients of more experienced surgeons have better survival rates (see Chapter 17: Traditional Approaches to Treatment). Insurance companies traditionally have not paid attention to this. They do not feel obligated to find you a qualified expert; their objective is, rather, to provide you with the lowest-cost professional possible. You must argue from your point of view and back it up with evidence to make your case.

Bottom Line To have your claim honored, you must understand how insurance companies process claims and the terms that they use.

2. How are referrals to specialists handled? What paperwork or approvals are needed?
3. Do I select from a list of contract physicians or from the staff of a group practice?
4. What is the procedure to change doctors, if I decide that I want someone else?
5. How are referrals to specialists handled?
6. Which services are covered or excluded?

Brain tumor treatment is complex and requires different specialists. Will the HMO or PPO provide occupational and speech rehabilitation training after surgery? If so, will it be provided in the hospital, at home, or at a far-away rehabilitation center? Location is essential if you are immobile.

Different states have specific laws for coverage of cancer and other conditions. You can find the exact coverage of your specific state on this website: http://www.insure.com/health/lawtool.cfm.

7. Which hospitals are available through the HMO or PPO? What if their provider does not offer the services or expertise that I need?

An editor, Lloyd, called me the other day about his father-in-law.

Dad has excellent insurance coverage in a modest city in northern California. He has emphysema, requires full-time oxygen, and underwent repair of a heart aneurysm 10 years ago. Now, he has a brain tumor, diagnosed by MRI scans, which could be a metastasis or primary brain tumor. His physicians wish to operate in a small community hospital that has a general ICU for post-operative care.

The family now needs answers to these questions:

- Is the individual who is in charge of the ICU knowledgeable about post-operative care for such patients?
- Do the anesthesiologists have experience with such complex cases?
- How many patients of this type has the neurosurgeon seen?

8. What arrangements and coverage does my HMO or PPO offer for emergency care at home or out of town?

9. Are there limits on coverage for medical tests, out-of-hospital care, prescription drugs, or other services that may be ordered by specialists?

10. Is there a per-visit cost for seeing PPO doctors? Other co-payments for services?

11. What is the difference in cost between using doctors inside vs. outside the network?

12. What is the deductible and coinsurance for care outside the HMO or PPO?

13. Is there a limit to the maximum expenses that I will have to pay out-of-pocket?

14. What is maximum total money that the PPO can apply toward my health care?

15. Whom do I contact to question or appeal denials?

As a person with a brain tumor, the care that you need is expensive and requires coordination among neurosurgical, oncologic, medical, endocrine, rehabilitation, neuropsychological, and other well-trained specialists. You will be in a stronger position to negotiate with your health insurance company, if armed with information. Answers to the 15 important questions above will help to empower you to get the best care possible.

OTHER TYPES OF PRIVATE INSURANCE

HOSPITAL INDEMNITY INSURANCE

Hospital indemnity insurance pays a fixed amount for each day spent in the hospital up to a maximum number of days, but the amount you receive will usually be less than the cost of a hospital stay. This type of insurance may also be used to cover medical or other health-related expenses. Some hospital indemnity policies will pay a specified daily amount, even if you have other health insurance. Other policies may coordinate benefits so that the money you receive does not equal more than 100 percent of the hospital bill.

DISABILITY INSURANCE AND MEDICAL INSURANCE

Disability insurance replaces lost *income* from long-term illness or injury. This is an important type of coverage for working-age people to consider; however, disability insurance will not pay the cost of rehabilitation, if you are injured. Check your medical insurance policy to see if it you are covered for disability. Ask if your employer offers group disability insurance automatically or as a choice; this may be one of the benefits where you work. You may also be eligible for some government-sponsored programs that provide disability benefits.

Many different kinds of individual disability insurance policies are available.

- Short-Term Disability Insurance typically covers the continuation of a salary for up to one year. It can provide a gross (before taxes) benefit of 40 to 100 per cent of your gross salary prior to disability, or a flat dollar amount. The net (take-home) benefit is calculated by deducting tax contributions and sick leave income from the gross benefit.

> Short-Term Disability Insurance typically covers continuation of salary for up to one year.

- Long-Term Disability Insurance pays benefits for several years or until retirement age. It can provide a gross benefit of 40 to 70 per cent of your gross salary prior to disability, or a flat dollar amount. As with short-term disability insurance, the net take-home benefit is calculated by deducting tax contributions and sick leave income from the gross benefit. Individual policies exist but are difficult to obtain, if there is a pre-existing condition within the past 10 years. The *Consumer's Guide to Disability Insurance* explains disability insurance and sources of disability income to help you decide if you need this coverage. It will also help you compare your choices of policies (see Table 23A-3).

> Long-Term Disability Insurance pays benefits for several years or until retirement age.

PURCHASING LONG-TERM CARE INSURANCE

Unfortunately, the decision to get the insurance must be made *before* one is ill. Long-term care insurance is designed to cover the costs of nursing home care, which can be several thousand dollars each month. Long-term care is usually not covered by health insurance carriers, except in a very limited way. Medicare covers very few long-term care expenses. There are many plans that vary in cost and services covered; each has its own limitations. There is detailed information in two free booklets: *A Shopper's Guide to Long-Term Care Insurance* and *The Consumer's Guide to Long-Term Care Insurance* (see Table 23A-3).

MEDICARE

When Am I Eligible for It?

Medicare is the federal health insurance program for Americans age 65 and older and some Americans who are disabled for 29 months or more (see definition for *disability**).

Medicare covers hospitalization, skilled nursing, home health, and hospice care and requires *deductibles** and *co-payments**. If you are receiving outpatient (not in hospital) care, Medicare will cover 80 per cent of allowable outpatient medical services, after a $100 deductible. You are responsible for 20 per cent of the charge (co-payment, co-insurance) regardless of the cost.

If you are eligible for Social Security or Railroad Retirement benefits and are age 65, you and your spouse (even if he/ she is under 65) automatically qualify for Medicare. If you are already getting Social Security retirement or disability benefits or railroad retirement checks, Social Security will contact you a few months before you become eligible for Medicare and give you the information you need to register. If you are not already receiving checks, you should contact Social Security at (800) 772-1213 about three months before your 65th birthday to sign up for Medicare. They also have a TTY phone connection at (800) 325-0778.

You should sign up for Medicare even if you don't plan to retire at age 65, or you may be penalized a 10 percent premium surcharge for each year past age 65 that you do not have Medicare. However, if you are age 65 or older and are covered under a group health plan, either from your own employment or you are covered from your spouse's employment, you may delay enrolling in Medicare medical insurance (Part B) without having to wait for a general enrollment period or need to pay the late enrollment surcharge. The rules allow you to enroll in:

- Medicare Part B any time while you are covered under the group health plan, or
- Part B during an eight-month special enrollment period that begins with the month your group health coverage ends or the month employment ends, whichever comes first.

Medicare Parts A and B – What Do They Cover?

Medicare has two parts: hospital insurance ("Part A") and outpatient coverage ("Part B").

Part A covers:
- Hospitalization and Hospice care
- Skilled nursing and Home health
- No premiums are required

Part B provides:
- 80 per cent of allowable payment to doctors for outpatient services after $100 deductible.
- You are responsible for 20 per cent of the charge, regardless of the cost.
- Services and supplies ordered by doctors.
- You must pay $78.20/month (in 2005) premiums, plus deductibles and co-payments.

Medicare does <u>not</u> cover, as of June 2005:
- Most nursing home care or services in the home.
- Many long-term care expenses.
- Prescription drugs (The Bush Plan [2005] will allow some coverage).

One proposal is that low-income seniors who want to remain in Medicare's traditional fee-for-service system would receive a $600 subsidy each year toward prescription drug costs. Seniors remaining in the existing set-up also would get assistance with high overall drug bills, although the Bush administration was not providing specifics of what constitutes a high bill.[3,4]

> Medicare does *not* cover outpatient prescription drugs unless administered in a doctor's office or an outpatient clinic.

Seniors who agree to move into managed care would get larger drug coverage although it was not immediately clear how sizeable this would be.

Medicare includes two deductibles:
- $840 for an inpatient hospitalization under Part A Medicare.
- $100 for services under Part B.

In most cases, a beneficiary must pay the deductible before Medicare covers any costs of medical care or services. The Part B premium is generally subtracted from an individual's Social Security benefit. Thus, beneficiaries will receive a smaller increase in their Social Security check than the amount of the cost-of-living increases.

HMOs are now available to Medicare enrollees in some locations. The best source of information on Medicare is the *Medicare Handbook*. It explains how Medicare works and your benefits. (For contacts see Table 23A-3). You can also contact your local Social Security office for information (http://www.ahrq.gov/consumer/insuranc.htm).

FIVE MAJOR CHALLENGES FOR BRAIN TUMOR PATIENTS COVERED UNDER MEDICARE

1. Medicare beneficiaries will spend 30 percent of after-tax income on health care by 2025.
2. Medicare has had a 35 per cent increase in premiums, and it will probably continue to rise.
3. Changes to outpatient oral drugs from hospital-based inpatient intravenous preparations may put more financial burden on the patient for drug payment.
4. Medicare operates on a fee-for-service basis.
5. There are special rules on payment if you have employer group health insurance coverage through your own job or that of a spouse.
   > If you are disabled and cannot function at your place of employment, your company's insurance becomes the secondary payer and Medicare becomes the primary.
   > If you are covered through your spouse's employment – their insurance is primary and Medicare is secondary.

EXTENDING MEDICARE COVERAGE

> HMOs are now available to Medicare enrollees in some locations.

Medicare does *not* cover outpatient prescription drugs, unless they are administered in a doctor's office or an outpatient clinic. Therefore, many people choose to enroll in Medicare HMOs or buy relatively inexpensive private health insurance supplements (MediGap, AARP) to reduce their out-of-pocket costs (see Table 23A-3 for a comparison of plans). If you cannot afford to buy private health insurance, you might be able to supplement your Medicare with Medicaid

| HICAP counselors can help you understand Medicare. |

(Medi-Cal in California). For more information or assistance with Medicare, you can contact The Health Insurance Counseling and Advocacy Program (HICAP) at (800) 303-4477.

MEDIGAP SUPPLEMENTAL INSURANCE TO COVER OUT-OF-POCKET MEDICAL EXPENSES

Medigap is a private insurance program that pays medical bills that are *not* covered under your Medicare Program such as:

- Deductibles for Medicare
- Co-insurance for Medicare
- Health services not covered by Medicare.

There are 10 standard plans within Medigap from which to choose. (Some states may offer fewer than 10.) You are eligible to buy *only* one Medigap policy. Shop carefully before deciding on the best policy for your needs. The AARP, formerly known as American Association of Retired Persons has a website and free booklets, *Guide to Health Insurance for People with Medicare. The Consumer's Guide to Medicare Supplement Insurance* will help you make the right choice. (See Table 23A-3.)

GETTING HELP TO UNDERSTAND MEDICARE AND THE SUPPLEMENTAL PLANS

The Health Insurance Counseling and Advocacy Program (HICAP) provides information to seniors and other people on Medicare. HICAP counselors can help you understand Medicare, compare private Medicare supplemental plans, review Medicare HMOs, develop a system to organize your doctor and hospital bills, file Medicare and private insurance claims, and prepare Medicare appeals or challenge claim denials. All HICAP services are provided free of charge. To speak to a HICAP counselor, call (800) 303-4477.

MEDICAID

Medicaid is a program that is funded by the federal government. Each state determines its own eligibility standards and scope of health services offered. Medicaid provides health care coverage for some low-income people. Eligible people may be:

- Aged or blind,
- Disabled or living below the poverty line with dependent children.

GUIDELINES IN APPLYING FOR GOVERNMENT AID:

1. Expect to have your application rejected the first couple of times.
2. If you draw $1.00 from Supplemental Security Income (or SSI – see "Getting my social security and state disability benefits" below), you automatically qualify for Medicaid.
3. If out-of-state treatments are required, check with the treating facility to see if they accept your state's Medicaid.
4. They make appointments either by phone or in person.
5. The official date of your application is the date of your first phone or in-person contact with them, if you get your written application in within six months of that date.
6. Go to www.ssa.gov to obtain all the rules and forms.
7. Many states give automatic Medicaid with SSI.
8. The only way you can be denied is in writing that includes a specific reason for denial.
9. See Medicaid Fact Sheet (see Table 23A-3).
10. I will use the California version of Medicaid, called MediCal, as examples that may apply to your state.

> Expect to have your government aid application rejected the first couple of times.

MEDICAID WITH NO BRAIN TUMOR TREATMENT SPECIALISTS IN YOUR STATE

If you can convince your local Medicaid worker that no physician in your state can perform the surgery, Medicaid will approve out-of-state treatments. You need to ask the physicians in the center where you wish to have treatment to write and fax you letters. They must use very strong language, describing the diagnosis, what has to be done, and why there is no local doctor qualified to do it. A social worker and financial person from the treatment center can help you accomplish this. The doctor and center also will have to accept the out-of-state payment level. Take those letters to Medicaid along with one of your own, requesting that they approve surgery.

> Local American Cancer Society offices can arrange car transportation for your doctor's visits or treatments.

Medicaid Reimbursement for Caretaker and Transportation Expenses

Caretaker payments and a standard rate (cents per mile) for travel can be reimbursed by Medicaid on a monthly basis. They provide a form that must be completed. (Medicaid in several states also provides van transportation to medical appointments.)

SOCIAL SECURITY (SSI AND SSDI) AND STATE DISABILITY (SDI)

Many public insurance benefits rest on a definition of *disability* and these have standard definitions adapted from Social Security and state disability programs.

Social Security Benefits (SSI and SSDI): The Definition of a "Disability"

Social Security defines *disability*:

a physical or emotional impairment that is severe enough to keep a person from working for a continuous period of not less than 12 months or that can be expected to result in death.

Important Differences Between SSI and SSDI

The Social Security Administration oversees two programs that pay disability benefits to legal residents of the United States: the Supplemental Security Income (SSI) program and Social Security Disability Insurance (SSDI) program.

> SSI is a supplementary benefit based only on income, not impairment status.

Supplemental Security Income (SSI) is a supplementary benefit based only on *income*, regardless of impairment status.

- **Supplemental Security Income** (SSI) provides a minimum monthly income to those without other resources. To receive SSI, you must *first* apply for other disability benefits if eligible, such as Social Security Disability Income (SSDI) and State Disability Insurance (SDI). In order to qualify, your assets can be no greater than $2,000. The home in which you are living is exempt, as is your car if it is valued at or below $4,500 *or* used to get to and from your medical appointments. You should check your eligibility for SSI as soon as possible after becoming disabled, in order to establish an *onset date* and start the application process.

Social Security Disability Income (SSDI) is awarded based on impairment, *regardless* of family income. Thus, for SSDI, *any* brain tumor is an impairment appearing in the Social Security List of Impairments.

- **Social Security Disability Insurance** (SSDI) provides a benefit based on an individual's Federal Insurance Contributions Act (FICA) contributions. Under FICA, 12.4 percent of your earned income up to an annual limit was paid into Social Security, and an additional 2.9 percent into Medicare. There are no income limits on Medicare taxes. If you're a wage or salaried employee, you paid only half the FICA bill (6.2 percent for Social Security + 1.45 percent for Medicare), and your employer paid the other half.

> SSDI is awarded based on impairment, not family income.

- SSDI requires that you must have paid into Social Security for at least 20 of the last 40 quarters (5 of the last 10 years) for individuals age 31 or older. SSDI requires a *full* five-month waiting period (unpaid). Eligibility begins in the sixth month, and payment is received at the seventh month to cover the previous month. This program has no asset limits and is solely based on contributions to FICA and medical eligibility.

- When you fill out your SSDI application, take your time and think it out carefully. Your position is that your impairment from a brain tumor disables you from your last and all your past employment. Let's say, for example, that you suffered a back injury. Your current occupation is in construction work, but your previous occupation was as a cashier. If your back injury disables you from heavy lifting, then clearly you can't go back to your current occupation, but it might not disqualify you from work as a cashier. If you are having problems with memory, coordination or sitting, then you could not be a cashier, either.

> On your SSDI application, mention that your impairment from a brain tumor may disable you from your last and all your past employment.

To apply for disability benefits, call the Social Security Administration at (800) 772-1213 to find a local office or see their website at http://www.ssa.gov.

SSI Calculations for Minors

SSI is based on parents' income. If yours exceeds the limits, states like Pennsylvania have Medical Access care, which covers everything that primary insurance does not. Each state is different. In some states, Medical Access care benefits are based on diagnosis, and income is not considered.

State of California Benefits (SDI)

The State of California administers a program called State Disability Insurance (SDI). This is a 52-week program, which issues payments every two weeks. You have paid your premium for this program through your employer, unless your employer has opted out and has a superior coverage. To be eligible you must have contributed into SDI via a California employer for at least 12 months for the full 52-week benefit. Statewide, toll-free number (800) 480-3287 and website is http://www.edd.ca.gov/fleclaimdi.htm. Check your own state's office for specific information.

VIATICAL SETTLEMENTS

Life insurance policies typically are used to benefit a beneficiary when the policyholder dies. Recent laws have made it possible for individuals with a catastrophic or terminal illness to sell their life insurance policy while they are still *alive*. Called *viatication*, it enables individuals with a terminal disease to access a crucial source of money while they are still alive. You can use the money to get additional treatment or to pay bills. Companies offering viatication services typically pay between 35 to 85 per cent of the policy's face value.

It is important to plan ahead for the continuation of the policy once you stop working, so that you have this option at a later date. Remember, you will only receive a *percentage* of the (discounted) face value of your life insurance policy. Another option is to contact the insurer of your policy to see if the company offers an accelerated benefits program. (See Table 23A-3.)

> Viatication enables individuals with a terminal disease to sell their life insurance policy while they are still alive.

THE FAMILY AND MEDICAL LEAVE ACT (FMLA) OF 1993

To What Amount of Leave Am I Entitled?

For the person with a brain tumor or family member caring for him or her, FMLA entitles eligible employees to take up to 12 weeks of unpaid, job-protected leave in a 12-month period for specified family and medical reasons.

Table 23A-2 Family and Medical Leave Act (FMLA) Guidelines
1. The employee (family member) must have a serious health condition.
2. The employee must work for a specific type of organization (employer).
3. The employee must have worked for a specified period of time and number of hours within an organization of a particular size and locale.
4. The employee must have specified reasons for taking leave.
5. The employee must take leave in acceptable ways.
6. The employee must work with a legitimate health care provider.

Terms of Eligibility

It is up to the employer to define "12-month period" as any of the following:

> FMLA allows you to take unpaid leave.

- Calendar year,
- Fiscal year,
- 12-months following commencement of leave,
- 12-months preceding the end of leave, or
- Fixed 12-week leave regardless of when it is taken.

Examples of Rules and Solutions in Using FMLA

1. The Employee (Family Member) Must Have a "Serious Health Condition."

A brain tumor must fit under federal guidelines of a "serious health condition," which means an illness, injury, impairment, or physical or mental condition that involves:

- Any period of incapacity or treatment connected with inpatient care (i.e., an overnight stay) in a hospital, hospice, or residential medical-care facility.
- Any period of incapacity or subsequent treatment in connection with such inpatient care.
- Continuing treatment by a health care provider, which includes any period of incapacity (i.e., inability to work, attend school or perform other regular daily activities) due to:
    1. a permanent or long-term condition (e.g., Alzheimer's disease, a severe stroke, terminal cancer). Only supervision by a health care provider is required, rather than active treatment.
    2. multiple treatments for restorative surgery or a condition that would likely result in a period of incapacity of more than three days if not treated (e.g., chemotherapy, radiation).

2. The Employee Must Work for a Specific Type of Organization (Employer).

Organizations that meet this condition include:
- Public agencies, including federal, state, and local employers, such as local schools.
- Private-sector employers, who have employed 50 or more employees in 20 or more work weeks in the current or preceding calendar year and who are engaged in commerce.
- Any industry or activity affecting commerce, including joint employers (two jobs) and successors of covered employers.

3. The Employee Must Have Worked for a Specified Period of Time and Number of Hours, Within an Organization of a Particular Size and Locale.

The employee must have:
- Worked for the covered employer for a total of 12 months.
- Worked at least 1,250 hours over the previous 12 months.
- Work at a location in the United States or in any territory possessed by the United States, where at least 50 employees are employed by the employer within a 75-mile radius.

4. The Employee Must Have Specified Reasons for Taking Leave.

Acceptable reasons include:

- Caring for an immediate family member (spouse, child, or parent) with a serious health condition, and
- Taking medical leave because of a serious health condition that renders the employee unable to work.
- Two spouses employed by the same employer can only take a combined total of 12 work-weeks of family leave to care for a parent who has a serious health condition.

5. The Employee Must Take Leave in Acceptable Ways.

Employees may:

- Take family medical leave intermittently, which means taking leave in blocks of time or reducing the normal weekly or daily workload.
- Choose to use accrued paid leave (such as sick or vacation leave) to cover some or all of the leave.
- The latter requires the approval of employers; the employer is responsible for determining whether an employee's use of paid leave counts as FMLA leave, based on information from the employee.

> FMLA entitles eligible employees to take 12 weeks of annual unpaid, job-protected leave for family illness.

6. The Employee Must Work with a Legitimate "Health Care Provider."

Approved health care providers include:

- Doctors of medicine or osteopathy who are authorized to practice medicine or surgery by the state in which they practice.
- Podiatrists, dentists, clinical psychologists, optometrists, and chiropractors.
- Nurse practitioners and clinical social workers who are authorized to practice and perform within the scope of their practice, as defined by state law.
- Christian science practitioners listed with the First Church of Christ, Scientist in Boston, Massachusetts.
- Any health care provider recognized by the employer or the employer's group health plan benefits manager.

Family medical leave is not always honored in the way one would expect, as illustrated by the following report from a caregiver who wanted time off to go fishing with the patient.

Hello, all! To make a long story short, what my boss is doing is harassing me. I was advised to take detailed notes and keep everything...Human Resources [HR] called me in to a meeting with my boss on Wednesday of this week, and we discussed the fishing trip...HR said that as long as I get a doctor's note stating it would be beneficial, I could go. I guess we cancer families aren't eligible for "vacations." We can only be there for the fun stuff like chemotherapies, surgeries, and doctor appointments.

Darla, wife of Alex, malignant Oligo. Marietta, GA

The same caregiver describes the ambivalence that she sensed from her co-workers during her leave:

Pardon my sarcasm. Although my fellow employees have been very supportive, there's an underlying "we are doing you a favor" tone about the place. It's not a favor! It's the law and any time they want to trade places with me, even for a day, the offer is open!

It sounds harsh, but we all know that there is fear around disease and cancer. In general, employers like to give the appearance of supporting their employees, but that inclination seldom surpasses the requirements of a sincere fight for life and a long-term battle against chronic diseases. Darla.

THE HEALTH INSURANCE PORTABILITY AND ACCOUNTABILITY ACT (HIPAA) AND PEOPLE WITH A BRAIN TUMOR

The Health Insurance Portability and Accountability Act (HIPAA) is a privacy law that prevents doctors from giving out private medical information without permission from the patient. The Act is a set of standards to protect patients, given the widespread availability of electronic information on patients. It was purportedly designed to protect against researchers looking at data on patients for purposes other than health care. Scientists can use such data as long as it is *de-identified*, so that it cannot be traced to the original source.

> The HIPAA law presents serious communication issues for patients with brain tumors and their families and doctors.

This law presents serious issues for patients with brain tumors and their doctors. It was not well thought out before implementation. Although you may not want your employer to know about your medical issues, the law is so stringent that it prevents health care professionals from having *any* communication regarding your case, without your prior approval, even if it would be helpful to you.

The Health Insurance Portability and Accountability Act was first introduced in 1996 and is only now going into effect. It mandates large fines up to $250,000 or imprisonment for violations, and most health care agencies are scared of the consequences. The reality is that few health care facilities are able to understand what they can and cannot release. For better or worse, many misinterpret the 100+ page manifesto.

Hospitals are mandated to provide employee training in the implementation of HIPAA. All staff (which means everyone who works in a hospital, including the cleaning crew) must attend an hour of training. The training includes a video, with different situations about how a patient's confidentiality could be violated (talking in an elevator, reading a computer screen that you pass, telling a friend about a case, and so forth).

The original version of the Act was so restrictive that:

- Doctors' offices could not use waiting room sign-in sheets.
- Hospital charts could not be kept at bedside.
- Doctors could not talk to patients in semi-private rooms.
- Doctors could not confer at nurses' stations without fear of being overheard and reported.

HIPAA does not apply when your records are used for:

- Patient care or government reporting (national statistics, cancer registries, etc.)
- Debt collection or internal hospital review of practice (quality assurance).
- The Act has now been amended to modify these restrictions, but the Act still affects how your doctor can communicate with you or your loved ones. The following example reflects the typical response since enactment of HIPAA:

I called my mom's neurosurgeon to discuss her condition after surgery. He refused to talk to me because of the new HIPAA rules. My mom hadn't seen him since the rules went into effect on April 15. Before he releases information or talks to anyone, my mom have to show up in person and sign a paper at his office. Faxes are not allowed, because I could fake them.

That means about three hours of driving for me and, with everything else going on, I don't have the time right now, so we are doing without the consultation. Tell me again how HIPAA is supposed to help patients?

Lloyd. Son. St Louis, MO.

Chris poses the following solution that worked for her:

Under HIPAA: We filled out a power of attorney when HIPAA was implemented earlier this year. We also had our social worker type up a form stating I, as John's caretaker, can have access to all labs, MRI's, etc. of John's information. John signed it and the social worker notarized and we have 10 copies of each. Carry it with you always. Even some of the nurses gave me a hard time when I asked for John's lab results during his last hospitalization. They shove these HIPAA forms in front of you and say "sign." We also added to the HIPAA forms my name but it doesn't matter because those forms go to medical records and no one can access them when you call and say "Can I get a copy of so and so's MRI? A down side to HIPAA.

Chris, Santa Monica, CA

CONCLUSION

Our healthcare systems are complex and have many components to master. This chapter has outlined the basic organization. In chapter 23B, I will show you how to use your new knowledge to ensure that you receive all your insurance benefits that will help you to heal maximally and have the best chances for a longer life.

THE GLOSSARY OF IMPORTANT HEALTH INSURANCE TERMS[5,6]

Co-insurance

The amount you are required to pay for medical care in a fee-for-service plan after you have met your deductible. The co-insurance rate is usually expressed as a percentage. Example, if the insurance company pays 80 percent of claim, you pay 20 percent.

Coordination of Benefits

A system to eliminate duplication of benefits when you are covered under more than one group plan. Benefits under the two plans usually are limited to no more than 100 percent of the claim.

Co-payment

A sharing of medical costs. You pay a flat fee every time you receive a medical service (example, $5 for every visit to the doctor). The insurance company pays the rest.

Covered Expenses

Most insurance plans, whether they are fee-for-service, HMOs, or PPOs, do not pay for all services. Some may not pay for prescription drugs. Others may not pay for mental health care. Covered services are the medical procedures that the insurer will pay for. They are listed in the policy.

Deductible

The amount of money you must pay each year to cover your medical care expenses *before your insurance policy starts paying.*

Disability

Most companies follow the Social Security definition: "physical or emotional impairment that is severe enough to keep a person from working for a continuous period of not less than 12 months or that can be expected to result in death."

Exclusions

Specific conditions or circumstances that the policy will not provide benefits.

Indemnity Insurance

With indemnity insurance, you can go to any doctor, hospital, or other provider and submit the bill to your insurance company.

HMO (Health Maintenance Organization)

Prepaid health plans. You pay a monthly premium, and the HMO covers your medical examinations, hospital stays, emergency care, surgery, checkups, lab tests, x-rays, and therapy. You must use the doctors and hospitals designated by the HMO.

Managed Care

Ways to manage costs, use, and quality of the health care system. All HMOs and PPOs, and many fee-for-service plans, have managed care.

Maximum Out-of-Pocket

The most money you will be required to pay per year for deductibles and co-insurance. It is a stated dollar amount set by the insurance company, in addition to regular premiums.

Medicare

The federal health insurance program for Americans ages 65 and older and some Americans who have been disabled for 29 months (see definition of disability). If you are eligible for Social Security or Railroad Retirement benefits, and are age 65 or over, you and your spouse automatically qualify for Medicare.

Non-cancelable Policy

A policy that guarantees you can receive insurance as long as you pay the premium. It is also called a guaranteed renewable policy.

Out of pocket

Money that you pay for which there is no insurance coverage.

Preferred Provider Organization (PPO)

A health care plan combination of traditional fee-for-service and HMO. When you use the doctors and hospitals that are part of the PPO, you can have a larger part of your medical bills covered, as in an HMO. You can use other doctors, but at a higher cost.

Point-of-Service (POS) Plan

Many HMOs offer an indemnity-type option known as a POS plan. The primary care doctors in a POS plan usually make referrals to other providers in the plan. Members can refer themselves outside the plan and still get some coverage. If the doctor makes a referral out of the network, the plan pays all or most of the bill. If you refer yourself to a provider outside the network and the service is covered by the plan, you will have to pay co-insurance.

Pre-existing Condition

A medical condition diagnosed or treated before joining a new plan. In the past, health care for a pre-existing condition was often not covered until after a waiting period. The <u>Health Insurance Portability and Accountability Act</u> (HIPAA) has changed the rules, however. A pre-existing condition is now covered without a waiting period when you join a new group plan, if you have been insured the previous 12 months. This means that if you remain insured for 12 months or more, you will be able to go from one job to another, and your pre-existing condition will be covered — without additional waiting periods — even if you have a chronic illness. If you have a pre-existing condition and have not been insured the previous 12 months before joining a new plan, the longest you will have to wait before you are covered for that condition is 12 months.

Premium

The amount you or your employer pays in exchange for insurance coverage.

Primary Care Doctor

Usually your first contact for health care. This is often a family physician or internist, but some women use their gynecologist. A primary care doctor monitors your health, diagnoses and treats minor health problems, and refers you to specialists if another level of care is needed.

Provider

Any person (doctor, nurse, dentist) or institution (hospital, clinic) that provides medical care.

Third-Party Payer

Any payer for health care services other than you. This can be an insurance company, an HMO, a PPO, or the federal government.

Viatical Settlement Company

A private enterprise that offers a terminally ill person a percentage of the policy's face value. It is not considered an insurance company. The *viatical settlement company* becomes the sole beneficiary of the policy in consideration for delivering a cash payment to the policyholder and paying the premiums. When the policyholder dies, the *viatical settlement company* collects the face value of the policy.

Viatication

A process which allows the holder of a life insurance policy to sell the rights to and interests in the benefits that will become available upon his or her death (along with the responsibility for subsequent premium payments) to someone else in exchange for money now.

Table 23A-3 Web Resources for Understanding Insurance and Health Care

Type of Information	Contact Information/ Website	
50 States mandated coverage	Consumer Insurance Guide	http://www.insure.com/health/lawtool.cfm
A chat group for financial information	http://groups.yahoo.com/group/Brain-Finance To start , simply send email to Brain-Finance@yahoogroups.com	
A Shopper's Guide to Long-Term Care Insurance	National Association of Insurance Commissioners, 120 W. 12th Street, Suite 1100, Kansas City, MO 64105.	http://www.longtermcareinsurance.org/
The Consumer's Guide to Long-Term Care Insurance.	Health Insurance Association of America, 555 13th St., N.W., Suite 600 East, Washington, D.C. 20004. (800) 582-3337 or TTY: (800) 843-3557	http://www.opm.gov/insure/ltc/
Access to medications	http://www.helpingpatients.org/	
Arguments/ assistance to protest denial of coverage for Clinical Trials	http://www.mcman.com	
Medical Care Ombudsman Program (MCOP), an independent referee. NCI office of Education and Special Initiatives	http://www.nci.nih.gov/aboutnci/oesi	
Checkup on Health Insurance Choices.	AHCPR Publication No. 93-0018, Dec1992. Agency for Health Care Policy /Research, info@ahrq.gov 540 Gaither Road , Rockville, MD 20850, Telephone: (301) 427-1364	http://www.ahrq.gov/consumer/ insuranc.htm http://www.about-disability-insurance.com

Denial of care (A case study) of denial	http://www.consumerwatchdog.org/healthcare/st/st000339.php3
Denial of coverage (Legal rights)	http://tcdc.uth.tmc.edu/candlaw/CAL98.html
Denial Settlement (Aetna)	http://www.usatoday.com/money/industries/insurance/2003-05-22-aetna_x.htm http://www.ama-assn.org/amednews/2003/06/16/prl10616.htm http://www.aetna.com/about/press/dec19_00c.html
Evolution of American Health Insurance	http://www.braintumorfoundation.org/hmos.htm
Family Medical Leave Act FMLA	U.S. Department of Labor, Frances Perkins Building, 200 Constitution Avenue, NW, Washington, DC 20210 1-866-4-USWAGE	http://www.dol.gov/esa/regs/compliance/whd/printpage.asp?REF=whdfs28.htm
Glossary of Financial and Medical Terms	http://www.oncolink.com/resources/article.cfm?c=6&s=28&ss=73&id=124
Health care term definitions	http://www.therapistfinder.net/glossary/managed-care.html http://www.aarp.org/healthcoverage/medicare/Articles/a2003-05-06-glossary.html http://tcdc.uth.tmc.edu/candlaw/CAL98.html
HICAP counselor	in California call (800) 303-4477.	http://www.inlandagency.org/html/hicap_home.htm and in other states
Medicare Assistance, appeals	Other states	http://hiicap.state.ny.us/home/link08.htm.
Insurance defined. How each system works: benefits, downsides	http://urac.org/ABCsHealthCoverage.pdf

Table 23A-3 Web Resources for Understanding Insurance and Health Care (Continued)

Medicaid Fact Sheet. Health Care Financing Administration. Publications, N1-26-27,	Centers for Medicare & Medicaid Services 7500 Security Blvd., Baltimore, MD 21244-1850. Toll-Free: 877-267-2323 TTY Toll-Free: 866-226-1819 For Medicaid eligibility and services contact State office.	http://cms.hhs.gov/ http://www.sccgov.org/scc/assets/ docs/413132mc.pdf or http: //www.dhs.cahwnet.gov/mcs/medi-calhome/MC210.htm or http: //www.dhs.cahwnet.gov/mcs/medi-calhome/CountyListing1.htm your area.
Medi-Cal HIPP- pays insurance premiums	To apply for Medi-Cal HIPP (800) 952-5294	http://www.apla.org/apla/benefits/ MEDICAL.HTM
Medicare Handbook. How the Medicare program works and your benefits. Free copy	Health Care Financing Administration, Publications, N1-26-27, 7500 Security Blvd., Baltimore, MD 21244-1850. Local Social Security office	http://www.ahrq.gov/consumer/ insuranc.htm
Medi-Gap Information Guide to Health Insurance for People with Medicare. The Consumer's Guide to Medicare Supplement Insurance.	Health Care Financing Administration, Publications, N1-26-27, 7500 Security Blvd., Baltimore, MD 21244-1850. American Association of Retired Persons (AARP). Health Insurance Assoc. of America, 555 13th St., N.W., Suite 600 East, Washington, D.C. 20004.	http://www.aarp.org/healthcoverage/ www.aarp.com
Social Security disability/ SSDI forms	Social Security (800) 772-1213 to find a local office	http://www.ssa.gov
States mandating Clinical Trial coverage	http://www.insure.com/health/lawtool	

The Consumer's Guide to Disability Insurance. Explains insurance, sources of income	Health Insurance Association of America, 555 13th St., N.W., Suite 600 East, Washington, D.C. 20004.	http://www.about-disability-insurance.com
Viatical Assignment-Insurance		http://www.opm.gov/insure/life/FAQs/ FAQs-10.asp http://www.quackwatch.org/ 02ConsumerProtection/viatical.html http://www.viatical-expert.net http://hopedc.org/viatical.html
Viatical Settlement-cautions		http://www.lsalliance.com/ExCo/agents_ examples.html

CHAPTER 23B

Receiving Health Care Benefits from Your HMO or Insurance Company – Challenges a Brain Tumor Patient Must Face

There have been many times - I admit - that I desperately wanted to surrender. Through the strength of my family, I battled as hard as the "beast" was battling me. Education is my power, my source of control. If you know your enemy, you can fight.

Sheryl R. Shetsky, Founder & President, Florida Brain Tumor Association

RECEIVING HEALTH CARE BENEFITS FROM YOUR HMO OR INSURANCE COMPANY

BASIC RULES TO OBTAIN YOUR INSURANCE BENEFITS

Arm yourself with knowledge.

Identify an advocate-representative to help you negotiate the system

Understand your policy, entitlements, and what is (and what is not) covered.

Know what can be negotiated, even if it is not covered.

Know the important federal rules that can protect and help you.

Do not assume they will understand your plight. You must make a strong case and be prepared to fight for your cause

EXAMPLES OF DENIALS THAT MUST BE CHALLENGED

FREQUENTLY ASKED QUESTIONS ABOUT BRAIN TUMORS & HEALTH INSURANCE

Denial of Social Security Disability Income (SSDI)? What you can do.

How do I obtain insurance with a pre-existing brain tumor?

Can my spouse/partner be eligible for coverage on my policy?

What help can I get if military insurance and SSI is not enough?

How do I cope with unexpected changes in program coverage?

How can my health insurance provider (HMO, PPO) help me?

What are the important considerations in using a case manager?

How do I fight a denial for home rehabilitation equipment, like a bed?

What if I do not challenge the HMO or insurance company's denial?

Can I get life insurance after I am diagnosed with a brain tumor?

What is Medicaid (Medi-Cal) and how does my state (California) define eligibility for it?

Can I have Medicaid if I already have private insurance?

COMMON PROBLEMS AND SOLUTIONS

Hidden costs to getting a second opinion

Assistance programs for rehabilitation

Covering local and out-of-state transportation costs

State and private funds to attend patient conferences

Regulations on voluntary fund raising to pay for medical bills
Medical expenses and tax deductions

🔑 Key search words

- HMO
- state programs
- SSI, SSDI
- disability
- health insurance
- transportation

- PPO
- medicare
- clinical trial
- family medical leave act
- medication
- private insurance

- POS
- medicaid
- social security
- FMLA
- consultations
- case manager

Cancer accounts for $60.9 billion in direct medical costs and $15.5 billion for indirect hardship costs.[1] For people with brain tumors, average monthly costs are about $5000 and indirect costs to employees averaged $945, the result of an average monthly loss of two workdays and five days due to short-term disability. This economic burden of cancer makes it imperative that insurance and other health coverage pay their appropriate portion to alleviate this hardship.

This financial weight can be exacerbated by denial of your first insurance claim. You may re-experience helplessness, loss of independence, and feelings of being overwhelmed. In addition to having to fight for your life, your financial stability is now in question. But you, too, can play the insurance game. Chapter 23A described how these Byzantine organizations work. Here you will find out how to negotiate to receive your benefits. It should not be this difficult, but that is the reality. The companies intend to keep the premiums that you have sent to them. For those interested in how this situation came to be, the website for the New York University Department of Neurosurgery offers an interesting historical perspective on insurance and HMOs.[2]

BASIC RULES TO OBTAIN YOUR INSURANCE BENEFITS

There are six principles for action you must understand to get your needs and services (see Table 23B-1). Actual techniques and the appeal process are outlined in Table 23B-2 (and examples #1-4 below). Insurance terms in this chapter are marked ♣ and are in the special glossary at the end of Chapter 23A.

Health plan groups manage common diseases, like diabetes and heart disease, much better than brain cancer. Neurooncology is a narrow specialty area that costs money and resources. Frankly, HMOs and prepaid health plans lack the motivation to provide this expertise. Nonetheless, there are often dedicated and skilled medical professionals within these groups, who get little or no attention for their expertise. Accept the challenge to seek them out. (See Chapter 6: Experts and Second Opinions.[3]) Much of the responsibility for getting the care that you need is in your own hands; it is you against *the system*.

Managed care policies are less expensive than other forms of insurance. Why? Managed care regulates how much health care you use, so that costs for your care can be controlled. For example, one type of managed care requires that you obtain written approval from your insurance company *before* you are admitted to a hospital. This is to make sure that the hospitalization is necessary. If you go to the hospital without this approval, you may not be covered for the hospital bill.

1. ARM YOURSELF WITH KNOWLEDGE

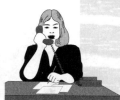

The first denied insurance claim can be shocking and intimidating. Feelings of being overwhelmed and helpless can come flooding in. To convince insurance companies to honor your claim (and not deny it), you must understand who they are, their view of you as the consumer, how they process claims, and the terms that they use.

Insurance is a business. As a business, the company has a mandate to manage your care *effectively* (Some may say to limit care.) in order to provide a profit to its shareholders. A brain tumor client is an *outlier* (i.e. a money drain). Insurance companies know that in the marketplace your total therapy package could run upwards of $450,000. You are now viewed as a high cost item to be surveyed and have been flagged for more scrutiny. Your minimal past expenses for routine care went under the radar screen. The company will not pay its share or provide care... unless you provide the information and are prepared to fight for your case (see Table 23B-1 and Table 23B-2).

Table 23B-1 Six Basic Rules to Obtain Your Insurance Benefits
1. Arm yourself with knowledge.
2. Identify an advocate-representative who will help you negotiate with the system.
3. Understand your policy, your entitlements, and what is (and what is not) covered.
4. Know what can be negotiated, even if it is not covered.
5. Know the important federal rules that can protect and help you.
6. Do not assume they will understand your plight. You must make a strong case and be prepared to fight for your cause.

Contact your local support groups and asked about others' experience with your HMO or insurance company. Go online and bring up the subject on all the brain tumor listservs or chat groups you may participate with (See Chapter 4: Searching the Web/ Internet and other resources.[6] The following website details what one family underwent following continuous denial of payments for brain tumor care by her HMO. See http://www.consumerwatchdog.org/healthcare/st/st000339.php3

2. Identify an Advocate-Representative Who Will Help You Negotiate with the System

Identifying an advocate to help you carry this burden is a must. This is a difficult battle. You may be on steroids or get less sleep than normal; after all, major changes have affected your life. It is difficult to provide detailed information and battle HMOs or insurance companies in this condition. The financial service person, social worker, or case manager at your hospital or clinic may be very helpful. Even a spouse who was previously unfamiliar with personal finances and insurance can become a formidable champion for details of claim refusals and clarifications. Finally your internist or primary care physician can be a powerful ally.

Identify an advocate to help you carry the burden.

3. Understand Your Policy, Your Entitlements, and What Is (and What Is Not) Covered

Health care in America has changed in the last 15 years. Most people in the United States used to have *indemnity insurance* coverage* (*term in Glossary at end of Chapter 23A). With indemnity insurance, you could go to any doctor, hospital, or other provider (who would bill for each service given); the insurance and the patient would each pay part of the bill.

Today, more than half of all Americans with health insurance are enrolled in some form of *managed care** plan or *health maintenance organization** (HMO), an organized way of providing (limiting) services and delaying payment for them. The organizational structures of such plans constitute a "word salad": *preferred provider organizations** (PPOs), health maintenance organizations (HMOs), and *point-of-service** (POS) plans. You've probably heard these terms before, but what do they mean, and what are the differences between them? (See Chapter 23A.)

For people with Indemnity and other Plans, there are ways to make the insurance dollars go even further.[4] This point relates to co-payments and deductibles. Any plan only pays up to its lifetime benefit. Cancer patients frequently exceed lifetime coverage limits. You can help yourself tremendously by comparing rates from different hospitals. All other things being equal (top-notch center, great expertise of your specialists etc), the lower the rates, the longer it takes to hit the maximum benefit limit and your dollar limit.

4. Know What Can Be Negotiated, Even if It Is Not Covered

How do you convince the insurance company to honor a claim? My suggestion: learn how to appeal all denials. Generally this requires a simple phone call or letter, yet only 30 per cent of claimants will appeal a denial. Remember, the insurance company is not expecting you to appeal. Times are changing, slowly. Aetna Insurance recently settled a $170,000 lawsuit and promised to interfere less with medical decisions and pay physicians more promptly (see Table 23B-2 and Aetna decision, Table 23B-3).

If your doctor orders an MRI scan, it might have to be "approved." Most often the person making this decision is not a physician. Unfortunately, the approval decision may not be based on your medical need, or even if your doctor thinks is necessary. Rather, the decision is usually made by a clerk who uses a checklist. If there is no code on his list or he does not understand, then it is denied. The guidelines may be out of date; and if so, a strong case can be made for coverage to avoid not just your litigation but a range of challenges. Guidelines may be commercial—in which case the company will probably tell you which ones they follow. However, in *all* cases you want the plan to explain the basis for the denial in detail and to point to the section of your policy, (in the booklet) that is used to support the denial. This makes it easier to challenge later.

If you get a turndown or restriction by message or phone, ask for it in writing. If they will not do this, then write an e-mail or letter memorializing what was said— make sure you always have the name and position of the persons contacting you. It is very important to record the health plan's grounds for denial. The if you can prove they erred on the original ground, they can't switch it to another.

A majority of states has mandated appeals for health coverage denials; you should take advantage of this. This gives you access to external independent review that for reasonable and necessary care can force coverage.

Dealing with plans that restrict physician access to those listed on their booklets.
If the care you need cannot be provided by experts, they have an obligation to let you have access to the level of care and expertise needed. For example, you should look at the resources available and check with your provider on what other resources have been accessible before; you then need to look up the physicians to whom you have uncontested recourse to see if they fill your need or not. In most

cases, once you get a medical director involved, you have a good chance to get the resources you need – not always, but usually.

Know the important federal rules that can protect and help you.
The Family and Medical Leave Act [FMLA] allows you to take unpaid leave (or vacation time) away from work in order to care for yourself, a dependent child, your spouse, or a parent (see FMLA, Chapter 23A). There are also federal and state assistance programs that provide money for medical and caregiver expenses, insurance premiums, and the like.

6. Do Not Assume *They* Will Understand Your Plight

The insurance company has a mandate to limit care to the minimum that they must deliver in order to provide a profit to their shareholders or sponsors. With brain cancer you are now a high cost "customer" to be contained; they have little sympathy for your plight. The company will not pay its share or provide care *unless* you provide the justification and are prepared to fight for your cause. The following is an example of what actions a patient took to prevail over her insurance company.

> *I very recently had a battle with a large insurance company. They raised our monthly rates to over $1000. I took this to Bill Nelson's office in Washington, D.C. He is a Florida senator who was the insurance commissioner for years. I asked ABC to do a story, and I contacted the largest paper in South Florida, the Sun-Sentinel; they ran a story. I won.*

> Name withheld

DENIALS THAT MUST BE CHALLENGED

When confronted with a denial of service, follow the five examples below:

Example #1

Denial of Coverage for a follow-up MRI.

Ask your doctor to write a "letter of necessity." The letter should state that it is within the guidelines of standard care that a follow-up MRI scan be performed at least every three months for the first two years following the diagnosis of a malignant brain tumor. The following is real advice from George who tackled this problem:

> *The way an HMO works is that your primary care physician has to request the MRI. If the doctor doesn't believe that you need it, he won't ask for approval. The insurance company should not deny a diagnostic test in a case such as yours! Talk to the doctor who placed the request to find out what went wrong. You may also have to talk to the local "IPA," or the umbrella organization that administers the HMO funds in your doctor's group. If that fails, file a written appeal with the insurance company and send copies to your doctor and IPA. You will get your MRI, if you push all of them. Threaten to hold them liable if progression of your tumor goes untreated because you failed to get proper follow-up.*

> George, Paradise Valley, AZ

You might want to draft a letter like the one below and give it to your doctor to put on his/ her office stationery:

> *At Duke, Cedars-Sinai Neurological Institute etc., and other brain tumor centers, the recommended follow-up MRI schedule is every three months for the first year, every four months in the second year, and every six months in the third year and thereafter. If your guidelines differ, can you provide me with the data to substantiate that decision? Otherwise we ask that you approve this reasonable request for routine monitoring for my brain tumor.*

Example #2

> Appeal all denials.

Your second opinion neurosurgeon states you will need intra-operative electrical mapping for a safe tumor resection. Your "plan" neurosurgeon does not perform this or other techniques.

Ask your consultant neurosurgeon to write a "letter of necessity" about *Standard of Care* to the Medical Director at the administrative address of your plan institution. Request to have your treatment covered by your out-of-network provider. If you are at a major Neurooncology institution, then you might use their trial or a cooperative group protocol that includes guidelines like these for a maximal tumor removal.

If this does not work, hire a lawyer or involve the local media (newspapers or television stations) in airing your plight. This can be a life-or-death situation, and you must act boldly to obtain the care you need and for which you have paid.

Stina writes about her husband:

> *And if all else fails don't forget the media. My husband's insurance plan was going to deny him treatment at an out-of-state center. I called one of the local broadcasters. If the insurance company did not approve of the surgery the network was going to do a story about us.*

> Stina, spouse of Carl, Malvern, PA

EXAMPLE #3

Denial of a second opinion.

You can usually get them to pay if there isn't a qualified expert inside your plan, whether they say they will pay or not. If they are "steering" you to just local care, then that is discriminatory. MCOP does medical record-based second opinions for a sliding-scale fee (See Table 23B-3).

EXAMPLE #4

Chemotherapy or anti-emetics are not covered under your plan.

Medications in common use are covered by most health insurance plans; however, chemotherapy drugs, especially those given as an outpatient, in pill or liquid form, are not always covered under these plans. Many insurance companies put chemotherapy in the same category as allergy medicine like antihistamines! Thus, when you consume the maximum, insurance pays no more. One course of chemotherapy will usually deplete the year's maximum for outpatient medications. Effective anti-nausea drugs used with Temodar (like Zofran or Kytril) are not usually covered and cost $7 to 20 per pill. The cheaper drugs that they do allow just do not work.

| The company will pay its share if you provide the justification and are prepared to fight for your cause. |

EXAMPLE #5

Denial for coverage in a Clinical Trial

This is a big one and you will have to bring out all your "big guns." It was made easier in 2001, when California joined seven other states in supporting clinical trials for cancer; Governor Gray Davis signed a law required health insurance companies to cover "routine services" of participating in Phase 1, 2, or 3 clinical trials. The covered costs include drugs, doctor visits, lab tests or hospitalizations as necessary. In 2004, at least 12 other states had the same law (see Table 23B-3 and (Chapter 21: Clinical Trials).

> Effective anti-nausea drugs used with Temodar (like Zofran or Kytril) may not be covered. Demand coverage!

In a highly publicized case seven years ago, the parents of a child refused care for an approved clinical trial lobbied the Department of Defense. The child's father was a military employee and the clinical trial was federally-sponsored. The parents won after seven months, using the Medical Care Ombudsman Program (MCOP), an independent referee. You can use this service to mount an argument against denials (http://www.mcman.com and see Table 23B-2, 23B-3). Here are the important components of a successful campaign to obtain coverage after it has been denied.[5]

Table 23B-2 Important Components of a Successful Reversal of Denial for Clinical Trial Treatment[5]
1. Obtain copies of your insurance company agreements and guidelines for clinical trial participation. (Some companies do not even have them!)
2. Identify contact persons at the NCI Office of Education and Special Initiatives (see http://www.nci.nih.gov/aboutnci/oesi) or Medical Care Ombudsman Program http://www.mcman.com).
3. Ask for form letters and guidance on appeals to your company.
4. In your letter, clearly state your purpose is to obtain coverage.
5. The label "clinical trial" may invoke initial denial because it is investigational. Call their bluff. If the trial is a Phase 3, the drug is not investigational.
6. For military type insurance like Champus-Tricare, know your rights.
7. The Department of Defense and NCI programs include follow up care. This is important to lessen your health care costs later on.
8. Regardless what happens, remember that the insurance company may be ignorant. Their responses are not "personal."

It is imperative on most appeals, at least on the second letter, that your physician provider includes letters from a variety of colleagues, in and out of state, people of stature, who support the specific treatment plan. If there have been two good clinical trials or articles, this might do the trick. These names might be obtained from co-investigators listed on the protocol. It is also imperative that your medical support team be available to participate at least by telephone in the hearing on the appeal if you can have more than just the letters—usually a doc who has gone the distance gets results.

If you are consistently denied service or coverage, you should appeal and threaten with newspaper or citizen advocates from radio or TV. Fortunately, there is a website that shows which drug companies and insurance companies have assistance plans (http://www.needymeds.com/).

FREQUENTLY ASKED QUESTIONS ABOUT INSURANCE & DISABILITY

I WAS REFUSED SOCIAL SECURITY DISABILITY INCOME (SSDI). WHAT CAN I DO?

We all may experience rejection as personal. What is normal is that SSDI applicants are often rejected on the first two to three attempts. Do not give up! Here are three people's stories about how they succeeded after rejection:

> They often turn you down the first time, but if you persevere, you will get it. They will send you the forms, and all of the rules are at www.ssa.gov. You also need to submit a letter from someone in charge of your care to itemize the deficits and the permanency of the deficits or the prognosis. With this information, you will get reviewed another time. Keep appealing, even three to four times if necessary. With brain cancer you will eventually be determined as disabled.

> SSDI applicants are often rejected on the first two or three attempts.

Susan, Naples, FL

> One parent applied for her 26-year-old son, telling them that he was unable to work, drive, go to school, or participate in routine daily activities. He was still denied disability! But you must re-submit. Your disability could be because you

have trouble focusing, reading, writing, and comprehending, and not actually from the brain tumor or the surgery. If your job required those skills (nurse, teacher, sales) then you would not be a candidate for other jobs either. You should be listed as never to work again and, as Social Security determines, 100 per cent disabled.

Miriam, Fargo, ND

It was almost a year after my diagnosis before I even learned I would be eligible to receive Social Security Disability Income (SSDI). I applied for it and, unfortunately, got a "jerk" to research my request file. You might get it approved easily, or you might not. It took me another year, two denials, and a lot of aggravation – but I got it. And I got it back-paid.

Here is some of my education on this. The amount you are eligible for depends on your past 10 years of employment and Social Security payments. Your spouse's employment or your financial situation do not affect this. You don't have to be "poor;" you are being paid for disability. This means you cannot both work and receive it. If you have not worked within 10 years, that can be a problem. Fill out the paperwork with as many words as you can find. Make sure you list every single problem that you have from the medical condition. My request was "start dated" when I had my first seizure.

Ronald, Thousand Oaks, CA

How Do I Obtain Insurance with a Pre-Existing Brain Tumor?

For people with brain tumors there are options for health insurance coverage, even with a pre-existing condition. HMO plans are required by law to cover pre-existing conditions immediately. Look into these possibilities:

- Professional Associations or Membership Organizations
  If you have a brain tumor and are having difficulty obtaining health insurance, you may be able to obtain group health insurance through a professional association that you might already belong to or may be able to join. The different associations include the your union, Bar Association, the Actors Association, Teachers' unions, the American Medical Association, and so on. Once you obtain health coverage through an association, you will have to pay the medical premiums yourself.

If you join an association and have a choice of health care plans, keep in mind that indemnity plans and PPO plans often have a period of up to six months before they will cover you for a pre-existing condition, if you have not had previous medical coverage.

- Health Insurance Plan of California (HIPC)
  HIPC offers coverage for people working independently or who work for small businesses. Since this plan pools together a large number of individuals, it offers many of the options previously available only to large businesses. As an HIPC member, you may be eligible to choose from many HMO or POS plans. To obtain more information, call (800) 255-4472. See if a similar program exists in your state.

- MRMIP: Major Risk Medical Insurance Program
  MRMIP is a state program that provides medical insurance for people who are unable to obtain medical insurance in the open market. If you have a pre-existing condition and have been denied coverage by private insurance companies and are not eligible for Medicare, you may be eligible for MRMIP. The program offers assorted plans with a wide range of medical providers and prescription drug coverage. The annual coverage limit is $75,000, with a lifetime maximum of $750,000. There is an annual *deductible** of $500, a required co-payment at the time of service, and a maximum out-of-pocket cost of $2,500 per year, as

> MRMIP state program provides medical insurance for those unable to obtain it in the open market.

of 2004. In 2004 there was a twelve-month wait for enrollment in MRMIPP. More information can be obtained by calling the California MRMIP phone number at (800) 289-6574; or go to the website at http://cc.ucsf.edu/crc/insurance_overview.html.

CAN MY SPOUSE OR PARTNER BE ELIGIBLE FOR COVERAGE ON MY GROUP POLICY?

Each insurance policy is different. Your best bet is to look at your policy certificate to see what is covered. If you work for a company, call the Human Resources representative within your personnel department to inquire about adding people to your policy. You do not have to disclose your partner's condition is at this point. If you would prefer to bypass the human resources personnel, call the insurance company directly and ask the customer service representative about specific pre-existing conditions. You might not want to mention "brain tumor" at this point.

WHAT HELP CAN I GET IF MILITARY INSURANCE AND SSI ARE NOT ENOUGH?

Consider the following scenario:

Ralph is now three months post op and has started to eat this week. The social worker at the hospital suggested that we apply for SSI. But they are telling us that we can only collect $30 a month and then only if Ralph is in the hospital. Does that sound correct? Is it based on the amount of money that the parents earn?

We know there are other services out there that we don't know about. My husband is retired military so Tricare pays 80 per cent of our medical expenses, but that 20 per cent adds up. I cannot tell the group how much it has helped me to read what everyone else is doing and going through.

Mary, Spouse of Ralph, Athens, GA

This is exactly the situation in which the social worker attached to your hospital or clinic can help. Or the Tricare Insurance representative or Medicaid Health Insurance Premium Payment program (HIPP) might help you pay for the continuation of your private insurance while you are on Medi-Cal. (See HIPP program details below.)

HOW DO I COPE WITH UNEXPECTED CHANGES IN PROGRAM COVERAGE?

The hoops and battles with Medicare, Medicaid, Social Security, and private insurance are only one part of the challenge faced by families of a brain tumor patient. There are many consequences that are difficult to anticipate, as illustrated by the example below:

Medicare covered Barbara and she had Medicaid until recently. We were served notice that she was "dropped" from Medicaid because she was out of state for more than 30 days. She was "out of state" because she was being treated at a major brain tumor center that was unavailable in our state!

We have appealed, and I believe that the negative decision has been overturned after an all-day effort yesterday. I arrived home from the long drive from Duke (North Carolina) and had to fight the Medicaid battle immediately upon my arrival. It took an act of congress. I have a meeting with them tomorrow morning to make it official. Hopefully, it will go without a hitch...

Bob, the Spouse, Albany, NY

CAN MY HEALTH INSURANCE PROVIDER (HMO, PPO) HELP ME?

The system is not all bad news. The organization's structure and economical orientation can help you. Your insurer might assign a *case manager* to coordinate your care, often a nurse or social worker who is experienced with brain tumors or general Neurology. This person can be your liaison to facilitate your care. Below are true patient testimonials:

Case #1

I am an adult with metastatic medulloblastoma to the abdomen. When the company I worked for changed insurance companies, they assigned a case manager to me mainly for the stem cell transplant; but she takes care of lots of other problems. This is a good thing... it is nice to know you have someone on the inside. This person knows your details, can go to bat for you, and can get the insurance company to take care of things that you need.

Adrien, Wichita, KS

Case #2

We had a case manager when Kyle was first diagnosed. It was nice...one person handles your case; if you have questions, you ask that person. It really cuts down on the red tape and telephone tag...not to mention not having to repeat yourself 100 times. It made getting things he needed much easier and much more personal.

Georgette, Mother, Atlanta, GA

WHAT ARE THE IMPORTANT CONSIDERATIONS IN USING A CASE MANAGER?

If your insurance company offers you case management service, ask the following questions before getting involved:

Bottom Line ▸ A case manager can be a great help to coordinate your care; this is often an experienced nurse or social worker.

- Can you leave the program if it does not work out for you?
- Can you switch to another case manager, if there is a personality conflict?
- Can you get a copy of the policy explaining (in writing) how this will change your situation? What benefit is there to you for choosing this program?

The Case Manager may negotiate with your health insurance carrier for a reduced price on drugs you need that are not considered as part of its pharmacy offerings. Also, check with your plan to see if it provides neuropsychological evaluations, rehabilitation equipment, and other things that you may need. If not, then use the tactic for denial of claims earlier in this chapter. Know what can be negotiated, even if it is not covered.

How Do I Fight a Denial for Home Rehabilitation Equipment, Like a Bed?

There are many different levels or features of hospital beds. One type can actually turn the patient at different intervals, blow air out slowly from the mattress to keep the person cool, and shift weight, and give massages to prevent blood clots in the leg. It is more expensive than the standard levels of beds that insurance usually wants to pay for.

Alice, Wife, Richardson TX.

Here, your primary physician or specialist could help you write a letter, or you could prepare it to send it out on the appropriate stationery. You would describe the special needs of the patient: brain tumor, predisposition to blood clots, weakness or paralysis, other rehabilitation exercises, time spent in bed, and how this could prevent expensive complications like bed sores and blood clots. This technique actually resulted in a patient victory! You should not have to work this hard to get needed equipment, but in the real world, this is how it happens. See Chapter 23A and Tables 23B-1 and 23B-2.

Look into aid organizations that will provide the needed equipment free or arrange for it at a deep discount; depending on whether equipment is owned or rented. You might find families who would be happy to recycle materials at a prorated cost or free after it has served it purpose; ask on chat rooms or local support groups.

What if I Do Not Challenge the HMO or Insurance Company's Denial of Care?

This is an example of the ugly consequences of inaction:

We had a client come in a few weeks ago wanting a will for himself and his wife. He told me that his wife had brain cancer. When I asked him which type, he handed me a piece of paper, and I read "glioblastoma multiforme." I asked where his wife was being treated, and he told me that they wanted to go to Moffitt in Florida, but her insurance company would not pay. Guess what? She worked for 12 years at the Clerk of the Court's Office in Tampa, FL!

He told me that she was diagnosed 2.5 months ago, had no treatment thus far, and was in St. Joseph's hospital. Immediately, I called and set up a no-charge consult with the senior neurosurgeon there. Moffitt was to start an appeal with her insurance company. He got her scans over to Moffitt and made the appointment, but she died two days later.

In a situation like this, you need help from an advocate who can present your case to the appropriate network. This might be a direct appeal to the insurance company. Or you can talk with one of the major brain tumor associations like the Brain Tumor Society, Ombudsman Programs, or Wellness Community to get information and a direction that others in your community, HMO, or insurance company have found successful (see Tables 23A-1, 23A-3, 23B-3).

Can I Get Life Insurance After I Am Diagnosed with a Brain Tumor?

Appeal all denials.

Most likely, the answer is "no." However, there are tactics that you can use to try to plead your case, as advised by an insurance company employee:

I work for an insurance company, and my husband has an oligodendroglioma-astrocytoma, grade II. We applied for term insurance before diagnosis, so luckily we have a small amount in place. However, I looked in the literature and read under brain tumors that malignant tumors definitely would be denied...<u>low grade tumors would be considered by the underwriter</u>.

So, there is a chance. I would get together with a life insurance agent who works with different companies. Have him choose a company that he feels has a good rating and will be around a long time, yet takes higher risk individuals. Sometimes the agent can even talk to the underwriter without going through the application process and get a hint as to whether it's worth it to apply. The application process is not too bad anyway, only takes about 1/2 hour for the agent to fill out the form and then a nurse comes to examine you at your home... So there is hope... you may have to visit with a few agents and weed through the companies.

RoseAnne, wife of Robert, Las Vegas, NM

What Is Medicaid (Medi-Cal)? How Does California Define Eligibility?

Medi-Cal is federally sponsored, state managed and distributed Medicaid coverage. Each state has its own program and rules on financial guidelines for people who meet the same disability standards as recipients of Social Security Disability Income (SSDI). Medicaid pays health care bills (at a reduced rate) incurred up to three months before the application date. Here are three examples for how you may become eligible:

- If you apply and qualify for Supplemental Security Income (SSI), you will automatically receive Medi-Cal coverage; the two programs are linked.
- If your monthly disability income (unearned income) exceeds SSI limits, but is not greater than $966.00, or $1,298.00 for a couple (as of 02/01/01), then you can apply for "Aged and Disabled" Medi-Cal coverage.

> The major disadvantage of MedicAid is that not all doctors will accept new MedicAid patients.

- If your disability income is above SSI limits and "Aged and Disabled" limits in the paragraph above, then you can apply for the "Medically Needy" Medi-Cal coverage, which may require a monthly co-payment called "share of cost." The "share of cost" begins if your disability income is more than $620.00 ($954.00 for a couple) per month (2003 figures).

The major disadvantage of Medi-Cal is that not all doctors will accept new patients with this coverage, because they pay the doctor such a small amount for service. There may be limitations on treatments and covered prescription drugs. For "Aged and Disabled" or "Medically Needy" Medi-Cal, you need to contact the County Welfare Office (Department of Human or Social Services) (see Table 23B-3).

Can I Have Medicaid if I Have Private Insurance?

If you have private insurance at the time that you become disabled, you may be able to enroll in the Medi-Cal/Health Insurance Premium Payment program (HIPP), which will help you pay for the continuation of your private insurance while you are on Medi-Cal. See if your state has such a program. In order to participate in the Medi-Cal/HIPP program:

- You must be eligible and enrolled in Medi-Cal, but not enrolled in any of the Medi-Cal HMO programs or Major Risk Medical Insurance Program (MRMIP), the state program for those who cannot get insurance in the open market.

> Local American Cancer Society offices can arrange car transportation for your doctor's visits or treatments.

  - You must also be insured under a private health insurance plan that does not exclude your serious medical condition.

- If you are eligible, Medical/HIPP will allow you to keep your private health insurance while you are on Medi-Cal. Unlike Medi-Cal, Medi-Cal/HIPP will not make retroactive payments.
- To apply for Medi-Cal HIPP, call the Medi-Cal HIPP office at (800) 952-5294.

SOLUTIONS TO VARIOUS PROBLEMS

Hidden Costs of Getting a Second Opinion

There may be several costs in getting a second opinion. The actual doctor's fee is only one of these. For example, a consultation at a university or large clinic might include a *facility* fee. This is a charge that the center makes in order to pay for their space and operating expenses; it often comes as a surprise to those seeking a consultation. Sometimes these fees are not insignificant, as you can see from the testimonial below:

> Ask, "What are all the costs of a consultation or second opinion?"

Our insurance will not cover out-of-state opinions. We have had major problems dealing with the financial department at MD Anderson. We live in Arizona and wanted a second opinion about chemotherapy from MD Anderson in Houston, Texas. As stated on their website, my mom paid $500 the day of the visit. We met with a doctor for an hour and discussed chemotherapy options. Nothing extravagant was done other than a traditional appointment.

A month or two later, MDA sends my mom a bill for $350 owed. They claim that the fee that they charged us the day of the visit only covered the doctor, not the facility charge.

Lucille. Scottsdale, AZ

This surprise might have been avoided if the initial inquiry had included the question "What are *all* the costs of getting a consultation?" or the confirmatory correspondence had been read carefully. If this information was not included, then you may have an argument for getting the institution to eliminate its charge.

OUT OF STATE OPINIONS

Patty, a very verbal brain tumor survivor, has helped me clarify the out of state opinion issues. For example, she has United Healthcare. On their web site you can look up any physician in the US. If they are on the list, you can fly there and pay the $15 co-pay. However, a plan like "NJ Plus" only has NJ Dr.'s listed.

ASSISTANCE PROGRAMS FOR REHABILITATION

Finding resources is a challenge. The brain tumor chat rooms and list servers are a great source for information. Groups like the Shriner's and Lion's Clubs can also help. The social worker at your center is usually a reliable resource.

In Texas, we have an organization called Texas Rehab. They organize occupational therapy to aid the brain damage my son got because of surgery for his oligodendroglioma tumor. They will test his cognitive and gross/fine motor skills to help him towards independent living.

Corporate Angels will fly you to doctors in distant cities.

Ann Marie. Mother to Shannon
with malignant ependymoma.
Austin, TX

Resources for Covering Local and out-of-State Transportation Costs

Your local American Cancer Society office can arrange car transportation for your doctor's visits, treatments and such. Large volunteer groups donate their time and often provide daily service when necessary. For those seeking second opinions or treatment at distant centers, there are some cost-saving options to get there.

- Passenger service representatives of major airlines may offer lower priced tickets on short notice or for trips that do not involve a Saturday layover.
- Corporate angels will fly you to doctors in distant cities. These private corporations provide their airplane for you, when their executives don't require it, or when they can fit more people in going to the same place. You must plan for these, but they are entirely free. Most social workers are aware of local and national groups that may provide this service (see Chapter 7, Table 7-6). The corporate angel program can be reached by calling (877) AIR-LIFE and for Air Care Alliance is (800) 296-1217.

> Caretaker payments and a standard rate (cents per mile) for travel can be reimbursed by Medicaid.

State and Private Funds to Attend Patient Conferences

There are many conferences around the nation for survivors of brain tumors. Sometimes they offer financial assistance or scholarships. In addition, some states offer support. In the example below, one parent cites some resourceful ways in which she met her needs:

In the state of Massachusetts, a Developmental Disability Council budgets $500 per family per year to attend workshops on their child's particular disability. My son has a non-verbal learning disability due to his right-sided, low grade astrocytoma. I explained this in writing, and we were pre-approved for reimbursement, which covered hotel, airfare, and registration fees for a regional conference in Maryland on learning disability.

On one of my growth hormone deficiency lists, a family wanted to attend the July national convention on growth deficiency in Chicago (see www.magicfoun dation.org). They wrote requests detailing their child's disability and their need to the Elks, Lions Club, and other service organizations in their local phone book. Within a week, they had three organizations offering to cover airfare, hotel, and conference costs in full for their family."

Ned, Father to Jamie, with low-grade astrocytoma, Plymouth, MA

REGULATIONS ON VOLUNTARY FUND RAISING TO PAY FOR MEDICAL BILLS

Here are some hints on managing voluntary funds to streamline the process and prevent problems with Internal Revenue Service audits:

1. Never...I say never...start fund raising in your own name. Have some one else do it and have payments for care go directly to the professional. That way it does not count as income (taxable!) to you.
2. People will try to claim a tax deduction for their donation. If the funds are not attached to a specific non-profit organization, this could lead to an investigation.
3. Make sure that you do not misrepresent the need. If you raise funds for a specific treatment and that treatment is not completely delivered, you might have to return the funds.
4. Do not raise funds for a person who might be receiving other forms of assistance. Raise the funds for the immediate family to cover out-of-pocket expenses, otherwise support for the patient might be withdrawn and cause a net loss.
5. Keep a separate bank account and a clear ledger for funds. Never put funds in your personal account.
6. Keep a photocopy of all contribution checks, accompanying cards, and addresses.
7. Provide an official "thank you" reply, including a receipt that clarifies the tax-deductible status of the contribution.

> Raise funds for the immediate family to cover out-of-pocket expenses. Do not put funds in your personal account.

The following is an example of what one parent did:

I set up a medical fund for Kenneth's insurance payments and premiums. The CEO of my credit union came through for Kevin when things were very difficult. We went to a lawyer so that everything was done legally, and the fund is overseen by the CEO. I had to file with the IRS, but the account is not taxable."

Bottom Line ▸ Be careful and follow the rules about voluntary fund raising to pay for medical bills.

I had a fundraiser for Kevin last year and received enough for 10 insurance payments, plus a bit extra; the total might have been around $11,000, and none of it was taxed. This has worked for us. Unfortunately, I had to cover lots of bases, as there are people out there who lie and pretend to have diseases. A woman from South Boston collected $40,000 in donations for herself. She was a fraud and cast a dark cloud on those who really need to do this type of thing. I always included letters and contacts in case a question came up.

Dad to Kevin, Struggling with a medulloblastoma, Detroit, MI

MEDICAL EXPENSES AND TAX DEDUCTIONS

You may deduct the portion of your medical expenses that *exceed* 7.5 per cent of your adjusted gross income. For example, if you earned $10,000, you could deduct any medical expenses that go over $750. Therefore, if your medical expenses were $1,000, only the portion beyond $750 would be deductible, that is $250.

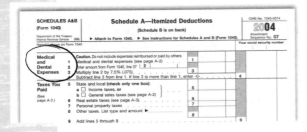

Accordingly, if you earned $100,000, you could deduct the part of medical expenses that exceeds $7,500. If your medical expenses were $10,000, only the portion beyond $7,500 could be deducted; that is $2,500. The exception is if you are subject to alternative minimum tax. For more information, see the websites for the Internal Revenue Service (see Table 23B-2).

CONCLUSION

Chapters 23A-23B were probably the most difficult chapters for me to write. The insurance issues are complex, even for physicians. I am especially indebted to Patty Adorno, and Ruth Hoffman and Grace Powers Monaco of Candle Lighters for their insights and detailed suggestions and Ted Schreck from Tenet Health.

Table 23B-3 Web Resources for Understanding Insurance and Health Care

Type of Information	Contact Information/ Website	
50 States mandated coverage	Consumer Insurance Guide	http://www.insure.com/health/lawtool.cfm
A chat group for financial information	http://groups.yahoo.com/group/Brain-Finance To start , simply send email to Brain-Finance@yahoogroups.com	
Checkup on Health Insurance Choices	Agency for Health Care Policy /Research, (AHCPR) Publication No.93-0018, Dec1992 info@ahrq.gov 540 Gaither Road , Rockville, MD 20850 Telephone: (301) 427-1364	http://www.ahrq.gov/consumer/ insuranc.htm http://www.about-disability-insurance.com
Denial of benefits: A case study.	http://www.consumerwatchdog.org/healthcare/st/st000339.php3	
Denial of coverage for Clinical Trials Medical Care Ombudsman Program (MCOP), an independent referee. NCI office of Education and Special Initiatives	http://www.mcman.com (MCOP Services) http://www.nci.nih.gov/aboutnci/oesi	
Denial of coverage- Legal rights	http://tcdc.uth.tmc.edu/candlaw/CAL98.html	
Denial of Coverage Settlement- Aetna	http://www.usatoday.com/money/industries/insurance/2003-05-22-aetna_ x.htm http://www.ama-assn.org/amednews/2003/06/16/prl10616.htm http://www.aetna.com/about/press/dec19_00c.html	
Evolution of American Health Insurance	http://www.braintumorfoundation.org/hmos.htm	

Table 23B-3　Web Resources for understanding Insurance and Health Care (continued)

Family Medical Leave Act FMLA	U.S. Department of Labor, Frances Perkins Building, 200 Constitution Avenue, NW, Washington, DC 20210 1-866-4-USWAGE	http://www.dol.gov/esa/regs/compliance/whd/printpage.asp?REF=whdfs28.htm
Glossary of Financial, health care and Medical Terms	http://www.oncolink.com/resources/article.cfm?c=6&s=28&ss=73&id=124 http://www.therapistfinder.net/glossary/managed-care.html http://www.aarp.org/healthcoverage/medicare/Articles/a2003-05-06-glossary.html	
HICAP counselor Medicare Assistance, appeals	in California call (800) 303-4477. http://www.inlandagency.org/html/hicap_home.htm and in other states http://hiicap.state.ny.us/home/link08.htm .	
Insurance defined. How each system works, benefits, downsides	http://urac.org/ABCsHealthCoverage.pdf http://tcdc.uth.tmc.edu/candlaw/CAL98.html	
Internal Revenue Service- medical deductions	http://www.irs.gov/individuals/page/0,,id per cent 3D13870,00.html and http://www.irs.gov/faqs/page/0,,id per cent 3D15757,00.html	
Medicaid Fact Sheet. Health Care Financing Administration. Publications, N1-26-27,	Centers for Medicare & Medicaid Services 7500 Security Blvd., Baltimore, MD 21244-1850. Toll-Free: 877-267-2323 TTY Toll-Free: 866-226-1819 For Medicaid eligibility and services contact State office.	http://cms.hhs.gov/ http://www.sccgov.org/scc/assets/docs/41312mc.pdf or http://www.dhs.cahwnet.gov/mcs/medi-calhome/MC210.htm or http://www.dhs.cahwnet.gov/mcs/medi-calhome/CountyListing1.htm your area.
Medi-Cal HIPP- pays insurance premiums	To apply for Medi-Cal HIPP (800) 952-5294	http://www.apla.org/apla/benefits/MEDICAL.HTM

Topic / Description	Source / Address	Web Address
Medicare Handbook. Publications, N1-26-27, How the Medicare program works and your benefits. Free copy	Health Care Financing Administration, 7500 Security Blvd., Baltimore, MD 21244-1850. Local Social Security office	http://www.ahrq.gov/consumer/insuranc.htm
Medications, Access		http://www.helpingpatients.org/
MediGap Information Guide to Health Insurance for People with Medicare. The Consumer's Guide to Medicare Supplement Insurance.	Health Care Financing Administration, Publications, N1-26-27, 7500 Security Blvd., Baltimore, MD 21244-1850. American Association of Retired Persons (AARP). Health Insurance Assoc. of America, 555 13th St., N.W., Suite 600 East, Washington, D.C. 20004.	http://www.aarp.org/healthcoverage/ www.aarp.com
Social Security disability/ SSDI forms	Social Security (800) 772-1213 to find a local office	http://www.ssa.gov
States mandating Clinical Trial coverage		http://info.insure.com/search/sitesearch.cfm?search=clinical%2btrial
The Consumer's Guide to Disability Insurance. Explains insurance, sources of income	Health Insurance Association of America, 555 13th St., N.W., Suite 600 East, Washington, D.C. 20004.	http://www.about-disability-insurance.com

CHAPTER 24

Heredity and Other Causes of Brain Tumors – Nature or Nurture?

My family history is full of cancer. My maternal grandmother and aunt had breast and cervical cancers; another maternal great aunt had colon cancer. My maternal grandfather had prostate cancer. Two paternal great aunts died of breast cancer. My great aunt's granddaughter (same generation as my son) was diagnosed with a PNET as a college freshman. She is 25 now, doing great, and in Physician's Assistant school at the University of Florida. I know this sounds awful, but all the people (except the cousin with a PNET and my dad, whose prostate cancer was found in his mid-50s) were rather elderly when their diagnosis was made. Only two did not recover with surgery or treatment.

Sue M, Santa Fe, NM

Key search words

• gene	• heredity	• mutation
• genetic	• cancer	• neurofibromatosis
• NF-1, NF-2	• acoustic neuroma	• astrocytoma
• medulloblastoma	• tuberous sclerosis	• polyps
• meningioma	• colon cancer	• cell phones
• nutrition	• cancer susceptibility syndrome	• HNPCC

The genes that you inherit are responsible for much of who you are. Surprisingly, a cancer of the brain can trigger the prevention or early diagnosis of cancer for other family members. The purpose of this chapter is to educate you about the causes of brain tumors and how this information can be helpful to you and your family.

FREQUENTLY ASKED QUESTIONS ABOUT HEREDITY AND BRAIN TUMORS

CAN I CATCH A BRAIN TUMOR FROM SOMETHING OR SOMEONE ELSE?

No. You can catch an infection, like a cold or even HIV from someone else. But you cannot *catch* any known form of brain cancer from another person. The major causes of most brain tumors remain unknown. Some have proposed that cellular phones might cause brain tumors. It is more likely that combinations of genes and/or toxic environmental exposures through air, food or water are the culprits (see Table 24-1). Brain tumors are on the rise. The reason does not appear only to be better diagnosis (example: MRI scans.[1])

Table 24-1 Known Risk Factors for Brain Tumors	
Cause	**Frequency**
Unknown	95%
Heredity: Single gene Gene combinations	1-5% Probably common
At risk populations	
Electrical workers	20% increased risk
Pesticide applicators	30% increased risk
Eating cured meats during pregnancy	Increased risk
Cell phones	Unproven as yet
Radiation to the head	15% lifetime risk
Father's occupation in oil/ chemical refining, farming, paper-pulp, painting, printing, pig and horse farming	Increased risk
Mother's exposure to flea and tick poisons	Increased risk

What Is "Genetics"?

Genetics is the study of heredity or the passing of characteristics (such as height, eye color, or tendency to get a tumor) from one generation to the next. Changes in the genes that occur inside a tumor over time are called *mutations*. They can make a tumor more malignant and resistant to therapy when it does grow back, but these changes will not be passed on to your children.

Exactly What Is a Gene?

Genes are the blueprints for our characteristics. Each gene sits on a DNA (deoxyribonucleic acid) "fence." The genetic code is an alphabet of four different compounds called purines or pyrimidines, each of which has code letters (A, C, G and T). Two of these code letters are always paired up, and they are called "base pairs." Different combinations of these base pairs create codes for different amino acids, which in turn make up different proteins like the ones found in blood cells, skin, and muscle.

We all have inherited two copies of every gene, one from our mother through her egg and one from our father through his sperm. Altogether, we have about 30,000 genes. These genes are located inside the center (nucleus) of our cells in structures called *chromosomes*, which also come in pairs. We have 46 chromosomes or 23 pairs.

> Most cancer genes are caused by a change – mutation – in the genetic program. A few are inherited.

Genes have two functions: to replicate themselves as cells divide or to code for proteins. Some genes make proteins that slow growth of the cell, while others serve to hasten growth. Other proteins signal the cell to perform specific functions, including when to die.

Genes write the *programs* that our cells follow. Many genes code for proteins that prevent cancer from forming. When a mutation (change in a gene that causes a new and different protein) occurs, there is a greater chance that a cancer might form. Mutations can happen by chance, or they can result after an exposure to a carcinogen (cancer-causing agent) like tobacco smoke. For example, two goldfish mate and you get more goldfish. Every once in a while one of the baby goldfish has a white spot, longer fins, or larger eyes. Either different combinations of genes or a mutation in a single gene is the cause for this new feature.

In 2003, scientists completed the project of the sequencing the complete DNA library in human beings.[2] We now know all or most of the base pairs making up 30,000 genes. However, we do not know what most of them do! We know what the sentences say but we do not know what they mean. Thus, the next decades will focus on understanding what different genes do and how they communicate with each other. For you, the patient, it means that there is a limit as to how much genetic information is available to help you.

If I Have Cancer, Does This Mean I Have "Bad" Genes?

No. Genes are morally neither good nor bad. All genes serve to make proteins that are responsible for maintaining life, such as building tissue like skin, or regulating functions like the body's ability to fight infection, or secreting a hormone. Some people think that movie stars inherited "good" proteins that gave them their trendy appearance, but these individuals can get cancer just like anyone else.

> Genes are the code or program for how our cells divide, produce proteins, or die.

Most cancers begin in one cell. Mutations occur in genes that regulate cell division or repair cell mutations. These mutations are sometimes repaired, similar to the "spell check" function in your word processing program. But when such uncorrected mutations accumulate in a cell (perhaps six to 12 of them), a cancer can occur. Rarely (probably about 5 per cent of the time), one of the mutations that can lead to cancer development is passed to the next generation through the egg or sperm. We have no control over which genes are passed on to our children.

Are Most Brain Tumors Inherited?

The answer is a qualified no. A recent study from Iceland on more than 2,000 people with cancer showed that for most gliomas patients there was no greater tendency to have another cancer in the family. In other words, the patient did not appear to have inherited a "glioma gene."[3]

The prevailing scientific view is that only one to five percent of all brain tumors have a known single gene cause. Like most other cancers and chronic diseases, the remaining 95 to 99 percent are probably due to an interaction between predisposed genes or mutations and non-genetic factors, such as exposures in the environment, diet, or other behaviors.

What Are the Common Hereditary Conditions Associated with Brain Tumors?

As of 2005, there are about 12 known single gene conditions which are strongly associated with human brain tumors. Each gene has been identified and *genetic tests* are available to detect them. This does not mean that everyone with an inherited susceptibility to one of these mutations will develop a brain tumor. It just means that the *likelihood* of developing a brain tumor is greater. In Table 24-3 you will find a description of common hereditary conditions associated with brain tumors, along with websites, organizations, and descriptive words for further web searches.

> At least 12 inherited genes can cause brain tumors and other cancers in the family.

GENES AND ME

What Good Will It Be to Know about a Genetic Cause? I Already Have a Brain Tumor.

To answer this question, here is an example from my own family. I have a 70-year-old third cousin who has prostate and colon cancer. His sister and two aunts also had colon cancer and a grand parent had breast cancer. Another great grandparent was said to have had a brain tumor. There are seven young adult children in their thirties and forties in the extended family and all have very young children. This could be a coincidence, or a mutation in the gene for TP53 (Li- Fraumeni syndrome) or hereditary non-polyposis colon cancer (HNPCC), a mismatch repair gene. A blood test is available that might diagnose this tendency.

Is There a Way to Prevent Cancer in the Family?

Yes. For example, individuals at higher genetic risk of colon cancer should undergo an annual, painless screening for blood in the stool. Likewise, people with familial polyposis (FAP), or HNPCC, could decrease their odds of dying from colon cancer by having a colonoscopy every two years starting at 20 or 30 years of age, rather than waiting until their 50s. Someone with a family history of cancer in any part of the body should press for an immediate head CT scan, if he or she has a seizure; don't assume that the seizure is "ordinary" or "febrile" in nature. Similarly, brain MRI scanning is recommended to begin in childhood for individuals prone to von Hipple-Lindau syndrome or brain hemangioblastomas.

There is actually a well-known association of gliomas with colon cancer, called Turcot Syndrome (see Table 24-3). Extended family members of someone with Turcot syndrome are predisposed not only to this syndrome but additionally to bowel, breast, leukemia, muscle and bone tumors. There are not one, but two Turcot Syndromes. One is associated with the APC gene, which leads to medulloblastoma; the other is caused by a *mismatch repair gene* that predisposes people to the development of glioblastoma. With the discovery of the APC gene, early diagnosis and preventive surgery for non-symptomatic individuals became possible.[4]

> Knowing if you have a cancer susceptibility gene can prevent cancer in other family members.

Screening and treatment at an earlier age is generally recommended for those with increased genetic risk. In addition, individuals in families with a history of cancer should visit a *clinical geneticist* to see if any blood tests for specific genes that increase cancer risk should be performed. To find a genetic counselor see Table 24-2.

WHAT IS IMPORTANT TO KNOW ABOUT MY FAMILY HISTORY?

Making a family tree is often the first step toward understanding your family's medical history. Your extended family history (blood relatives like parents, siblings, children, aunts, uncles, cousins, grandparents, etc.) of cancer is important to share with your primary physician or oncologist for two reasons. First, when a person has an *inherited* mutation in a cancer susceptibility gene, it is likely that there will be a family history of specific types of cancers. Second, the specific pattern of cancer types in a single individual or family can be a strong indicator of a single gene mutation, or *hereditary cancer* syndrome. Some of these patterns can feature brain tumors. (See Table 24-3 for the 12 common ones.) The following website can help you put together your family tree. http://genetics.faseb.org/genetics/ashg/educ/007a.shtml

The pattern in which cancers occur (childhood, young adulthood, or older age) helps in making the diagnosis. For example, gliomas

> Brain tumors, colon or breast cancer, and birth marks can be clues to cancer susceptibility genes.

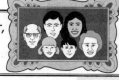

in the same family can be due to a mutated Neurofibromatosis (NF-1) gene, a condition in which grape-like tumors appear along the nerves in the arms, legs and spine. An inherited mutation in another gene called TP53 causes Li-Fraumeni syndrome, which features early onset breast cancer, muscle tumors (sarcomas), leukemia, lymphoma, adrenal cancer, or brain tumors in childhood.

Neurofibromatosis 2 (NF-2) features neuromas of the hearing nerve *and* meningiomas of the spine. It is important to note that cancer, particularly in the brain, lung, or liver, may represent a metastasis or spread from somewhere else. Whether or not the cancer is hereditary depends upon the original tumor type, not its location in the brain.

If you are concerned because of cancers in your family, consult a *medical geneticist* at a major cancer center for help. This person will evaluate the patterns in detail and advise you as to whether it looks like a trend of bad luck or a hereditary syndrome.

FACTS ABOUT GENETIC BLOOD TESTS

Should I get my blood tested for genetic (inherited) *risk* of a brain tumor? Most people want a "yes" or "no" answer to the question of their *risk* for a brain tumor, if there has been one brain tumor in the family. We do not know all the genes for brain tumors. In fact, we only know of a dozen and have the blood tests for these. Even for known genes, interpretation of the tests can require an expert's explanation.

A blood test for a cancer gene is a serious step. Consulting with a genetic counselor can be very helpful.

Before discussing your case with a geneticist or having your blood tested for genetic risk of brain cancer, it is important for you to answer the following questions:

1. Is it an accurate, proven test?
2. Will it identify the people at risk in the family?
3. Is there any action that will follow, if I know the results?
4. Do I really want to know the results, even if the answer is "maybe"?
5. Should we have the test done?

The result of most tests is usually one of the following:

a. Normal
b. Detects the presence of a disease-related mutation
c. Not normal, but "a variant of uncertain clinical significance"

The clear answers are a) and b), but often the answer is c). It is for this reason, that I strongly advise my patients to obtain the services of an expert clinical geneticist, so that correct interpretations and advice can be given. Many Internet sites offer a "genetic blood test" for cancer. But their "hype" may not be helpful to you when you get the result.

I have advised three families who obtained a genetic test on their children via the Internet. Each received a test result called a "variant." They assumed that this meant that they all had a cancer susceptibility gene mutation, since they were not properly counseled about the meaning of their test result or treatment options. They assumed there was no possible treatment and they were left feeling guilty, highly anxious and expectant of an early death.

> Genetic analysis of tumors can sometimes tell to which treatments they will respond

This conclusion was not true, however. After genetic counseling, it was explained that their "variant" was a "normal variant" and that they had no greater chance of having a cancer than the general population. In fact, the family history usually will be the best indicator of risk in these cases.

There are several reasons *not* to get a blood test for inherited risk:

1. Often the results may not answer the question of risk. If a tumor is discovered through the screening process, we do not know yet if early detection will improve survival chances, although it seems logical that it would. Remember also that there is no pill to correct the condition and it may mean living with uncertainty.
2. If there are no living children or relatives, then results of genetic testing are not useful.
3. Lastly, you must assess whether you are an "information seeker" for whom knowledge is comforting, or whether you are an "information avoider" for whom too much information causes anxiety.

CAN GENETIC ANALYSIS PREDICT TUMOR BEHAVIOR?

"Genetic Analysis" or "Genetic Testing"?

There is a practical difference between these for you as the patient. *Genetic analysis* is the technique that researchers use to study the genes and the proteins for which they code. *Genetic testing* is the procedure or test that is used on a patient's blood or tissues to determine the presence of a *known* inherited gene that might predispose a person to brain cancer or place their children at increased risk.

Oligodendroglioma tumors can now be tested using *genetic analysis* for the 1p/ 19q chromosome deletion to see if they are chemotherapy-sensitive or chemotherapy-resistant.[5] This test is done on the tumor and has nothing to do with passing the gene on to family members.

Two recent studies using *genetic analysis* showed that identifying "fingerprints" of brain tumors can improve diagnosis and predict long-term survival. These are the first steps in helping doctors distinguish between tumors that will respond successfully to standard treatments and tumors that require more aggressive or experimental treatments.

Dr. Scott Pomeroy of Children's Hospital in Boston used a "gene chip" to identify genes that were active in tumors from patients with medulloblastomas and other childhood brain tumors. They accurately distinguished between medulloblastomas and other types of tumors based on the combination of active genes in each tumor. Their *genetic analysis* also distinguished between children at higher and lower risk for recurrence of medulloblastoma. Several active genes in lower risk *desmoplastic* medulloblastoma involved a protein called "sonic hedgehog" (SHH) that is also important during brain development. Finally, the researchers predicted which children would be successfully treated for medulloblastoma based on the pattern of gene activity at the time the tumors were diagnosed.[6]

Ian F. Pollack, M.D. of the University of Pittsburgh Medical Center, found mutations in a gene called TP53, whose activity was associated with survival for malignant gliomas. Children with gliomas that had low p53 activity were more likely (than those with high p53 levels) to survive for 5 years without tumor progression. Higher-grade gliomas generally have a poor prognosis. However, estimating p53 levels allowed Dr. Pollack to distinguish between children whose tumors tended to recur early versus others whose tumor did not recur and survival was better. However, it is important to emphasize that in any one case, this marker does *not* confirm a favorable or unfavorable outcome, merely a trend. Accordingly, this marker is *not* used as a genetic test to determine how aggressively an individual person's tumor should be treated.[7]

WHAT IS GENE THERAPY?

Gene therapy is an experimental treatment technique in which a gene (as a segment of DNA on a chromosome) is transferred into a patient's tumor cells. Often, a virus is used as the "transport vehicle" for delivering the gene into the

DNA of a tumor cell. While in the tumor cell, the new gene attempts to reverse the cause of excessive cell division and growth, or selectively destroys the tumor cell. The challenges for gene therapy are formidable:

- Directing the virus to transmit information only into tumor cells;
- Getting the virus to attach and enter enough tumor cells;
- Determining what information from the gene needs to be integrated into the tumor cell or host in order to stop tumor growth; and
- Sparing of normal brain cells.

This experimental treatment was first performed with glioblastoma patients about eight years ago and is currently in clinical trials. This is a "magic bullet" or "smart bomb" approach. For example, the gene for enzyme TK, which is critical for survival, is carried within a virus called "herpes simplex." The tumor cells are metabolically active and take up the gene before the virus is killed; thus, the only cells in the brain that should carry the TK gene are the tumor cells. After the virus has delivered the gene into the tumor cells, an anti-herpes drug called Ganciclovir is injected intravenously. Theoretically, all tumor cells carrying the TK gene should be killed. This therapy has been tolerated surprisingly well and has benefited some individuals.

> Gene Therapy is an experimental treatment for brain tumors.

Not all tumor cells take up the gene, however. In those cases, either the virus does not attach or the gene is not inserted. Furthermore, even if only a proportion of tumor cells take up the gene, many of them are killed after the administration of Ganciclovir due to the release of cytokines that kill adjacent tumor cells. This is called the "innocent bystander" effect.

Another approach, demonstrated in rats by Dr. Alfred Yung at MD Anderson Hospital in Houston, Texas, attempts to re-program the brain tumor cell. Dr. Young and his colleagues inserted into the tumor a controlling agent for growth factors like EGF and VEGF, as well as the anti-oncogene, p53. Dr. Yung found that inserting the normal p53 gene into glioma cells resulted in tumor cell death. The researchers used an adenovirus (a common cold virus) as a carrier of the normal gene into the cells. Theoretically, the normal gene replaces the abnormal one, restoring normal gene function and, thus inducing programmed cell death.

A new Phase I clinical study using this technology will begin in conjunction with the North American Brain Tumor Consortium and the New Approaches to Brain Tumor Therapy Central Nervous System Consortium (NABTT). The National

Cancer Institute and RPR Gencell, Inc., a biotechnology company, will fund the study.

WHAT ARE SOME CAUSES AND RISKS FOR BRAIN TUMORS?

Only five percent of all brain tumors are due to a single, known, inherited susceptibility gene. What about the rest? The most basic truth is that we have *not* identified any one factor that causes a brain tumor in any given individual. Electric blankets, cell phones, and artificial sweeteners are not the sole culprits. When tumors appear in families, *environmental exposure* plus *susceptibility* genes are the likely cause.

Do Cell Phones Cause Brain Tumors?

Over the past few years, it seems like there has been weekly television and newspaper coverage on the role of cell phones in causing brain tumors. In April 2000, a neurologist filed an $800 million lawsuit against the cellular phone maker, Motorola, Inc., as well as eight telecommunication companies. He claimed that his cell phone caused a malignant brain tumor, since he developed his tumor on the side that he held the phone, and he was a frequent user.

A British report, published in April 2000, said that earpieces could triple the amount of electro-magnetic radiation reaching the brain. That study, published in the independent British Consumers Association magazine, Which?[8] It measured electromagnetic intensity, but not how much radiation was actually *absorbed* near the ear. A Finnish study showed that radio waves from cell phones heat the brain but to very low levels. Swedish researchers found that brain tumors were more likely to occur on the side of the head more often in contact with mobile phones. Based on these reports, the British government in late 2000 urged parents to limit children's use of mobile phones. Newspapers and then the Internet spread the word quite rapidly. With that introduction and touch of hysteria, let's state what is known about cell phones and cancer:

Cell phones have not yet been proven to cause brain tumors.

- All levels of mobile phone radiation — with or without hands-free kits — fall comfortably within guidelines set by British and international organizations.

- Hands-free kits (external speaker) for mobile phones further reduce the amount of radiation that users are exposed to, compared with normal use of mobile phones.[9]
- There is no definitive scientific evidence that frequent cell phone use can cause cancer or other medical problems.[10]

Should you use an earpiece because it might prevent a brain tumor? Sure, that is wise, as we know that the follow-up time of these studies demonstrating "no effect" is relatively brief (less than five years of use). We do not know if children are more susceptible to these effects.

An association of cell phones with an eye tumor called *uveal melanoma* (that can spread to the brain) was reported recently. Dr. Andreas Stang examined 118 people with uveal melanoma and obtained details about their use of digital mobile phones. He compared them with a control group of 475 people without disease. To prevent bias, the researchers were not told as to whether the person they were examining suffered from cancer or was healthy. They found that uveal melanoma patients had a much higher rate of mobile phone use.[11] This study needs confirmation.

How might a cellular phone affect the eye? The watery contents of the eye assist the absorption of radiation. Cells called melanocytes found in the uveal layer of the iris (the colored part of the eye) grow and divide more rapidly when exposed to microwave radiation. Since uveal melanoma starts with such cells, mobile phone radiation might help to *initiate* cancer, especially in those with a genetic predisposition.

HOW ARE RISK FACTORS DETERMINED? DO STATISTICS APPLY TO ME?

Confusion exists about the interpretation of statistics and causes of cancer. Terms like *risk factor* also cause confusion. For example, a study of electrical workers concluded that their *risk* for a brain tumor was increased by 0.2 (20 per cent).[12] This does *not* mean that 20 per cent of electrical workers will get a brain tumor. It does mean that if the baseline risk says that 10 out of 100,000 people will get a brain tumor, then the chance for electrical workers is increased by 20 percent.

The calculation goes: 20 per cent x 10 [the baseline risk] = 2 + 10 = 12 = 12 out of 100,000. Yes, the risk is greater, but it is still a rare event.

Studies do suggest associations or risk factors for brain tumor development (see Table 24-2).[13] There has been much discussion of industrial and other work exposures in causing brain tumors. A summary of more than 33 studies of pesticide applicators found a possible 30 per cent increased risk, but whether it was directly due to the chemical or suppressed immunity to infection is unknown.[14]

X-ray radiation therapy to the head is *definitely* associated with risk for developing both meningiomas and glial tumors, but not everyone who has radiation to the head will get a brain tumor. Children with leukemia who were treated with head radiation were shown to have a 15 percent lifetime risk of developing a brain tumor.[15] This does mean that of 100 cured children, 15 will probably get a brain tumor in their lifetime.

Diet has also been linked to the cause and prevention of cancer. Exposure to cured meats (nitrites and nitroso- compounds) during pregnancy may be associated with an increase risk of a brain tumor in the unborn child.[16] Some foods also contain antidotes to these carcinogenic compounds, such as natural antioxidants that can be found in fruits and vegetables.

A father's occupation in oil or chemical refining, farming, paper-pulp, painting, printing, or pig and horse farming was shown by one study to increase his offspring's risk of developing a brain tumor.[17] Another study found no such association.[18] A mother's exposure to flea and tick poisons[19] also has been suggested as a risk factor for brain tumor development in her children;[20] however, her intake of alcohol or cigarettes was *not* found to be associated with brain tumors (see Table 24-1).[21]

The relative role of carcinogens and antidotes is unclear. Caution in the use of "natural" antioxidants like beta-carotene, and vitamins A and E is warranted.[22] For example, in a recent clinical trial on prevention of lung cancer in smokers, the group taking beta-carotene had a *higher* rate of lung cancer. The study had to be stopped![23,24]

A risk factor does NOT mean you will get a cancer, just that your chances are greater to have one. Even if you have a risk factor, however, your chance of dying from a brain tumor may be less than dying from in a car accident if you are drinking alcohol, or as a result of smoking cigarettes. Risk factors should not be assumed or overestimated without information.

Bottom Line ➡ A risk factor does NOT mean you will get a cancer, just that your chances are greater to have one.

How Can I Find Reliable Genetic Information on the Internet?

There are several websites where you can obtain general information about specific genetic conditions, locations of genetic counseling centers around the world, and up to date availability of testing.

I advise *against* obtaining a blood or urine test via a commercial site without arranging for subsequent genetic counseling. Many of the tests are not sensitive or specific, and the results can be confusing. A professional interpretation by someone who knows your specific case will be most helpful to you.

The American Board of Medical Genetics, American College of Medical Genetics, and National Society of Genetic Counselors all have websites. More information about genetic testing and help in finding a genetic counselor can be found in Table 24-2. You can also get some leads by asking your specialist or calling your local university medical center, too.

Table 24-2 Internet Resources for Brain Tumor Causes & Heredity

Content	Website
Cell Phones	http://www.protectingourhealth.org/newscience/learning/2003/2003-0129salfordetal.htm http://www.medscape.com/viewarticle/408066
Family History Tree	http://genetics.faseb.org/genetics/ashg/educ/007a.shtml
General Information, Testing, Human Genome	http://www.genetests.org/servlet/access?id=8888891&key=EX5CzITTuA6mZ&fcn=y&fw=adAl&filename=/concepts/conceptsindex.html http://www.roswellpark.org/document_1180_267.html (terminology) http://www.ornl.gov/techresources/human_genome/medicine/assist.html (general) http://www.ncbi.nlm.nih.gov/genome/guide/human (Genome Project) http://www.ornl.gov/sci/techresources/Human_Genome/publicat/genechoice/index.html (choices) http://www.genetests.org (gene tests)
Genetic Counseling	http://www.nsgc.org http://www.ornl.gov/sci/techresources/Human_Genome/publicat/genechoice/index.html (choices) http://www.nsgc.org/consumer/index.asp (general)
Genetic Testings, Locations, Counseling Clinics	http://www.genetests.org/servlet/access?id=8888891&key=UNAI33FaCvWbz&fcn=y&fw=ZvOZ&filename=/ http://www.bccancer.bc.ca/PPI/Prevention/Hereditary/default.htm (prevention)
NF-1 General	http://www.understandingnf1.org http://gslc.genetics.utah.edu/units/disorders/nf1/diagnosis
Tuberous Sclerosis: Resources and diagnosis	http://www.tsalliance.org http://www.ninds.nih.gov/health_and_medical/disorders/tuberous_sclerosis.htm http://www.title14.com/ts/tssites.html (many sites) http://www.emedicine.com/derm/topic438.htm

Table 24-3 Common Hereditary Conditions Associated with Brain Tumors

Tumor type	Findings/ Tumors	Birth marks	Child/ adult	Genetic Condition	Gene affected	Websites, Contact Information
Brain stem gliomas, low grade. Optic pathway gliomas Glioblastoma multiforme (GBM)	Skin fibromas "Bright objects" on MRI	Brown patches; Freckles in armpit	Both	Neurofibroma-tosis Type 1 [NF-1]	NF-1, Neurofibromin	http://www.understandingnf1.org http://www.cdc.gov/genomics/hugenet/reviews/NF1gene.htm
GBM Astrocytomas PNET	Breast, colon, lung, sarcomas, leukemia melanoma, prostate, adrenal		Both	Li Fraumeni	TP53, tumor suppressor	http://www.rush.edu/rumc/page-P07253.html
GBM Astrocytomas	Polyps, colon cancer		Both	FAP (familial adenomatous polyposis	APC gene codon 1309 develops cancer 10 years earlier	http://www.rush.edu/rumc/page-P07209.html
Glioma Medulloblastoma Ganglioglioma Ependymoma	Colon cancer, Family history of polyps	Skin patches	Both	Turcot's Brain tumor-Intestinal Polyposis Syndrome (type 1)	mismatch repair gene develops glioblastoma; HNPCC gene	http://cmgs.org/BPG/Guidelines/2002/HNPCC.htm

Table24-3 Common Hereditary Conditions Associated with Brain Tumors (continued)					
GBM Astrocytomas	Colon , rectal cancer		Hereditary non –polyposis colorectal cancer [HNPCC]	HNPCC	http://www.genetic health.com/CRC_HNPCC_ Other_Cancers_in_ HNPCC.shtml http://mybestcare.com
Giant cell astrocytomas (low grade)	Skin patches, facial skin tumors, rectal polyps, heart kidney-myomas	Yes	Tuberous sclerosis	TSC1/ TSC2 (tuberin)	http://www.tsalliance. org/WhatIsTSC/genetics.asp
Acoustic Neuroma (2 sides) Meningioma	Cataracts, multiple meningiomas, gliomas, skin schwannomas	Brown patches	Neurofibro-matosis type 2 [NF-2]	NF-2, Merlin	http://www.webcrossings.c om/nf2crew/links.html http://neurosurgery.mgh. harvard.edu/NFR/nf2.htm
Medulloblastoma	Colon cancer, > 100 polyps; high risk for familial medulloblastoma		Turcot's (Brain Tumor-Intestinal Polyposis Syndrome, type 2)	APC gene	
Medulloblastoma	Melanoma, meningiomas	Dark large birthmark	Gorlin's Syndrome- Basal nevus	Sonic Hedgehog [SHH, PTCH genes]	http://www.whonamedit. com/synd.cfm/2212.html http://health.allrefer.com/ health/basal-cell-nevus-syndrome-info.html http://www.emedicine. com/ped/topic1592.htm

Note: The "Adults / Both / Child" classification column appears between the fourth and fifth text columns:
- Giant cell astrocytomas — Adults
- Tuberous sclerosis — Both
- Turcot's — Both
- Gorlin's Syndrome — Child

			Child			
Pineal gland PNET	Retinoblastoma, Osteosarcoma			Trilateral Retinoblastoma	RB-1 (Tumor suppressor)	http://www.ncbi.nlm.nih.gov/entrez/query.fcgi?cmd=Retrieve&db=PubMed&list_uids=10391573&dopt=Abstract http://jncicancerspectrum.oupjournals.org/cgi/medline/pmid;11545631
Gangliocytoma Hamartoma of cerebellum			Both	Lhermitte-Dulcos; Cowden's syndrome	PTEN 1	http://cpmcnet.columbia.edu/news/journal/journalo/archives/jour_v17n1_0011.html http://www.ispn.org/Meetings/Aalborg/Poster05.htm
Angioma of meninges	Port-wine stain upper face	Port-wine stain upper face		Sturge-Weber	Unknown	http://www.sturge-weber.com http://www.ninds.nih.gov/health_and_medical/disorders/sturge_doc.htm http://www.rarediseases.org/search/rdbdetail_abstract.html?disname=Sturge%20Weber%20Syndrome
Hemangioblastoma of spine, cerebellum	Renal cell, pheochromocytoma		adult	Von Hippel-Lindau	vhl, Hamartin (a tumor suppressor)	http://www.vhl.org http://www.ninds.nih.gov/health_and_medical/disorders/vonhippe_doc.htm http://www.geneclinics.org/profiles/vhl http://www.ncbi.nlm.nih.gov/disease/VHL.html

CHAPTER 25

Your Legacy

All trials force the question, "Who are you, really?"
It's up to each of us to get very still and say,
"This is who I am."
No one else defines your life. Only you do.

Oprah Winfrey, O Magazine, October, 2000

Key search words

- legacy
- narrative
- end of life
- dying
- pain
- Picasso

- family
- communication
- advance directive
- hospice
- prognosis
- Matisse

- storytelling
- living will
- palliative care
- insurance
- immortality

"Your Legacy" must seem like an unusual name for a chapter in a book about brain tumors. I had not planned on writing this chapter, but I have some thoughts that did not seem to fit in other portions of the book. These ideas are about relationships; quality and meaning of our lives; what we want to tell those who have been important to us; and sometimes preparation for dying. A close friend and oncology nurse, Leslie, reminds me that it is important to take charge of your life – all the way – until the moment of passing and not to let "the system" or others dictate plans against your wishes. The Terri Shiavo case in March 2005 forced this question on to the American consciousness.

HOW DO YOU WANT TO LIVE YOUR LIFE?

In January 2005, I had just returned from giving the closing keynote address at the Florida Brain Tumor Association, a meeting of more than 300 survivors. One might surmise that this would be a depressing experience – a group of people, stuck together for three days, waiting to die from their brain tumors? It was quite the opposite. This was a celebration of life…and loving. Everywhere I went, people talked about how much they *gained* from having cancer. The tumor was a wakeup call – that whatever time remains of life needs to be lived fully. While David Bailey (a *glioblastoma multiforme* long-term survivor), played the guitar, Samantha and others were spontaneously dancing to his award-winning rhythms.

We make decisions about work, spouse, and schools, yet most of us put off dealing with how we want to die. We concentrate on living, as if the unspoken will take care of itself. With a brain tumor or any serious illness, active decisions need to be made about how we might live *and* die.

HAS YOUR BRAIN TUMOR CHANGED YOUR LIFE?

Probably. Was any of it for the better? Your *response* to your brain tumor is part of the story that you leave behind for others.

- Some people's lives will be consumed by the tumor.
- Some will be propelled by the tumor to help others in an unforeseen way; for example, they may participate in a clinical trial to help themselves and others; or they may choose to answer questions on Internet chat groups..
- Some will experience life as usual. Beth completes her e-mails with the following signature:

I am a 60-year-old female in good health...except for the occasional brain tumor.

Thank you - Beth.

Let's take a different worst-case scenario. In 1995, Jean Bauby, Editor of *Elle*! Magazine in Paris, was at the top of the fashion world – large house, sports cars, fame – until he had a brain stem stroke and was "locked in" – alive but only able to move his left eyelid. He wrote a short book about his experience with the help of a companion and a lettered communication board.[1] It literally was written one letter at a time. In the book, he tells of his life in a narrative, and relationships discovered *after* losing his ability to communicate. This story was his gift to family and the rest of the world. At times he is very blunt:

My present life is divided between those who knew me before...and all the others. What kind of person will those who know me now, think I was? I do not even have a photo to show them.[1]

The following passage illustrates Ruth's narrative about her husband:

Sometimes, I feel I would give anything to be back in our days of normal living, in the spaces of time between the first three surgeries that John had during our marriage. Other days, I feel alive right now in a way that I never did when things were normal, like somehow I am more awake than I ever was before.

Ruth, husband to John, Victoria BC, Canada

Noelle's inspiration is her mother, Georgina, who became a quadriplegic after treatment for a meningioma:

Today is my mom's 25th anniversary of diagnosis and also my brother's birthday. After three surgeries, radiation, spinal plating, a shunt, etc., she is still around and making it through each day. She was diagnosed in 1977 with a brainstem/skull base meningioma. She is a "quad," unable to move except for her right arm and her head a little bit. Still she has her tracheotomy and a respirator and feeding tube. She knows exactly what's going on.

She is my strength, and I'm so grateful to have her for my mom. She has always taught us what was important in life – friends and family. She may not be able to walk, but she can't fall...The biggest challenge is communication because she has to mouth everything; and I have not mastered reading lips, yet. But we work really hard to be sure we understand her correctly.

I'm so proud of her. She has worked so hard to do so many things that she was told were impossible. She is my best friend and my greatest cheerleader. She gives so much more than I could ever give her. Because of her, I'm grateful to have all of you to learn from and to share the ups and downs of brain tumors.

Noelle, daughter of Georgina,
"who I'm so proud to be just like!"
diagnosed with meningioma in 1977...
still smiling and smelling roses

WHAT ARE THE STORIES ABOUT YOUR LIFE THAT YOU WISH TO LEAVE BEHIND?

Groucho Marks, the comedian, used to say, "None of us is getting out of this thing alive!" So, if we are going to die someday, what legacy do we choose to leave behind? Consider these questions:

- What do we want to say to our spouse, loved ones, children, friends, or colleagues, that we have postponed saying?
- What lessons have we learned?
- How can we structure our lives so that we can do the things we would like to do and say the things that we would like to say?

Each of us has an important story, our own *narrative* that is our life.[2] This narrative represents the threads in the fabric of our being: family circumstances, siblings, incidents, adventures, people you met, things that happened to

> Narrative – our own important story, that is our life; it represents the threads of our fabric.

you, decisions that you made, and how all of these things influenced who you are. If you do not tell the story, then it dies with you and there is no immortality. Children of all ages need to know these stories to understand themselves and their parents. This theme was poignantly developed in the movie "Big Fish" (2004), where the adult son (Billy Crudup) goes on a mission to understand his father (Albert Finney) and distinguish the myth that he grew up with from reality.

We must talk to each other as much as we can. When one of us dies, there will be some things the other will never be able to talk of with anyone else.[3]

This quotation could have been a conversation between two long time lovers separated by illness. In fact, it was spoken between two of the greatest artistic rivals of the 20th Century – Pablo Picasso to Henri Matisse during their declining years. It reaffirms the fundamental importance of meaningful communication, beyond illness and brain tumors.

If you are a family member of someone with a brain tumor, you have an opportunity to help your loved one complete his or her story with greater meaning and dignity and to add to the depth of your own story as well. The following exchange on "letting go," shows how important our narrative continues to be until the very end.

I was wondering if anybody had any advice on how to reassure my dad that it is ok to let go. He has been in the nursing home for two weeks after becoming paralyzed on his right side and losing all his communication. Hospice says he is only a few days away from passing away, but he keeps hanging on for some reason. He will become agitated and suddenly grab on to the bed rail or whatever is in his reach. They say he is doing this because for some reason he is not ready to go.

Robert L, Chicago, IL

Hi Robert: My husband Mitchell experienced the same things as your dad during this stage. It is harder for younger people to find comfort with the end of life, as they have unfinished business and find it more difficult to part with their loved ones. This 'stage' was as hard on me as it was on Mitchell, as I struggled with needing to let him go, but not really wanting to. I eventually stopped encouraging him to 'let go' and just began to instill comfort to him and allow him the time to find his own way. We would touch, hold him, hold his hand, use comforting words like 'I love you,' 'we are all here,' 'you're o.k.' I can only imagine how hard it would be for me to let go of my life.

My advice to you is to give your dad a final gift...allow him to take his time, find his way and, once again, regain some control of his life. Take care and enjoy the moments you have left with your dad.

Mary

Telling your story can allow a type of inner healing to occur. This healing can manifest as a positive feeling about your life that counteracts fear, anxiety, shame, guilt, anger, and depression. The positive feelings that come from telling your story will, in turn, free you to tell more important stories. This can have a powerful impact on those who are closest to you.[4] If you do not tell the stories now...then when will you?

IS THERE A GOOD SIDE TO HAVING A BRAIN TUMOR?

Sounds like a ridiculous question, doesn't it? Steve DePesa was diagnosed with a *glioblastoma multiforme* as a young adult.[5] He coined the phrase "the good side to having a brain tumor" and wrote a survival guide for people with brain tumors.[6] In it, he wrote a few lines about how having a brain tumor changed his awareness, for the better. I have spoken to thousands of brain tumor survivors. Most tell me that Steve's words echo true for them, too. Steve cites the following things as being the good side of having a brain tumor:

1. You wake up to life.
2. You appreciate everything about life, but especially family and friends.
3. You become very humble very fast, which is timely since the feeling that there is a God watching over us suddenly becomes very, very real.
4. You are without a doubt going to face the toughest battle anyone on earth has ever faced.
5. Keep your chin up and come out swinging; people will acknowledge your spirit, your courage, strength and stamina.
6. The purpose of this life may in fact be a) to experience life and b) to learn our hard lessons about the battles between good and evil.

COMPLETING YOUR LIFE – THE TO-DO LIST

Doctors and patients see *end of life* and even what constitutes a *good death* quite differently.[7] There is danger in letting only your physicians, who typically offer a concrete, disease-oriented perspective, guide you about these meanings. Yet, patients and families see psychosocial and spiritual issues as equally important as physiologic or disease concerns. Table 25-1 outlines key areas that have been identified as important by patients and families in end-of-life care. The rest of this chapter focuses on how to best complete these tasks.

Bottom Line ▶ Doctors and patients see end of life and even what constitutes a good death quite differently.

Table 25-1 Completing Your Life – The To-Do List

Task	Responsible Party
1. Clear decision making - a living will	1. Patient and family
2. Pain and symptom management	2. Patient, health professionals, family, hospice
3. Affirmation of myself as a whole person	3. Patient and family and hospice
4. Telling my Story	4. Patient
5. Contributing to others	5. Patient

A decision to make a *living will* or have hospice care is not a decision for a quick dying. Rather, it means that you are paying attention to important items about your life that may have been overlooked. It also calls for some clear decision-making. Not having pain and being in a comfortable place can allow these steps to take place.

WHAT IS A "LIVING WILL"?

A *living will* is a legal document that makes sure that your wishes about living and dying are carried out. (See Table 25-2 for resources on living wills.) Do you want to be placed on a life support system? Do you want to spend your final days at home or in intensive care (ICU) connected to tubes and monitors?

> *Living will* – a legal document that ensures your wishes about living and dying are carried out.

A living will tells your doctor and family about your desires for medical care, if you are unable to relay them yourself. *Advance Directives* are the actual orders in the hospital or care facility records that put into action what your living will document says. Specifically, the directives that you decide on will dictate the degree to which doctors should go to keep you alive in the event that you become incapacitated. There are prepared forms which you can download from the Internet (Chapter 4) that will guide you on how to do this.[8,9] (See also Table 25-2.) Your choice of an "advocate," a person who speaks for you, is important in making sure your wishes are carried out.

> Advance Directives – the actual orders in the hospital or care facility records that put into action what your living will document says.

Question: My 80-year-old mother was operated on for a glioblastoma *multiforme*. However, nine days have passed since the surgery and she has not regained consciousness and is on ventilator support. What do we do now?

Answer: This is a very difficult problem that has no right or wrong answers. You and the surgeons obviously wanted to help her and give her some good quality life by removing the tumor. Unfortunately, 80-year-olds have less reserve than younger people do to undergo the stress of surgery and manipulation of the brain. At this point, you must ask the surgeons and medical physicians if there is any meaningful chance for recovery. If not, is support merely prolonging her death or her life? In this situation, many people would consider taking her off life support.

If this woman had instructed her son how to direct her care in the event she became unable to do so, then there would be no question about what should be done. This is the purpose of a living will.

A growing number of cancer patients receive aggressive treatments, even when they are near death.[10] Consequently, more patients than ever are admitted to emergency rooms and intensive care units during the last few weeks of life. One could specify in a living will, for example, that end-of-life care take place in a *hospice* setting or at home. Hospice services and related medical resources could reduce the chance that a patient receives overly aggressive treatment at the end of life. This could improve the quality of care for many terminally ill patients. You have choices about what will happen to you and your family.

WHAT IS HOSPICE?

In medieval times, a hospice was a place where the sick or wounded could find rest and comfort. In the

Hospice today is a model of care, not just a specific place.

1960s, Dr. Cicely Saunders of St. Christopher's Hospice in London pioneered the concept of hospice as a pain-free and comfortable final journey. Hospice today is a *model of care*, not just a specific place.

To accomplish its goals, the contemporary hospice emphasizes strict attention to *comfort* rather than cure. Hospices offer *palliative care* in four major areas of life: physical, spiritual, psychological, and social. The preponderance of care provided by palliative service at the end of life is aimed at symptom management (breathing difficulties, pain, stomach and intestinal complaints, delirium). Both the patient and family are included in the care plan. Support is based on the patient's wishes and family's needs. Research shows that only 8 per cent of patients who died in *hospice* experienced pain, compared with 20 per cent of those in hospital and 29 per cent of those at home without hospice support.[11] The choice to reside in hospice usually means making the decision to spend one's final weeks, months, or years at home or in a homelike setting.[12]

We all fear the possibility of suffering and pain, especially near the end of our lives. Hospice affirms life and regards dying as a normal process. It is not part of any religious movement, and its methods neither hasten nor postpone death. It provides a personalized and caring community that enables patients and families to make necessary end-of-life preparations. Hospice also aids in the bereavement process.

> Hospice emphasizes strict attention to comfort rather than cure in four major areas: physical, spiritual, psychological, and social.

What Is Palliative Care?

Palliative care extends the principles of hospice care to a larger population that can benefit from receiving this type of care; typically, it could begin earlier in the illness. No specific therapy is excluded from consideration. Trained volunteers can offer respite care for family members as well as meaningful support to the patient. Useful website resources can be found in Table 25-2.

> Palliative care: extends a principle of hospice care and typically begins earlier in the illness. No specific therapy is excluded.

Which Specialists Are on the Hospice Team?

The hospice team includes physicians, nurses, social workers, counselors; hospice certified nursing assistants, clergy, therapists, and volunteers. In addition, hospice provides medications, supplies, equipment, hospital services, and home aides, when needed.

> *Of all the agonizing decisions we had to make regarding Jacqueline's care, we had no second thoughts about this one. The end of her life was better because she had – our whole family had – hospice care. It's not just medical; it's social work support as well, supporting the family psychologically as they go through this horrific experience. Having that support from someone familiar with what we were going through, helped me to replenish my emotional energy enough to*

deal...to be more "present" and less dizzy with mental pain in my moments with Jacqueline, than I might otherwise have been.

Sam, husband of Jacqueline, Quebec CANADA

How Is Hospice Paid for?

Hospice coverage is widely available and provided by Medicare nationwide, by Medicaid in 39 states, and by most private insurance providers. Medicare covers all services and supplies for hospice care related to terminal illness. In some hospices, the patient may be required to pay a 5 per cent or $5 *co-payment* for medication and a 5 per cent co-payment for respite care (see Chapters 23A and 23B). Hospice will assist families in finding out whether the patient is eligible for coverage. Barring this, most hospices provide for anyone who cannot pay using money raised from the community, memorial, or foundation gifts.

CHAPTER 25
Your Legacy

> Hospice team: physicians, nurses, social workers, counselors, hospice certified nursing assistants, clergy, therapists, and volunteers.

WHAT KIND OF AFFIRMATION WILL YOU NEED AT THE END OF LIFE?

When we are ill, the totality of our needs must be affirmed. These might be summarized in seven example areas:

1. Enough medication to be pain-free, even if the amount necessary is above "average." (Inattention to prolonged or unrelieved pain could prevent you from achieving your goals in the last years of life.[13,14])
2. Home cooking instead of hospital food.
3. Comfort foods like sorbet or popcorn, or old movies at 2:00 a.m.
4. Moments of candor, laughter, and reminiscing with close friends and family.
5. Time to fiddle and adjust the electric hospital bed without getting a whiplash.
6. Straightforward answers to questions like "Will I walk again?" "Why am I retaining all this fluid?" "Do I still need my usual medications?"

It is your right to have these needs met.

We also want our uniqueness and contributions affirmed; we want to feel valued.

We want to know that our lives have made a difference to others. Sheryl's story about getting her needs met was just as dynamic before her tumor diagnosis, as after it; only it took a different pathway. Here, she tells it like it is in March 2004 (and she won't let me shorten it):

When I started the Florida Brain Tumor Association (FBTA), I had absolutely no vision of what we would have today – a national, strong activist organization that helps many and perhaps changes survival outcomes of people's lives. As for myself, I had no idea I would grow from my brain tumor experience; after all, I was 'entitled' to be miserable. But secretly, I also envisioned getting completely well. Hard work for me always solved any problems.

I was very successful (in my pre-brain tumor life) in Chicago; life was good. I was an aggressive, 23-year-old, a driven advertising and marketing/executive diva – a different kind of diva. I had no perception when I was diagnosed in 1989 that I would learn so much about life…and death. That I would lose so many dear friends to the disease that has been tearing me down little by little. I never anticipated that I would be asked to speak all over the country at conferences and even be selected to speak in Washington D.C. this year at a congressional breakfast. I am honored to have been chosen as the patient activist to represent brain tumor patients in this country. Believe me they will see/hear my passion, no matter how I'm feeling physically.

I need to do more. I've been blessed with so much extra time – been "pulled out of line." My prognosis was two to three years back in '89. I'm determined to be productive with my time, in addition to having two incredible sons (that's another chapter – being a mother/parent during crisis). It never ends.

When we feel well, none of us wants our life's journey to end. Yet, the end is a reality. Making the most of our lives, expressing important things to those we care about, and exercising some control over how our lives will end surely make this transition easier. This is one of the lessons that I have learned from my patients. Never as a practicing physician did I expect to hear any patient say that on balance he/she gained more from having a brain tumor than was lost because of it. But this has been true for so many.

N.B. Sheryl organized and successfully put on the Florida Brain Tumor Conference, January 21-23, 2005

Table 25-2 Internet Resources for Legacy Issues

Resource	WEB Address
Decision making	http://www.elca.org/dcs/endoflife.html http://www.jcaho.org/general+public/ making+better+choices/helping+you+choose/hc.htm
"End of Life Resources"	http://www.growthhouse.org http://www.athealth.com/Consumer/newsletter/FPN_4_25.html http://www.lastacts.org http://www.npr.org/programs/death (NPR Radio Program)
Hospice Information	http://www.hospicenet.org http://www.americanhospice.org http://www.hospicefoundation.org
National Hospice and Palliative Care Organization	http://www.nhpco.org
Hospice & Palliative Care Associates (NY)	http://www.hospicecny.org
National Association for Home Care & Hospice,	www.nahc.org
Hospice Association of America	www.hospice-america.org
Living Will	http://www.tchospital.org/AddDir/Living%20Will.htm http://www.ces.ncsu.edu/depts/fcs/frm/docs/fcs364.html ex: N. Carolina http://www.agingwithdignity.org/news.html http://www.uslegalforms.com/living-will-forms.htm (All States)
Palliative Care	http://www.promotingexcellence.org http://cancer.gov/BenchMarks/archives/2003_06/feature_article.html

CHAPTER 26

Summary for Brain Tumors –
Leaving the Garden of Eden

The original and companion book, *Brain Tumors: Leaving the Garden of Eden: A Survival Guide to Learning the Basics, Getting Organized & Finding Your Medical Team* will empower you!

This book offers you guidance on how to find experts, assess your current team & the roles of and questions to ask each expert. There are 30 black-and-white illustrations and 350 websites/other contacts.

This chapter contains the summary and outline of every chapter in *Leaving the Garden*. In this way you can see if you wish to have this important source of information at your fingertips. You can also see excerpts of each chapter, live, and download any chapter on the web at www.survivingbraincancer.com

Leaving the Garden has what you need to be a successful and surviving patient. It begins with the basics – from brain anatomy to *high tech* tests (Chap 2); shows you how to get organized (Chap 3); get up to date info about your brain tumor that your doctor might be unaware (Chap 4); provides specific questions to ask each of 20 specialists who could be caring for you (Chapter 5); how to find experts & get the best care at "high tech" brain tumor centers of excellence (Chap 6, 7). There is a chapter on each common tumor: gliomas, metastases, germinomas, meningiomas pituitary, PNET... and more. Also there is a medication chapter: taking steroids, monitoring your pain relief & precautions about seizure medications

BRAIN TUMORS – LEAVING THE GARDEN OF EDEN: A SURVIVAL GUIDE TO LEARNING THE BASICS, GETTING ORGANIZED & FINDING YOUR MEDICAL TEAM

- Rehabilitation specialist (Physiatrist, Occupational Therapist, Physical Therapist, Speech Therapist)
- Finances and Rehabilitation
- Neuropsychologist, Psychologist, Psychiatrist

- Endocrinologist
- Ophthalmologist
- Dentist
- Nurse
- Tumor Board

CHAPTER 6
EXPERTS AND SECOND OPINIONS

CHAPTER 26
Brain Tumors:
Leaving the
Garden of Eden

CHAPTER 11
TUMORS ORIGINATING IN THE BRAIN – MEDULLOBLASTOMAS, PNETS AND EPENDYMOMAS

APPENDIX

Child & Adult World-Wide Brain Tumor Centers

Apendix 1: MAJOR (COG#) CHILDRENS BRAIN TUMOR CENTERS

Legend — • Available expertise, ¤ Not available

Columns: 1 = NEW BT PATIENTS per YR, 2 = MULTIDISCIPLINARY, 3 = NEUROSURGERY, 4 = RADIATION, 5 = NEURO-ONCOLOGY, 6 = REHABILITATION, 7 = NEUROPSYCHOLOGY, 8 = ENDOCRINE, 9 = TUMOR BOARD, 10 = CLINICAL TRIALS

STATE	Institution Name/ address & Best "Who to" info	Telephone / Email / Website	1	2	3	4	5	6	7	8	9	10
AK	**Pediatric Hemato/Oncology Arkansas Children's Hospital** 800 Marshall Street Little Rock, Arkansas 72202 *Robert L. Saylors, MD*	**Tel:** 501-364-1494 **Email:** saylorsrobertl@uams.edu **Web:** www.archildrens.org	30	•	•	•	•	•	¤	•	•	•
AL	**Univ. Alabama, Children's Hospital of Alabama Neuro-Oncology Division** 1600 7th Avenue, South, ACC 512 Birmingham, AL 35233 *Alyssa T. Reddy, MD*	**Tel:** 205-939-9285 **Web:** www.chsys.org	60	•	•	•	•	•	•	•	•	•
AZ	**Phoenix Children's Hospital** 1919 E. Thomas Road Phoenix, AZ 85016 *Michael M. Etzl, Jr. MD*	**Tel:** 602-546-0920 **Email:** metzl@phoenixchildrens.com jboklan@phoenixchildrens.com **Web:** www.phoenixchildrens.com	40	•	•	•	•	•	•			•
CA	**Children's Hospital of Orange County** 455 S Main Street Orange, CA 92868 *Violet Shen M.D.*	**Tel:** 714-516-4348 **Email:** vshen@choc.org or jmiller@choc.org **Web:** www.choc.org/institutes/ neuroscience2.cfm	75	•	•	•	•	•	•			•
CA	**Jonathan Jaques Children's Cancer Center at Miller Children's Hospital,** 2801 Atlantic Avenue, Long Beach CA 90806 *Mark Robert, MD*	**Tel:** 562-933-8600 **Email:** wmroberts@memorialcare.org **Web:** www.jjccc.com	12-15	•	•	•	•	¤				•

State	Institution	Contact	#												
CA	**The Neural Tumors Program Childrens Hospital Los Angeles,** 4650 Sunset Boulevard, Mail Stop #54 Los Angeles, CA 90024 *Jonathan L. Finlay, MD*	**Tel:** 323-906-8147 **Email:** jfinlay@chla.usc.edu **Web:** www.childrensheadstart.com	120	•	•	•	•	•	•	•	•	•	•	•	•	•
CA	**Children's Hospital & Research Center Oakland** 747 52nd Street Oakland, CA 94609	**Tel:** 510-428-3272 **Email:** jtorkildson@mail.cho.org **Web:** www.childrenshospital oakland.org	25	•	•	•	•	•	•	•	•	•	•	•	•	•
CA	**City of Hope** 1500 E Duarte Rd, MOB 4 Duarte CA 91016 *Karla Wilson, RN*	**Tel:** 626-471-7170 626-359-8111 x63989 (direct) **Email:** kwilson@coh.org	10	•	•	•	•	•	•	•	•	•	•	•	•	•
CA	**Loma Linda University** Coleman Pavilion A-1120 11175 Campus Street Loma Linda, CA 92354	**Tel:** 909-558-8626 **Email:** abedros@ahs.llumc.edu	42	•	•	•	¤	•	¤	¤	•	•	•	•	•	•
CA	**Sutter Neuroscience Medical Group** 2800 L Street, suite 500 Sacramento, Ca 95816 *Dr. Nora W. Wu*	**Tel:** 916-454-6850 **Email:** Wunw@sutterhealth.org **Web:** http://checksutterfirst. org/neuro	30	•	•	•	•	•	•	•	•	•	•	•	•	•
CA	**UCSF Pediatric Brain Tumor Center** 505 Parnassus Ave, M779 San Francisco CA 94143 *Mitchel Berger ,MD*	**Tel:** 415-353-3933 **Email:** Bergerm@neurosurg.ucsf.edu **Web:** http://neurosurgery. medschool.ucsf.edu/index.html	30	•	•	•	•	•	•	•	•	•	•	•	•	•
CT	**Yale University School of Medicine, Dept. Pediatrics** 333Cedar St New Haven CT 08520-8064 *Jack van Hoff, MD*	**Tel:** 203-785-4640 **Email:** jack.vanhoff@yale.edu	14	•	•	•	•	¤	•	•	•	•	•	•	•	•
DC, WASH	**Dept. of Neurology Children's National Med Ctr** 111 Michigan Ave., NW Washington, DC 20010 Deborah LaFond *Roger J. Packer, MD*	**Tel:** 202-884-2120 202-884-3659 **Email:** rpacker@cnmc.org dlafond@cnmc.org **Web:** www.dcchildrens.com	120-150	•	•	•	•	•	•	•	•	•	•	•	•	•

STATE	Institution Name/ address & Best "Who to" info	Information (Telephone / Email / Website)	1 NEW BT PATIENTS per YR	2 MULTIDISCIPLINARY	3 NEUROSURGERY	4 RADIATION	5 NEURO-ONCOLOGY	6 REHABILITATION	7 NEUROPSYCHOLOGY	8 ENDOCRINE	9 TUMOR BOARD	10 CLINICAL TRIALS
DE	A. I. duPont Hospital for Children 1600 Rockland Road Wilmington, DE 19899 Andrew W. Walter, MS MD	Tel: 302-651-5500 Email: awwalter@Nemours.org Web: www.kidshealth.org	20	•	•	•	•	•	•	•	•	•
FL	Children's Hospital of SW Florida/Lee Memorial Health System 9981 S. Healthpark Dr. #156 Ft. Myers, FL. 33908	Tel: 239-432-3333 Email: emad.salman@ leememorial.org Web: www.leememorial.org	3	•	¤	•	•	•			•	•
FL	All Children's Hospital Pediatric Heme/Onc Assoc. 880 Sixth St. So., Suite 140 St. Petersburg, FL 33701 Jerry Barbosa, MD	Tel: 727-767-4176 Fax: 727-767-4379 Web: www.allkids.org/resources/cancercare/index.htm	16	•	•	•	¤	•	¤		•	•
FL	Children's Center Cancer Florida Hospital Cancer Inst. 2501 N. Orange Ave # 589 Orlando, FL 32804 Clifford A Selsky, PhD MD	Tel: 407-303-2080 Email: Clifford.Selsky.md@flhosp.org Web: www.flhosp.org www.kidsdocs.com	60	•	•	•	•	•	•		•	•
FL	Nemours Children's Clinic Pediatric Oncology 5153 N. Ninth Ave Pensacola, FL 32504 Jack Kelleher, MD	Tel: 850-505 4790 Email: jfkelleh@nemours.org Web: www.nemours.org	8-15	•	•	•	•	•			•	•
FL	Tampa Childrens Hospital 3001 W. Dr. MLK Jr. Blvd. Tampa FL 33607 Cameron K. Tebbi, MD	Tel: 813-870-4252 Email: Cameron.Tebbi@baycare.org Web: www.stjosephschildrens.com	10	•	•	•	•	•			•	•

Legend: • AVAILABLE EXPERTISE   ¤ Not available

State	Hospital	Contact	#									
FL	**Univ. Florida, Shands Children's Hospital** 1600 SW Archer Road, Hematolog/Oncology HD 209, Gainesville Florida 32610. *Amy Smith, MD*	**Tel:** 352-392-5633 Email : smithaa@peds.ufl.edu	45	•	•	•	•	¤	•	•	•	•
FL	**University of Miami/ Holtz Children's Hospital** 1611 NW 12 Ave ACC West 5A Miami, FL 33136 *Dr. Antonello Podda*	**Tel:** 305-585-5635 Fax: 305-325-8387 **Email:** apodda@med.miami.edu **Web:** www.med.miami.edu	12	•	•	•	•	•	•	•	•	•
GA	**Children's Healthcare of Atlanta, Brain Tumor Prog.** 5455 Meridian Mark Rd #400 Atlanta, GA 30342 *Claire Mazewski MD* *Anna Janss, MD PhD*	**Tel:** 404-785-6171 Fax: 404-785-3511 **Email:** Patricia.mcelfresh@choa.org michele.drummond@choa.org **Web:** www.choa.org/cancer	80-95	•	•	•	•	•	•	•	•	•
IA	**Div Ped. Hemato/ Oncology, Children's Hospital of Iowa** 200 Hawkin's Drive Iowa City, IA 52242 *Sue O'Dorisio, MD PhD* *Rajev Vibhakar, MD PhD*	**Tel:** 319-356-7873 **Email:** sueodorisio@uiowa.edu Rajeevvibhakar@uiowa.edu **Web:** www.uihealthcare.com/ depts/med/pediatrics/divisions/ hemonc/index.html	17	•	•	•	•	•	•	•	•	•
IL	**Neurooncology Program, Children's Memorial Hospital** 2300 Children's Plaza, Box 28, Chicago, IL 60614	**Tel:** 773-880-3792 **Email:** wastellpflug@ childrensmemorial.org **Web:** www.childrensmemorial.org	150	•	•	•	•	•	•	•	•	•
IL	**University of Chicago Comer Childrens Hospital** 5841 S Maryland Av MC4060 Chicago IL 60637 *Kelly Kramer RN, PNP or Charles M. Rubin, MD*	**Tel:** 773-702-6808 **Email:** crubin@uchicago.edu kkramer@peds.bsd.uchicago.edu **Web:** www.uchicagokidshospital.org	26	•	•	•	•	•	•	•	•	•
KY	**Kosair Children's Hospital** 231 E. Chestnut Street Louisville, Ky 40202 *Salvatore Bertolone, MD*	**Tel:** 502-629-7750 **Email:** sjbert01@louisville.edu	14	•	•	•	•	•	•	•	•	•

Legend: • AVAILABLE EXPERTISE ▢ Not available

STATE	Institution Name/ address & Best "Who to" info	Information (Telephone / Email / Website)	1 NEW BT PATIENTS per YR	2 MULTIDISCIPLINARY	3 NEUROSURGERY	4 RADIATION	5 NEURO-ONCOLOGY	6 REHABILITATION	7 NEUROPSYCHOLOGY	8 ENDOCRINE	9 TUMOR BOARD	10 CLINICAL TRIALS
KY	University of Kentucky Medical Center, 800 Rose St, Lexington, KY 40536, *Dr. M. Greenwood*	**Tel:** 859-323-0239 **Email:** jgeil@uky.edu **Web:** www.uky.edu	9			•	•	•	•	•	•	•
MA	Pediatric Brain Tumor Clinic Mass General Hospital for Children, 55 Fruit St, Yawkey 8B, Boston, MA 02114 *Beverly LaVally, RN MS*	**Email:** blavally@partners.org **Web:** www.massgeneral.org/cancer/care/pediatric/brain.asp	65	•	•	•	•	•	•	•		•
MA	New England Medical Center #14, 750 Washington St, Boston, MA 02111	**Tel:** 617-636-5535 **Email:** ckretschmar@tufts-nemc.org **Web:** www.TuftsNEMC.org	25			•						•
MA	Pediatric Brain Tumor Program, Dana-Farber / Children's Hospital Cancer Care Room G331, 44 Binney Street, Boston, MA 02115 *Drs. Mark Kieran, Susan Chi, Dr. Christopher Turner*	**Tel:** 617-632-2680 **Email:** pedibraintumor@dfci.harvard.edu **Web:** www.dana-farber.org/braintumor	120	•	•	•	•	•	•	•	•	•
MD	National Cancer Institute Neuro-Oncology Branch, Bldg 82, Rm 219, 9030 Old Georgetown Road, Bethesda, Maryland 20892 *Kathy Warren, MD*	**Tel:** 301-402-6298 **Email:** warrenk@mail.nih.gov **Web:** http://home.ccr.cancer.gov/nob	500	•			•					•

State	Institution	Contact	No.													
MD	**Johns Hopkins University** CMSC-800 600 N. Wolfe St. Baltimore, MD 21287 *Kenneth J. Cohen, MD*	**Tel:** 410-614-5055 **Email:** kcohen@jhmi.edu **Web:** www.hopkinskimmelcancercenter.org	85	•	•	•	•	•	•	•	•	•	•	•	•	•
ME	**Maine Children's Cancer Program,** 100 Campus Drive Scarborough, ME 04074 *Virginia Hamilton MD*	**Tel:** 207-885-7565 **Email:** hamilv@mmc.org	11	•	•	•	•	•	•	•	•	•	•	•	•	•
MI	**DeVos Children's Hospital** 100 Michigan Ave NE MC85 Grand Rapids, MI 49503 *Albert Cornelius, MD*	**Tel:** 616-391-2086 **Email:** albert.Cornelius@spectrum-health.org **Web:** www.devoschildrens.org	25	•	•	•	•	•	•	•	•	•	•	•	•	•
MI	**Pediatric Neuro-Oncology University of Michigan Medical Center, L-3208 WH** 1500 E. Medical Center Dr. Ann Arbor, MI 48109-0203 *Patricia Robertson, MD*	**Tel:** 734-936-5062 **Email:** prob@umich.edu **Web:** www2.med.umich.edu/departments/mott/clinics/dsp_cliniclist.cfm?group_id=NEURO	100	•	•	•	•	•	•	•	•	•	•	•		•
MN	**Children's Hospitals & Clinics of Minnesota – Minneapolis Campus** 2525 Chicago Avenue S., Minneapolis, MN 55404	**Tel:** 612-813-5940 **Email:** Anne.Bendel@childrensmn.org **Web:** www.childrensmn.org/Communities/Hemonc.asp	20	•	•	•	•	•	•	•	•	•	•	•	•	•
MN	**Children's Hospitals & Clinics of Minnesota. St. Paul Campus** 345 N. Smith Ave. St. Paul, MN 55102	**Tel:** 651-220-6732 **Email:** Chris.Moertel@childrensmn.org **Web:** www.childrensmn.org/Communities/Hemonc.asp	20	•	•	•	•	•	•	•	•	•	•	•	•	•
MN	**Pediatric Hematology/Oncology Mayo Clinic,** 200 First Street SW Rochester, MN 55905 *Cynthia Wetmore MD PhD*	**Tel:** 507-284-2652 **Email:** wetmore.cynthia@mayo.edu **Web:** http://mayoresearch.mayo.edu/mayo/research/staff/wetmore_cj.cfm	45	•	•	•	•	•	•	•	•	•	•	•	•	•

STATE	Institution Name/ address & Best "Who to" info	Information (Telephone / Email / Website)	1 NEW BT PATIENTS per YR	2 MULTIDISCIPLINARY	3 NEUROSURGERY	4 RADIATION	5 NEURO-ONCOLOGY	6 REHABILITATION	7 NEUROPSYCHOLOGY	8 ENDOCRINE	9 TUMOR BOARD	10 CLINICAL TRIALS
MN	**University of Minnesota Children's Hospital – Fairview,** *MMC 484, 420 Delaware St. SE Minneapolis, MN 55455*	Jane Torkelson, RN: 612-273-8422 Joseph Neglia, M.D: 612-626-2778 **Email:** jtorkel1@fairview.org or jneglia@umn.edu **Web:** www.cancer.umn.edu/page/clinical/p_brain.html	20	•	•	•	•	•	•	•	•	•
MO	**The Children's Mercy Hospitals and Clinics** Div. Hematology/Oncology 2401 Gillham Road Kansas City, Missouri 64108	**Tel:** 816-234-3265 **Email:** mhethering@cmh.edu **Web:** www.childrens-mercy.org	37			•	•	•				•
MO	**St. Louis Children's Hospital Washington University School of Medicine,** One Children's Place # 8116 St. Louis, MO 63110 *Debra Spoljaric, PNP*	**Tel:** 314-454-6018 **Email:** spoljaric_d@kids.wustl.edu **Web:** www.stlouischildrens.org	40	•	•	•	•	•			•	•
MO	**Cardinal Glennon Children's Hospital/Saint Louis University Dept. of Pediatrics** 1465 South Grand Blvd. St. Louis, MO 63104 *William Ferguson, MD*	**Tel:** 314-577-5638 **Email:** ferguswss@slu.edu **Web:** www.cardinalglennon.com	15	•								•
NC	**Duke University Medical** Center DUMC, Box 3624 Durham NC 27710 *Sri Gururangan MRCP*	**Tel:** 919 684 3506 **Email:** Gurur002@mc.duke.edu **Web:** www.cancer.duke.edu/btc	500	•	•	•	•	•			•	•

Information legend: • AVAILABLE EXPERTISE   ¤ Not available

State	Center	Contact	#	Services
NE	**Children's Hospital/ Univ. Nebraska Medical Center, Pediatric Hemato/Oncology,** *8200 Dodge St. Omaha, NE 68114 Minnie Abromowitch, MD*	**Tel:** 402-955-3949 **Email:** pcoccia@unmc.edu or mabromowitch@chsomaha.org	31	• • • • • • • • • •
NV	**Comprehensive Cancer Centers of Nevada Sunrise Hospital for Children** 3196 S. Maryland Pkwy #400, Las Vegas NV 89119 *Jonathan Bernstein MD*	**Tel:** 02-732-0971 **Email:** jonbern1@aol.com	35	• • • • • □ • • • •
NY	**Memorial Sloan Kettering Cancer Center Brain Tumor Program (Peds)** *1275 York Ave. New York 10021*	**Tel:** 212-639-8292 or 212-639-5954 **Email:** Khakooy@mskcc.org pediatrics@mskcc.org **Web:** www.mskcc.org	63	• • • • • • • • • •
NY	**"Alfano Fnd Program in Pediatric Neuro-Oncology" Morgan-Stanley Children's Hospital of NY-Presbyterian** 161 Fort Washington Ave# 718 New York, NY 10032 *James Garvin MD PhD*	**Tel:** 212-305-5872 or Coordinator: 212-305-8685 **Email:** bec9013@nyp.org **Web:** www.herbertirvingchildren.com	50	• • • • • □ • • • •
NY	**The Children's Hospital at Montefiore** 3415 Bainbridge Avenue Bronx, New York 10467 *Adam Levy, MD*	**Tel:** 718-741-2342 **Email:** adlevy@montefiore.org **Web:** www.montekids.org	35	• • • • • • • • • •
NY	**New York Presbyterian Hospital-Weill Cornell** 525 East 68th Street, Box 99 New York, NY 10021 *Mark Souweidane, MD*	**Tel:** 212-746-2363 **Email:** mmsouwei@med.cornell.edu **Web:** www.cornellneurosurgery.org	45	□ □ □ □ • □ □ • •
NY	**University of Rochester Medical Center Dept of Pediatrics,** Box 777, 601 Elmwood Ave. Rochester, NY 14642	**Tel:** 585-275-2981 **Email:** david_korones@urmc.rochester.edu	20	• • • • • • • • • •

STATE	Institution Name/ address & Best "Who to" info	Information • AVAILABLE EXPERTISE ¤ Not available / Telephone Email Website	1 NEW BT PATIENTS per YR	2 MULTIDISCIPLINARY	3 NEUROSURGERY	4 RADIATION	5 NEURO-ONCOLOGY	6 REHABILITATION	7 NEUROPSYCHOLOGY	8 ENDOCRINE	9 TUMOR BOARD	10 CLINICAL TRIALS
NY	NYU Medical Center 317 E. 34th St. New York, NY 10016 *Jeffrey C. Allen MD* *Sharon Gardner MD*	Tel: 212 263-6725 Email: Jeffrey.Allen@NYUMC.org Sharon.Gardner@NYUMC.org Web: www.med.nyu.edu/pedho	90	•	•	•	•	•	•	•	•	•
NY	Schneider Children's Hospital, Pediatric Hematology/ Oncology 269-01 76th Avenue, CH255 New Hyde Park, NY 11040 *Dr. Mark Atlas* *Dr. Arlene Redner*	Tel: 718-470-3460 Email: matlas@lij.edu redner@lij.edu Web: www.schneiderchildrenshos pital.org	50	•	•	•	•	•	•			•
NY	Cancer Center for Kids Winthrop University Hosp. 400 Old Country Road # 440 Mineola, NY 11501 *Dr. Mark Weinblatt*	Tel: 516-663-9400 Email: mweinbl@yahoo.com	10	•	•	•	•	¤	•	•	•	•
OH	Children's Hospital Cleveland Clinic 9500 Euclid Avenue, S20 Cleveland, OH 44195 *Joanne Hilden, MD*	Tel: 216-444-8407 Email: hildenj@ccf.org Web: www.clevelandclinic.org/ childrenshospital	50		•	•	•	•				•
OH	Rainbow Babies & Children's Hospital Hematology/ Oncology 11100 Euclid Ave RB&C 340 Cleveland, OH 44106	Tel: 216-844-3345 Email: chad.jacobsen@uhhs.com	20	•	•	•	•	•				•

	Institution	Contact													
OH	**Columbus Children's Hospital, Hemato-Oncology** 700 Children's Drive Columbus, OH 43205 *Randal Olshefski, MD*	**Tel:** 614-722 -3583 **Fax:** 614-722-3699 **Email:** Olshefskir@chi.osu.edu	40	•	•	•	•	•	•	•	•	•	•	•	•
OK	**University of Oklahoma Health Sciences & OU Medical Center** Jimmy Everest Center 940 NE 13th, MR 3000 *Oklahoma City, OK 73104*	**Tel:** 405-271-5311 or **Email:** Rene-cNall@ouhsc.edu **Web:** www.OUphysicians.com	35	•	•	•	•	•	•	•	•	•	•	•	•
PA	**Children's Hospital of Pittsburgh, Neuro-Oncology,** *3705 Fifth Ave. Room 4B-220* Pittsburgh, PA 15213	**Tel:** 412-692-7056 **Email:** regina.jakacki@chp.edu **Web:** www.chp.edu	70	•	•	•	•	•	•	•	•	•	•	•	•
PA	**St. Christopher's Hospital for Children** **Section of Oncology** Erie Avenue at Front Street Philadelphia, PA 19134-1095 *Duncan Stearns, MD*	**Tel:** 215- 427-4447 **Email:** DUNCAN.Stearnsmd@ tenethealth.com **Web:** www.stchristophershospital. com	20-30	•	•	•	•	•	•	•	•	•	•	•	•
PA	**Penn State Children's Hospital, Hershey Med Cntr** 500 University Dr, PO Box 850 Hershey, PA 17033	**Tel:** 717-531-6012 **Email:** mac36@psu.edu **Web:** www.hmc.psu.edu/ hematology	20	•	•	•	•	•	•	•	•	•	•	•	•
RI	**Hasbro Children's Hospital** 593 Eddy Street Providence, RI 02903 *Peter Manley, MD*	**Tel:** 401-444-5171 **Email:** pmanley@lifespan.org **Web:** www. hasbrochildrenshospital.org	20	•	•	•	•	•	•	•	•	•	•	•	•
TN	**T C Thompson Children's Hospital,** 910 Blackwood St Chattanooga, TN 36403 *Manoo Bhakta, MD*	**Tel:** 423 -78-7289 **Email:** Manoo.bhakta@erlanger.org **Web:** www.erlanger.org	5	•	•	•	•	•	•	□	□	□			
TN	**St Jude Children's Research Hospital (Neuro-Oncology)** 332 N Lauderdale Memphis TN 38105 *Amar Gajjar, MD or Jennifer Havens, RN*	**Tel:** 901-495-5007 **Email:** braintumors@stjude.org **Web:** www.stjude.org/brain-tumors	145	•	•	•	•	•	•	•	•	•	•	•	•

STATE	Institution Name/ address & Best "Who to" info	Telephone / Email / Website	1 NEW BT PATIENTS per YR	2 MULTIDISCIPLINARY	3 NEUROSURGERY	4 RADIATION	5 NEURO-ONCOLOGY	6 REHABILITATION	7 NEUROPSYCHOLOGY	8 ENDOCRINE	9 TUMOR BOARD	10 CLINICAL TRIALS
TN	**Monroe Carell Jr Children's Hospital at Vanderbilt** 2200 Children's Way Nashville, TN 37232	Tele: 615-936-2938 **Email:** John.Kuttesch@Vanderbilt.edu **Web:** www.vanderbiltchildrens.com www.mc.vanderbilt.edu/vicc	40	•	•	•	•	•	•	•	•	•
TX	**Driscoll Children's Hospital** 3533 South Alameda St Corpus Christi, Texas 78411	**Tel:** 361-694-5311 **Email:** Dragutin.loncar@dchstx.org **Web:** www.driscollchildrens.org	10	•	•	•	•	•	•	•	•	•
TX	**Neuro-Oncology Program Children's Medical Center of Dallas,** 1935 Motor Street Dallas, TX 75235 *Daniel Bowers, MD*	**Tel:** 214-456-6139 **Email:** Daniel.Bowers@ utsouthwestern.edu **Web:** www.childrens.com/ccbd	90	•	•	•	•	•	•	•	•	•
TX	**Univ. of Texas MD Anderson Cancer Center, Div. Pediatrics Unit 87,** 1515 Holcombe Blvd Houston, TX 77030 *Joann Ater, MD* *Johannes Wolff, MD*	**Tel:** 713-792-6665 or 713-792-5410 **Email:** jater@mdanderson.org **Web:** www.mdanderson.org	65	•	•	•	•	•	•	•	•	•
TX	**Texas Children's Cancer Ctr** 621 Fannin St; CC 1410 Houston, TX 77030 *Murali Chintagumpala MD*	**Tel:** 832-822-1482 **Email:** mxchinta@txccc.org **Web:** www.txccc.org	90	•			•	•	•			•
TX	**The Howard A. Britton MD Children's Cancer Center CHRISTUS Santa Rosa Children's Hospital** 8th floor, 333 N. Santa Rosa San Antonio, Texas 78207	**Tel:** 210-704-3405 **Email:** shahs2@uthscsa.edu **Web:** www.pediatrics.uthscsa. edu/Hematology-Oncology	20				•	•	•	•		•

• AVAILABLE EXPERTISE
□ Not available

State	Institution	Contact	No.
UT	**University of Utah, Primary Childrens Hospital** 100 N. Medical Drive, Salt Lake City, UT 84113 *Carol Bruggers, MD*	**Tel:** 801-588-2680 **Email:** Carol.bruggers@ihc.com	66
VA	**Virginia Commonwealth University, Children's Medical Center**, Box 980121 1101 East Marshall Street Richmond VA 23298	**Tel:** 804-828-9605 **Email:** kgodder@vcu.edu **Web:** www.vcu.edu/pediatrics	25
VA	**University of Virginia Health System, Department of Neurosurgery** PO Box 800212 Charlottesville, VA 22908 *John A Jane Jr., MD*	**Tel:** 434-243-5749 **Email:** johnjanejr@virginia.edu **Web:** www.healthsystem.virginia.edu/internet/neurosurgery/	40
WA	**Children's Hospital and Regional Medical Center** 4800 Sand Point Way NE Seattle, WA 98105 *Russell Geyer, MD*	**Tel:** 206-987-2106 **Email:** russ.geyer@seattlechildrens.org **Web:** www.seattlechildrens.org	70
WA	**Sacred Heart Children's Hospital, Hemato/Oncology** 101 West 8th Ave Box 2555 Spokane, WA 99220-2555	**Tel:** 509.474.2777 or 1-800-541-0843 **Web:** www.shmcchildren.org	10
WI	**Midwest Childrens Cancer Center,** 8701 Watertown Plank Rd, Milwaukee WI 53226 *Sachin Jogal, MD*	**Tel:** 414-456-4170 **Email:** sjogal@mcw.edu **Web:** www.mcw.edu/display/router.asp?docid=2257	25
WI	**University of Wisconsin Children's Hospital K4/4CSC** 600 Highland Avenue Madison, WI 53792 *Diane Puccetti, MD*	**Tel:** 608-263-6200 **Email:** Puccetti@wisc.edu **Web:** www.pediatrics.wisc.edu	80
WI	**Pediatric Oncology. Marshfield Clinic** 1000 N. Oak Ave. Marshfield, WI 54449 *Michael J. McManus, MD*	**Tel:** 715-389-3050 **Email:** mcmanus.michael@marshfieldclinic.org **Web:** www.marshfieldclinic.org	5

STATE	Institution Name/ address & Best "Who to" info	Telephone / Email / Website	NEW BT PATIENTS per YR	MULTI-DISCIPLINARY	NEURO-SURGERY	RADIATION	NEURO-ONCOLOGY	REHABILITATION	NEURO-PSYCHOLOGY	ENDOCRINE	TUMOR BOARD	CLINICAL TRIALS
			1	2	3	4	5	6	7	8	9	10
AUSTRALIA	**Centre for Children's Cancer Sydney Children's Hospital** High Street, Randwick, NSW, Australia, 2031 *Richard Cohn, MD*	**Tel:** (0061) 2-9382-1730 **Email:** R.Cohn@unsw.edu.au **Web:** www.kids-cancer.org	25	•	•	•	•	•	•	•	•	•
AUSTRALIA	**Women's and Children's Hospital, Department of Haematology / Oncology** 72 King William Road, North Adelaide SA 5006	**Tel:** (0061) 8-8161-7411 **Email:** cywhs.oncsec@cywhs.sa.gov.au **Web:** www.wch.sa.gov.au	10	•	•	•	•	•	•	•	•	•
CANADA	**Alberta Childrens Hospital** 1820 Richmond Rd. SW Calgary AB T2T 5C7 *Douglas Strother, MD*	**Tel:** 403-943-7272 **Email:** Doug.strother@calgaryhealthregion.ca	20	•	•	•	•	•	•	•	•	•
CANADA	**McMaster Children's Hospital** 1200 Main St. W Hamilton, Ontario CANADA L8N3Z5 *Dr. I. Odame*	**Tel:** 905-521-2100 x73482 **Email:** odamei@mcmaster.ca **Web:** www.hamilton healthsciences.ca	10-15	•	•	•	•	•	•	•	•	•
CANADA	**CancerCare Manitoba** 675 McDermot Ave. Winnipeg MB R3E 0V9	**Tel:** 204-787-4643 **Email:** eisensta@cc.umanitoba.ca **Web:** www.cancercare.mb.ca	10	•	•	•	•	•	•	•	•	•
CANADA	**The Hospital for Sick Children** 555 University Avenue Toronto, Ontario M5G 1X8 *Dr. Eric Bouffet*	**Tel:** 416-813-8889 **Email:** eric.bouffet@sickkids.ca annie.huang@sickkids.ca **Web:** www.sickkids.ca/haematologyoncology	75-100	•	•	•	•	•	•	•	•	•

AVAILABLE EXPERTISE: • AVAILABLE EXPERTISE □ Not available

Country	Institution	Contact	#												
CANADA	**Neurosurgery, Room C-819 Montreal Children's Hospital** 2300 Tupper Street Montreal, Quebec H3H 1P3 CANADA *Dr. J. P. Farmer*	**Tel:** 514-412-4492 **Email:** jean-pierre.farmer@mcgill.ca	25	•	•	•	•	•	•	•	•	•	•	•	•
ENGLAND	**University of Nottingham Children's Brain Tumour Research Centre** Queen's Medical Centre Nottingham NG7 2UH, UK *Professor Richard Grundy*	**Tel:** (0044)-115-823-30620 **Email:** Richard.grundy@ nottingham.ac.uk	35-40	•	•	•	•	•	•	•	•	•	•	•	•
JORDAN	**King Hussein Cancer Center** Queen Rania Street P.O.BOX 1269 Al-Jubeiha Amman 11941 JORDAN *Dr. I Qaddoumi, MD*	**Tel:** 962-6-5300-460 **Email:** iqaddoumi@khcc.jo **Web:** www.khcc.jo	60	◻	•	•	◻	•	•	•	•	•	•	•	•
SWZ	**University Children's Hospital of Zurich,** Steinwiesstrasse 75, CH-8032 Zurich, SWITZERL.	**Tel:** (0041) 44-266-7111 **Email:** Michael.Grotzer@kispi. unizh.ch **Web:** www.kispi.unizh.ch	35	•	•	•	•	•	•	•	•	•	•		
SWZ	**Brain Tumor ProgramUniversity Childrens Hospital, Bern Inselspital,** CH-3010 Bern, SWITZERLAND *Roland Ammann, MD*	**Tel:** (0041) 31-632-1087 **Email:** Roland.ammann@insel.ch	10	•	•	•	•	•	•	•	•	•	•		

Listed centers are full or affiliate members of the Childrens Oncology Group (COG) and/ or Society for Neurooncology who responded to a request for institutional information January 26, 2006.

Appendix 2: MAJOR ADULT BRAIN TUMOR CENTERS

STATE	Institution Name/ address & Best "Who to" info	Telephone / Email / Website	1 NEW BT PATIENTS per YR	2 MULTI-DISCIPLINARY	3 NEUROSURGERY	4 RADIATION	5 NEURO-ONCOLOGY	6 REHABILITATION	7 NEUROPSYCHOLOGY	8 ENDOCRINE	9 TUMOR BOARD	10 CLINICAL TRIALS
CA	**City of Hope Medical Center** Department of Neurosurgery 1500 E. Duarte Rd. Duarte, CA 91010 *Tisha Cruz*	**Tel:** 626-471-7100 **Email:** tcruz@coh.org **Web:** www.cityofhope.org	55	•	•	•	•	•	¤	•	•	•
CA	**UCSF Brain Tumor Center** 505 Parnassus Ave Rm M779 San Francisco, CA 94143-0112 *Mitchel S. Berger, MD*	**Tel:** Ann 415-353-3933 **Email:** Bergerm@neurosurg.ucsf.edu **Web:** www.neurosurgery. medschool.ucsf.edu/index.html	450	•	•	•	•	•	•	•	•	•
CA	**UCLA Brain Tumor Program** 10833 Le Conte Avenue [CHS 74-145] Los Angeles, CA 90095 *Dr. Linda Liau* *Dr. Tim Cloughesy*	**Tel:** 310-825-5111(Neurosurgery) or 310-825-5321(Neuro-Onc) **Email:** neuroonc@ucla.edu or kvolpicelli@mednet.ucla.edu **Web:** www.neurooncology. ucla.edu or http://neurosurgery. ucla.edu/Programs/BrainTumor/ BrainTumor_Intro.html	400	•	•	•	•	¤	•	•	•	•
CA	**University of Southern California USC Norris Cancer Center** 1441 Eastlake Ave, Suite 3459 Los Angeles, CA 90033 *Thomas Chen MD PhD*	**Tel:** 323-865-3486 **Email:** TChen68670@aol.com or mcorwin@usc.edu **Web:** http://www.usc.edu/ schools/medicine/departments/ neurological_surgery	70	•	•	•	•	•	•	•	•	•
CA	**USC Neuro-Oncology Norris Compr Cancer Center** 1441 Eastlake Ave, #3440 Los Angeles, CA 90033 *Omid Hamid MD*	**Tel:** 323-865-0843 **Email:** onh@usc.edu **Web:** www.uscnorris.com	150	•	•	•	•	•	•	•	•	•

AVAILABLE EXPERTISE: • AVAILABLE EXPERTISE ¤ Not available

State	Center	Contact	#									
CA	**Sutter Neuroscience Medical Group** 2800 L Street, Suite 500 Sacramento, CA 95816 *Dr. Nora W. Wu*	**Tel:** 916-454-6850 **Email:** Wunw@sutterhealth.org **Web:** http://checksutterfirst.org/neuro	130	•	•	•	•	•	•	•	•	•
CO	**St. Anthony Hospital Central** 4231 W. 16th Ave. Denver, CO 80204 *Attn: Dr. Charles Mateskon*	**Tel:** 303-629-3610 **Email:** charlesmateskon@centura.org **Web :** www.stanthonyhosp.or	93	•	•	•	¤	•	•	•	•	•
FL	**Florida Hospital Cancer Institute (Neuro-Oncology)** 2501 N. Orange Ave, #249 Orlando, FL 32804 *Edward Pan MD* *Nicholas Avgeropoulos MD*	**Tel:** 407-303-2770 **Email:** Edward.panmd@flhosp.org Nicholas.avgeropoulosmd@flhosp.org dr-nick@neuro-oncology.net	150	•	•	•	•	•	•	•	•	•
GA	**Emory Winship Cancer Institute** 1365 Clifton Road NE Bldg C Atlanta, Georgia 30322 *Kristen Griener, PA-C, MS* *Surasak Phuphanich, MD*	**Tel:** 1-888-946-7447 **Email:** kristen.greiner@emoryhealthcare.org **Web:** www.winshipcancerinstitute.org	150	•	•	•	•	•	•	•	•	•
IA	**Depart. Neurosurgery and Radiation Oncology, University of Iowa Hospitals and Clinics,** 200 Hawkins Drive Iowa City, Iowa 52242 *Kelly Hochstetler, RN*	**Tel:** 319-356-3853 **Email:** timothy-ryken@uiowa.edu hochstetler@uiowa.edu	300	•	•	•	•	•	•	•	•	•
IL	**Evanston Northwestern Healthcare, Neuro-Oncology Program, Kellogg Cancer Care Center,** 2650 Ridge Ave Evanston, IL 60201 *Patricia Lada RN*	**Tel:** 847-570-2025 **Email:** plada@enh.org **Web:** www.enh.org	250-300	•	•	•	•	•	•	•	•	•
IL	**The University of Chicago Brain Tumor Center, The University of Chicago** 5841 S. Maryland Ave, MC 3026. Chicago, IL 60637 *Maciej S. Lesniak, MD*	**Tel:** 773-834-4757 **Email:** mlesniak@surgery.bsd.uchicago.edu **Web:** www.ucneurosurgery.org www.chicagobraintumors.org	150	•	•	•	•	•	•	•	•	•

STATE	Institution Name/ address & Best "Who to" info	Information	1 NEW BT PATIENTS per YR	2 MULTIDISCIPLINARY	3 NEUROSURGERY	4 RADIATION	5 NEURO-ONCOLOGY	6 REHABILITATION	7 NEUROPSYCHOLOGY	8 ENDOCRINE	9 TUMOR BOARD	10 CLINICAL TRIALS
IL	Univ. of Illinois at Chicago, 1801 W TaylorOCC M/C 821, Chicago, IL 60612, John Villano, MD, PhD, Maria Walker RN	Tel: 312-996-4922 Email: jvillano@uic.edu Web: www.hospital.uic.edu/	60	•	•	•	•	•	¤	•	•	•
MA	Tufts-New England Medical Center, Neurology & Neuro-oncology, Box # 314, 750 Washington Street, Boston, MA 02111, Jay-Jiguang Zhu, MD, PhD	Tel: 617-636-4856 or 5627 Fax: 617-636-8199 Email: jzhu@tufts-nemc.org Web: www.tufts.edu/med/neurosurgery/news.shtml	200	•	•	•	•	•	•	•	•	
MA	Lahey Clinic, Brain Tumor Center, Dept. Neurosurgery, 41 Mall Rd, Burlington, MA 01805, Rosemary Dolan	Tel: 781-744-1990 Email: rosemary.e.dolan@lahey.org Web: www.lahey.org	150	•	•	•	•	•	•	•		•
MA	Center for Neuro-Oncology Dana Farber/Brigham and Women's Cancer Center, SW430D, 44 Binney Street, Boston, MA 02115, Patrick Y.Wen, M.D.	Tel: 617-632-2166 Email: pwen@partners.org Web: www.dfci.harvard.edu	400-500			•	•	•				•
MA	Pappas Center for Neuro-Oncology Mass. General Hospital, 55 Fruit Street, Yawkey 9E, Boston, MA 02114, Tracy T. Batchelor, MD	Tel: 617-643-1938 Email: tbatchelor@partners.org Web: www.massgeneral.org/cancer/education/neuro.asp	400	•	•	•	•	•	•			•

AVAILABLE EXPERTISE
• AVAILABLE EXPERTISE
¤ Not available
Telephone
Email
Website

	Facility	Contact	#											
MI	**Detroit Medical Center Harper University Hospital** 4160 John R Ste 730 Detroit, MI 48201 *Lucia Zamorano, M.D.*	**Tel:** 248-7232477 **Email:** lzamoran@dmc.org **Web:** www.luciazamorano.com	120	•	•			•	•	•	•	•	•	•
MI	**Univ. of Michigan Hospital** 1914 Taubman Center/0316 Ann Arbor, MI 48109 *Larry Junck, M.D.*	**Tel:**734-936-9047 **Email:** ljunck@umich.edu **Web:** www.med.umich.edu/neuro/clinical/oncology.htm	300	•	•			•	•	•	•	•	•	•
MO	**Siteman Cancer Center Barnes-Jewish Hospital Washington University School of Medicine** St. Louis, MO *JoAnn Steel, RN, MSN*	**Tel:** 314-747-2125 **Email:** jsteel@im.wustl.edu **Web:** www.siteman.wustl.edu	160	•	•	□		•	•	•	•	•	•	•
NC	**Carolina Neurosurgery and Spine Associates** 225 Baldwin Road, Charlotte, NC 28204 *Peggy Boltes, RN*	**Tel:** 704-376-1605 **Email:** Peggy@CNSA.com **Web:** www.carolinaneurosurgery.com/index.html	250	•	•			•	•	•	•	•	•	•
NC	**Wake Forest University Baptist Medical Center,** Medical Center Boulevard, Winston-Salem, NC 27157 *Edward G. Shaw, M.D*	**Tel:** 336-713-6925 **Email:** statter@wfubmc.edu eshaw@wfubmc.edu **Web:** www1.wfubmc.edu/neurosurgery/Brain+Tumor+Center+of+Excellence	400	•	•			•	•	•	•	•	•	•
NJ	**New Jersey Neuroscience Institute at JFK Medical Center (Neurooncology)** 65 James Street Edison, N.J. 08818 *Joseph C. Landolfi, D.O.*	**Tel:** 732-321-7950 **Email:** jlandolfi@solarishs.org **Web:** www.njneuro.org	170	•	•			•	•	•	•	•	•	•
NJ	**Dept. of Neurosurgery, New Jersey Medical School** 90 Bergen Street, Suite 8100 Newark, NJ 07103 *Michael Schulder, MD*	**Tel:** 973-972-2907 **Email:** Schulder@umdnj.edu **Web:** www.theuniversityhospital.com/braintumor	200	•	•			•	•	•	•	•	•	•

STATE	Institution Name/address & Best "Who to" info	Information (Telephone, Email, Website)	1 NEW BT PATIENTS per YR	2 MULTIDISCIPLINARY	3 NEUROSURGERY	4 RADIATION	5 NEURO-ONCOLOGY	6 REHABILITATION	7 NEUROPSYCHOLOGY	8 ENDOCRINE	9 TUMOR BOARD	10 CLINICAL TRIALS
NY	**New York Presbyterian Hospital-Weill Cornell** 525 East 68th Street, Box 99 New York, NY 10021 *Susan C. Pannullo MD*	**Tel:** 212-746-2438 **Email:** scp2002@med.cornell.edu **Web:** www.cornellneurosurgery.org	250	•	•	•	•	•	•	•	•	•
NY	**Columbia University Medical Center** Room 434, 710 W 168th St New York, N.Y. 10032 *Jeffrey N. Bruce MD*	**Tel:** 212-305-7346 **Email:** jnb2@columbia.edu **Web:** www.cumc.columbia.edu/dept/nsg/NSGCPMC/specialties/braintumor.html	150	•	•	•	•	•	•	•	•	•
NY	**Memorial Sloan Kettering Cancer Center** Adult Brain Tumor Program 1275 York Ave., NY 10021	**Tel:** 212-639-7123 **Email:** deangell@mskcc.org **Web:** www.mskcc.org	500	•	•	•	•	•	•	•	•	•
OH	**Cleveland Clinic Brain Tumor Institute R20** 9500 Euclid Ave Cleveland, OH 44195	**Tel:** Patient appointments 800/223-2273 x 58971 Clinical Trial Info: 866/223-8100 **Web:** www.clevelandclinic.org/neuroscience/treat/brain www.clevelandclinic.org/neuroscience/treat/brain	529	•	•	•	•	•	•	•	•	•
PA	**Univ. Pennsylvania Health System, Dept. Neurosurgery** 3rd Floor Silverstein, 3400 Spruce Street Philadelphia, PA 19104 *Joanna Lopinto, BSN RN*	**Tel:** 215-615-4590 **Email:** JLopinto@uphs.upenn.edu **Web:** www.uphs.upenn.edu/neurosurgery	426	•		•		•	•			•

Legend: • AVAILABLE EXPERTISE   ▢ Not available

PA	Adult Neurooncology Serv. UPMC Cancer Center, 5th Fl **5150 Center Ave. Pittsburgh, PA 15232** *Frank S. Lieberman M.D.*	**Tel:** 412-692-2600 **Email:** f@upmc.edu	200	•	•	•	•	•	•	•	•						
TX	**The Methodist Hospital Neurological Institute** 6560 Fannin St., Suite 944 Houston, Texas 77030 *Pamela New M.D.*	**Tel:** 713-4412-3831 **Email:** pnew@tmh.tmc.edu **Web:** www.methodisthealth.com Select " centers of excellence" Then "cancer services"	194	•	•	•	•	•	•	•	•						
TX	**M. D. Anderson Cancer Center** 1515 Holcombe Blvd, Unit 442 Houston, TX 77030	**Tel:** 713-563-8749 **Email:** dbower@mdanderson.org **Web:** www.mdanderson.org/ departments/braintumor	1000	•	•	•	•	•	•	•	•						
VA	**University of Virginia Neuro-Oncology Center,** Box 800432 Charlottesville, VA 22908 *David Schiff, M.D. or Edward Laws M.D.*	**Tel:** 434-982-4415 **Email:** davidschiff@virginia.edu or el5g@virginia.edu **Web:** www.uvabraintumor.org	540	•	•	•	•	•	•	•	•						
WA	**Univ. Washington Medical Center,** 1959 NE Pacific St, Mailstop 356465, Room RR650 Seattle, WA 98195	**Tel:** 206-543-2340 **Email:** aspence@u.washington.edu **Web:** http://depts.washington.edu/neuroonc	200	•	•	•	•	•	•	•	•						
WA	**Virginia Mason Medical Center** 1100 9th Ave. Seattle, WA 98111	**Tel:** 206-341-0420 **Email:** neulpt@vmmc.org **Web:** www.virginiamason.org	60	•	•	•	•	•	•	•	•						
WA	**Swedish Cancer Institute** 1221 Madison Street 2nd Flr. Seattle, WA 98104 Henry Kaplan, M.D.	**Tel:** 206-386-2442 **Email:** patra.grevstad@swedish.org **Web:** www.swedish.org	44	•	•	¤	•	•	¤	•	•						
WI	**Medical College of Wisconsin Department of Neurology** 9200 W Wisconsin Ave Milwaukee WI 53226 *Hendrikus Krouwer M.D., PhD*	**Tel:** 414-805-5223 **Email:** hkrouwer@mcw.edu **Web:** www.mcw.edu	100-125	•	•	•	•	•	•	•	•						

Legend: • AVAILABLE EXPERTISE ¤ Not available

STATE	Institution Name/ address & Best "Who to" info	Information (Telephone / Email / Website)	1 NEW BT PATIENTS per YR	2 MULTIDISCIPLINARY	3 NEUROSURGERY	4 RADIATION	5 NEURO-ONCOLOGY	6 REHABILITATION	7 NEUROPSYCHOLOGY	8 ENDOCRINE	9 TUMOR BOARD	10 CLINICAL TRIALS
BRAZIL	**Instituto de Neurologia de Curitiba,** 300 Jeremias Maciel Perreto Curitiba, PR, BRAZIL, 81.210-310 *Mauricio Coelho Neto MD*	**Tel:** (0055) 41-3028-8580 **Email:** mcoelho29@yahoo.com / inc@inc-neuro.com.br **Web:** www.inc-neuro.com.br	156	•	•	¤	•	¤	•	•	•	¤
CANADA	**Calgary Brain Tumour Prog.** c/o **Tom Baker Cancer Centre,** 1331 – 29 St. NW Calgary, Alberta T2N 4N2	**Tel:** 403-521-3046 **Email:** maureenv@cancerboard.ab.ca **Web:** www.cancerboard.ab.ca	126	•		•	•	¤	•	¤		•
FRANCE	**Unité de Neuro-Oncologie CHU Timone** 264 rue Saint Pierre 13385 Marseille cedex 05, FRANCE	**Tel:** (0033) 49-138-6569 **Email:** olivier.chinot@ap-hm.fr **Web:**	200	•	•	•	•	•	•	•		•
HOLLAND	**Neuro-Oncology Unit Daniel den Hoed Cancer Center,** Groene Hilledijk 301 3075 EA Rotterdam the NETHERLANDS *Prof M.J. van den Bent*	**Tel:** (0031) 10-439-1415 **Email:** m.vandenbent@erasmusmc.nl	100	•		•	•	¤	¤	¤	•	•
ISRAEL	**Hadassah Hebrew University Hospital** P.O.Box 12000 Jerusalem 91120, ISRAEL *Prof. Tali Siegal M.D.*	**Tel:** 972-2-677-8854 **Email:** neuro-onco@hadassah.org.il **Web:** www.hadassah.org.il	250	•			•	•	•	•	•	•

Country	Center	Contact											
ITALY	Division of Neuro-Oncology University and San Giovanni Battista Hospital Via Cherasco 15 10126 Torino, ITALY R. Soffietti, M.D.	Tel: (0039) 11-633-4904 Fax: (0039) 11-696-3487 Email: riccardo.soffietti@unito.it Web: www.molinette.piemonte.it	100	•	•	•	•	•	•	•	•	•	•
ITALY	Neuro-Oncology Unit Istituto Oncologico Veneto - IRCCS Via Gattamelata 64 35128 Padova, ITALY	Tel: (0039) 49 -821-5622 Email: aa.brandes@yahoo.it	490	•	•	•	¤	•	•	•	•	•	•
ITALY	Dipartimento di Oncologia Medica Ospedale Bellaria AUSL Città di Bologna Via Altura 3 40100 Bologna, ITALY	Tel:(0039) 51-622-5334 Email: giovanna.cavallo@ausl.bo.it enrica.labanti@ausl.bo.it	•	•	•	•	•	•	•	•	•	•	•

The Centers listed in this Table responded to a "blast" email sent to members of the Society for Neurooncology on January 26, 2006, requesting information on their respective center.

Glossary

GLOSSARY

Advance directive

The actual orders in the hospital or care facility records that put into action what your living will document says.

Anticipatory nausea and vomiting

Anticipatory means vomiting at the thought of the drug, or even before arriving at the clinic or hospital. This can affect compliance with taking the drug.

Astrocyte

A brain cell that provides support, structure, nutrition to other brain cells.

Astrocytomas (Astro-sigh –TOE- maz)

The most common types in the brain tumor family are called "gliomas." They develop from star-shaped glial cells called astrocytes. Pathologists assign grades to an astrocytoma following biopsy Low-grade, well differentiated: Also called, grade I and II astrocytomas. Their cells look relatively normal and are less malignant than the other two grades. They grow more slowly and sometimes can be completely removed. They can still be life threatening, if they are deep within vital locations, mid-grade, anaplastic, or Grade III astrocytomas grow more rapidly than well-differentiated astrocytomas and contain cells with malignant traits. Surgery followed by radiation and chemotherapy contribute to very long survivals.

High-grade, grade IV or glioblastoma multiforme (GBM): These tumors grow rapidly, invade nearby tissue, and contain cells that are very malignant. GBMs are among the most common and serious primary brain tumors that strike adults. Doctors usually treat glioblastomas with surgery followed by radiation therapy. Chemotherapy may be used before, during, or after radiation. There are many experimental studies available.

Astrocytoma (Juvenile Pilocytic)

This is low-grade astrocytoma occurs in young children, most commonly near the cerebellum or 4th ventricle. Surgery is usually curative. When it occurs in other locations (near the hypothalamus or optic nerves or cerebrum) or in adults, it can be difficult to completely remove and may recur.

Benign cancer

A tumor that tends to grow slowly, if it grows at all.

Brain Stem Gliomas (BSG) or Gliomas of the Brain Stem

Named by their location at the base of the brain rather than the cells they contain, BSGs are more common in children and young adults. There are two types: intrinsic and extrinsic or exophytic. Each behaves very differently. Surgery usually is not helpful for the intrinsic types because of their critical location but has a role for the exophytic types. Radiation therapy often reduces symptoms and improves survival.

Cancer

Any tumor that has the potential to grow without treatment.

Cancer susceptibility gene

An inherited mutation that can lead to cancer.

Chordomas

More common in people in their 20s and 30s, develop from remnants which should have dissolved early in fetal development and is later replaced by the spinal cord. The tumors are often slow growing but can spread to other areas in the spine and brain. They typically are treated with surgery and radiation.

Choroid Plexus Carcinoma (CPC)

A rare and malignant tumor that is not curable with surgery alone but is treated with chemotherapy and sometimes radiation.

Choroid Plexus Papilloma (CORE-oid PLEX-us PAH-pee-LO-muh) (CPP)

CPP is a rare, benign tumor most common in children under the age of 12 years. CPPs grow slowly and eventually block the flow of cerebrospinal fluid causing hydrocephalus and increased intracranial pressure. CPP is most effectively treated with surgery which resolves the hydrocephalus in half of the patients. Patients can require a shunt in addition to re-section.

Clinical geneticist

A professional who uses your history and possibly blood tests to find out if you have for specific genes that increase cancer risk.

Clinical nurse specialist

Has expertise in subspecialty areas such as Neurosurgery or Neurooncology. Can assist physicians.

Craniopharyngioma

It is not cancer and technically is not a "brain" tumor, though it occurs inside the head. They commonly affect infants and children. Developing from cells left over from early fetal development, they are located just behind the nose, near the pituitary gland. Pressure from the tumor can cause headache or disturbance in the pituitary gland's function. Treatment usually includes surgery and, in some patients, radiation therapy.

CT or CAT scan Computerized Axial Tomography

An x-ray device linked to a computer produces an image of a cross-section of the brain. A special dye material may be injected into the patient's vein prior to the scan to help make any abnormal tissue more evident.

Cyst

A fluid filled sac. When not attached to a cancer, it is considered "benign." Benign cyst is different from a benign tumor. Cysts can be associated with a tumor.

DNET

Dysembryoplastic neuroepithelial tumor or desmoplastic cerebral astrocytoma. This is a variety of astrocytoma or mixed tumor, occurs in infancy or childhood and is extremely rare (less than 1 %). DNETs are often confused with a GBM by pathologists not familiar with childhood brain tumors. Surgery is often curative.

Ependymoma

Ependymomas usually affect children and develop from cells that line the hollow cavities of the brain (ventricles) and the canal inside the spine. About 85% of ependymomas are low grade but often are locally invasive. The pathologist's grade is not always predictive of their growth potential. Treatment usually includes surgery and then radiation therapy. Chemotherapy is used, especially for recurrent tumors.

Fellow

A graduate physician who has completed medical school, and residency training in an area of specialty such as internal medicine, pediatrics, or neurosurgery. The Fellow is the professor's right hand man.

Ganglioglioma

This is the rarest form of (mixed) glioma and contains both glial cells and mature nerve cells (neurons). They grow slowly in the brain or spinal cord. Gangliogliomas are usually treated with surgery. See MIXED GLIOMAS.

Gene therapy

An experimental treatment technique in which a gene (as a segment of DNA on a chromosome) is transferred into a patient's tumor cells.

Genes

The blueprints for our characteristics. Each gene sits on a DNA (deoxyribonucleic acid) "fence." They are located inside the center (nucleus) of our cells in structures called chromosomes that come in pairs. We have 46 chromosomes or 23 pairs.

Genetic analysis

The technique that researchers use to study the genes and the proteins for which they code.

Genetic testing

The procedure or test on a patient's blood or tissues to determine the presence of a known inherited gene.

Genetics

The study of heredity or the passing of characteristics (such as height, eye color, or tendency to get a tumor) from one generation to the next.

Germinoma

This family of tumor types that can occur anywhere in the body, usually in the midline (chest, ovaries, testicles, brain)as opposed to one side or the other. It can spread to the brain from anywhere else, or actually start to grow from there. Over the last 75 years, various names have been used for the different types: seminomas, germ cell tumors, teratomas, endodermal sinus tumor, choriocarcinoma (from the placenta), and non-germinomatous germ cell tumor.

In the brain, most do develop from the pineal gland and are called pineal region tumors (location). The tumor is made up of very primitive embryonic cells and sometimes can even contain teeth, muscle tissue or other glands (teratoma). Knowledge of the exact type is critical for your treatment success, as the different types require very specific therapies.

Glioma

A tumor from glial or astrocyte cells. Astrocytoma and glioma are interchangeable words in this book. There are a few gliomas that are called "benign," but they are more accurately named "low grade" (slow growing). High-grade gliomas are more malignant (faster growing). About half of all primary brain tumors are gliomas. Within the brain, gliomas usually occur in the lobes of the upper part of the brain; but they may also grow in other areas, especially the optic nerve, the brain stem, and particularly among children in the cerebellum. Gliomas are classified into several groups because there are different kinds of glial cells. See also ASTROCYTOMA and OLIGODENDROGLIOMA, mixed glioma.

Glioma of the brain stem

See BRAIN STEM GLIOMA.

Hemangioblastoma

A rare, non-cancerous tumor which arises from the blood vessels of the brain and the spinal cord. The most common form is linked in a small number of people as an inherited, genetic disorder called von Hippel-Lindau disease. Hemangioblastomas do not usually spread. Surgery can be curative. Kidney cancer, adrenal tumors and retinal abnormalities can also be present so a screening evaluation is recommended. (Derived from Brain Tumor Society, Bruce Cohen, & www.virtualtrial.com)

Hereditary cancer syndrome

The specific pattern of cancer types in a single individual or family; a strong indicator of a single gene mutation.

Hereditary non-polyposis colon cancer (HNPCC),

A mismatch repair gene that can lead to brain and colon cancer.

Hospice

Emphasizes strict attention to comfort rather than cure. It offers care in four major areas of life: physical, spiritual, psychological, and social. Hospice today is a model of care, not just a specific place.

Hospice team

Physicians, nurses, social workers, counselors, hospice certified nursing assistants, clergy, therapists, and volunteers.

Indemnity insurance

Allows you to go to any doctor, hospital, or other provider (who would bill for each service given); the insurance and the patient each pay part of the bill.

Insurance terms

See Chapters 23A and 23B.

Karnofsky score

It is a measure of your ability to perform activities of daily living likes getting dressed, feeding yourself. It measures how you are responding to treatments and can determine your eligibility and strength to enroll on a clinical trial.

Lesion

A catch-all "doctor speak" term for any tissue mass ("lump") in question.

Living will

A legal document that makes sure that your wishes about living and dying are carried out.

Malignant cancer

A tumor that has grown or is growing, usually rapidly, and will not stop without some type of therapy.

Medical student

In medical school, but is not part of the house staff and is not a hospital employee.

Medulloblastoma

Represents more than 25% of all childhood brain tumors and is a PNET. Other more rare PNETs include Neuroblastomas, Pineoblastomas, Medullo-epitheliomas, Ependymoblastomas. Because their malignant cells can spread by the spinal fluid, PNETs are more difficult to remove totally through surgery. Doctors usually remove as much tumor as possible with surgery, and then prescribe radiation and chemotherapy.

Meningioma

Meningioma is not a true brain tumor. It develops from thin membrane, or meninges, that cover the brain and the spinal cord. Meningiomas account for 25% of all brain tumors. They affect people of all ages, but are most common among those in their 40s. Meningiomas grow slowly, generally do not invade surrounding normal tissue, and rarely spread to other parts of the nervous system; most are benign. Surgery is the preferred treatment for meningiomas. Recurrent meningiomas may require additional treatment including radiation therapy.

Metastasis

A tumor that has spread from some other part of the body.

Metastatic Tumor

A tumor that has spread (to the brain) from elsewhere. Most frequently, the original sites are lung, colon, and breast cancer as well as melanoma. Therapy depends on the number of tumors, their size, and whether the primary tumor is under control, or not. There are many clinical trials using new treatments; several look promising.

Mixed Glioma

A tumor that contains more than one type of glial cell, usually astrocytes and oligodendroglial cells. Neuropathologists do not always agree on the difference between mixed gliomas and anaplastic oligodendrogliomas. New tests detecting lost genes (1p/ 19q) help predict which of these tumors will respond to chemotherapy and radiation. See also oligodendroglioma and ganglioglioma.

Mutation

Changes in the genes that occur (in a tumor) over time.

Narrative

Our own important story that is our life. It represents the threads in the fabric of our being.

Neurofibromatosis (NF-1),

A genetic condition in which grape-like tumors appear along the nerves in the arms, legs and spine, and sometimes in the brain and optic nerves.

Nurse Practitioner (CNP)

They are certified and licensed to examine, diagnose, and make independent treatment decisions in the absence of a physician.

Oligodendroglioma (O-lee-go-den-dro-glee-oma)

This tumor, a form of glioma (5-8% of all brain tumors) can often present with a seizure or a bleed inside the brain.. They arise from the special glial cells, oligodendroglia, that wrap around the nerves and insulate them. They occur most often in adults 30-55 years old and start within the brain's cerebral hemispheres. These tumors are treated with surgery. If completely removed and are low grade or benign, no further therapy is needed. The more malignant and recurring types can be very responsive to chemotherapy and radiation. Long term survivals are common.

Optic nerve gliomas

These astrocytomas or gliomas are found on or in the optic nerve and are particularly common in persons with Neurofibromatosis 1, also called NF-1. Treatment may include observation, surgery, radiation or chemotherapy. The most important factors affecting therapy decisions are vision preservation and damage to other parts of the brain.

Palliative care

Extends a principle of hospice care to a larger population; typically it begins earlier in the illness. No specific therapy is excluded.

Physician's Assistant (PA)

May have been a medic in the Armed Forces, an emergency medical technician (EMT) who has received two to three years of training and is licensed by the state. Physician's assistants work under the supervision and direction of a physician.

Pineal tumor

The pineal gland is a small structure deep within the center of the brain. Pineal tumors are very rare, about 1% of brain tumors. Surgery for a biopsy to confirm the tumor type is very important. Different types of tumors requiring different therapies can all look identical on the CT and MRI scans. The three most common pineal region tumors are gliomas, germ cell tumors, and primitive neuroectodermal tumors (PNETs). Radiation or chemotherapy, or both are used for malignant pineal tumors.

Pineocytoma

A rare tumor of the pineal gland that is usually removed by surgery and requires no additional therapy. A few are mixed with cells that are more immature and re-grow and can spread. Tumors that cannot be resected are commonly treated with radiation. Little data exists for any reliable chemotherapy. (See supratentorial PNETs).

Pituitary adenoma

Tumors that compriser about 10% of tumors in the head. Doctors classify pituitary adenomas into two major groups: 1) secreting Vs. non-secreting and 2) micro adenomas (<1.5 cm) Vs. macroadenomas (>1.5cm). Secreting tumors release unusually high levels of pituitary hormones, triggering one or many symptoms. These can include a) decreased sexual function or desire (impotence), b) loss of menstrual periods (amenorrhea), c) milk production in male or female breast (galactorrhea caused by prolactin), d) abnormal body growth (acromegaly), e) high blood pressure, f) sugar diabetes and fat deposits in the face and neck (Cushing's syndrome), or g) hyperthyroidism. Surgery and / or the drug bromocriptine or its newer drug successors treat prolactin-secreting pituitary adenomas. Larger, non-secreting adenomas are treated with surgery and radiation therapy.

Pituitary or "master gland"

A small oval-shaped structure located at the base of the brain, is just behind the nose. This "master gland' releases several chemical messengers called hormones, which control the body's other glands and influence the body's growth, metabolism, and sexual function and maturation.

Primitive Neuroectodermal Tumor or PNET

Primitive neuroectodermal tumors (PNETs) usually affect children and young adults. Their name reflects the belief held by many scientists that these tumors spring from primitive cells left over from early development of the nervous system. PNETs are very malignant; grow rapidly and about 35% spread easily within the brain and spinal cord. In rare cases, they spread outside the CNS. They used to be called Medulloblastoma when they occurred in the back of the brain, near the cerebellum.

Professor or consultant

Also called attending physicians (attendings). He/ she is "top of the ladder" for responsibility.

Risk

The chance or odds that an event can happen to you.

Schwannoma

A tumor that comes from the cells that form a protective sheath around the body's nerve fibers. They're usually benign and surgically removed when possible. One of the more common forms of this tumor affects the eighth cranial nerve, which contains nerve cells important for balance and hearing. Facial paralysis may occur if the tumor involves the adjacent seventh nerve. Also known as vestibular schwannomas or acoustic neuromas, these tumors may grow on one or both sides of the brain and are potentially curable with stereotactic radiosurgery. People with a different form of inherited Neurofibromatosis, NF-2, can have these and benign meningiomas as well.

Teaching hospital

Has a nationally approved educational program for Nursing or Medicine.

Teratoma, Malignant Teratoma

A member of the family of germ cell (germinoma) tumors. It is composed of two or more cell types and can contain teeth, skin and hair. The more slow growing ones are called teratomas. Malignant teratomas secrete "marker" proteins called AFP, and B-hG that are detected in the blood and spinal fluid. They are treated with a combination of chemotherapy and radiation.

Tumor or neoplasm

A solid "anything" that should not be there, before or after it is actually diagnosed.

UBO

Doctor-speak for "unidentified bright objects" on an MRI scan.

Vascular Tumor

A rare, non-cancerous tumor arising from the blood vessels of the brain and the spinal cord. The most common vascular tumor is the hemangioblastoma, often linked with a genetic disorder called von Hippel-Lindau disease. Hemangioblastomas do not usually spread and surgery provides the cure. A screening is recommended to rule out renal cancer, adrenal tumors and retinal abnormalities.

References

CHAPTER 17

1 Paul Zeltzer, *Brain Tumors – Leaving The Garden Of Eden: A Survival Guide To Learning The Basics, Getting Organized & Finding Your Medical Team* (Encino, CA: Shilysca Press, 2004).

2 R. Benveniste, and R.I. Germano, "Evaluation of Factors Predicting Accurate Resection of High Grade Gliomas by Using Frameless Image-Guided Stereotactic Guidance," *Neurosurgical Focus*, 14:2003.

3 L. Recht, et al., "Quantitative measurement of quality outcome in malignant glioma patients using an independent living score (ILS). Assessment of a retrospective cohort," *J Neurooncol*, 2003 Jan;61(2):127-36.

4 P.M. Zeltzer, et al., "Metastasis stage, adjuvant treatment, and residual tumor are prognostic factors for medulloblastoma in children: conclusions from the Children's Cancer Group 921 randomized phase III study," *J Clin Oncol*, 1999 Mar;17(3):832-45.

5 A.L. Albright, et al., "Effects of medulloblastoma resections on outcome in children: a report from the Children's Cancer Group," *Neurosurgery*, 1996 Feb;38(2):265-71.

6 J.A. Cowan, et al., "The impact of provider volume on mortality after intracranial tumor resection," *Neurosurgery*, 2003 Jan;52(1):48-53; discussion 54.

7 D.M. Long, et al., "Outcome and cost of craniotomy performed to treat tumors in regional academic referral centers," *Neurosurgery*, 2003 May;52(5):1056-63.

8 M.J. Glantz, et al., "Practice parameter: anticonvulsant prophylaxis in patients with newly diagnosed brain tumors; Report of the Quality Standards Subcommittee of the American Academy of Neurology," *Neurology*, 2000 May 23;54(10):1886-93, http://www.aan.com/professionals/practice/pdfs/gl0059.pdf

9 E.C. Nwokedi, et al., "Gamma knife stereotactic radiosurgery for patients with glioblastoma multiforme," *Neurosurgery*, 2002 Jan; 50(1): 41-6; discussion 46-7.

10 D.C. Shrieve, et al., "Treatment of patients with primary glioblastoma multiforme with standard postoperative radiotherapy and radiosurgical boost: prognostic factors and long-term outcome," *J Neurosurg*, 1999 Jan; 90(1): 72-7.

11 G. Berg, E. Blomquist, and E. Cavallin-Stahl, "A systematic overview of radiation therapy effects in brain tumours," *Acta Oncol*, 2003;42(5-6):582-8.

12 S.B. Tatter, et al., "An inflatable balloon catheter and liquid 125I radiation source (GliaSite Radiation Therapy System) for treatment of recurrent malignant glioma: multicenter safety and feasibility trial," *J Neurosurg*, 2003 Aug;99(2):297-303.

13 G. Akabani, et al., "Vascular targeted endoradiotherapy of tumors using alpha-particle-emitting compounds: theoretical analysis," *Int J Radiat Oncol Biol Phys*, 2002:54(4):1259-75.

14 D.A. Reardon, et al., "Phase II trial of murine (131)I-labeled antitenascin monoclonal antibody 81C6 administered into surgically created resection cavities of patients with newly diagnosed malignant gliomas," *J Clin Oncol*, 2002 Mar 1;20(5):1389-97.

15 T.A. Kaleita, et al., "Prediction of neurocognitive outcome in adult brain tumor patients," *J Neurooncol*, 2004 Mar-Apr;67(1-2):245-53.

16 A. Auperin, "Prophylactic cranial irradiation for patients with small-cell lung cancer in complete remission," *N Engl J Med*, 1999 Aug 12;341(7):476-84.

17 A. Muacevic, et al., "Stereotactic radiosurgery for multiple brain metastases from breast carcinoma," *Cancer*, 2004 Apr 15;100(8):1705-11.

18 International Radiosurgery Support Association, P.O. Box 60950, Harrisburg, PA, 17106 USA, 2002. (Phone: 717-671-1701, Fax: 717-671-1703, www.irsa.org).

19 M.D. Walker, et al., "Randomized comparisons of radiotherapy and nitrosoureas for the treatment of malignant glioma after surgery," *N Engl J Med*, 1980;303(23): 1323-9.

20 Retrieved February 28, 2005 at http://www.virtualtrials.com/temodar.

21 V.A. Levin, et al., "Phase III randomized study of postradiotherapy chemotherapy with combination alpha-difluoromethylornithine-PCV versus PCV for anaplastic gliomas," *Clin Cancer Res*, 2003 Mar;9(3):981-90. Additionally: S. Gundersen, K. Lote, and K. Watne, "A retrospective study of the value of chemotherapy as adjuvant therapy to surgery and radiotherapy in grade 3 and 4 gliomas," *Eur J Cancer*, 1998 Sep;34(10):1565-9.

22 M.D. Prados, et al., "Procarbazine, lomustine, and vincristine (PCV) chemotherapy for anaplastic astrocytoma: A retrospective review of radiation therapy oncology group protocols comparing survival with carmustine or PCV adjuvant chemotherapy," *J Clin Oncol*, 1999 Nov;17(11):3389-95.

23 S. Gundersen, K. Lote, and K. Watne, "A retrospective study of the value of chemotherapy as adjuvant therapy to surgery and radiotherapy in grade 3 and 4 gliomas," *Eur J Cancer*, 1998 Sep;34(10):1565-9.

24 R.A. Kristof, et al., "Combined surgery, radiation, and PCV chemotherapy for astrocytomas compared to oligodendrogliomas and oligoastrocytomas WHO grade III," *J Neurooncol*, 2002;59(3):231-7.

25 M.J. van den Bent, O.L. Chinot, and J.G. Cairncross, "Recent developments in the molecular characterization and treatment of oligodendroglial tumors," *Neuro-oncol*, 2003 Apr;5(2):128-38.

26 M.J. van den Bent, et al., "Second-line chemotherapy with temozolomide in recurrent oligodendroglioma after PCV (procarbazine, lomustine and vincristine) chemotherapy: EORTC Brain Tumor Group phase II study," *Ann Oncol*, 2003 Apr;14(4):599-602.

27 M. Westphal, et al, "A phase 3 trial of local chemotherapy with biodegradable carmustine (BCNU) wafers (Gliadel wafers) in patients with primary malignant glioma," *Neuro-oncol*, 2003; 5(2): 79-88.

28 R. Stupp, et al., "Promising survival for patients with newly diagnosed glioblastoma multiforme treated with concomitant radiation plus temozolomide followed by adjuvant temozolomide," *J Clin Oncol*, 2002 Mar 1; 20(5):1375-82. Comment in: *J Clin Oncol*, 2002 Jul 15;20(14):3179-80; discussion 3181-2.

CHAPTER 18

1 C.D. Myers, J. Bergman, and L.K. Zeltzer, "Complementary and alternative medicine use in children with cancer," excerpted from *Psychosocial Aspects of Pediatric Oncology*, edited by S. Kreitler and M.B. Arush (New York: Wiley, 2004).

2 P.M. Wolsko, D.M. Eisenberg, and R.B. Davis, "Insurance coverage, medical conditions, and visits to alternative medicine providers: results of a national survey," *Arch Intern Med*, 2002 Feb 11;162(3):281-7.

3 D.M. Eisenberg, R.B. Davis, and S.L. Ettner, "Trends in alternative medicine use in the United States, 1990-1997: results of a follow-up national survey, et al., *JAMA*, 1998 Nov 11;280(18): 1569-75.

4 Paul Zeltzer, *Brain Tumors – Leaving The Garden Of Eden: A Survival Guide To Learning The Basics, Getting Organized & Finding Your Medical Team* (Encino, CA: Shilysca Press, 2004).

5 Retrieved March 1, 2005 at http://cis.nci.nih.gov/fact/4_13.htm. Additionally: G.S. Omenn, et al., "Risk factors for lung cancer and for intervention effects in CARET, the Beta-Carotene and Retinol Efficacy Trial," *J Natl Cancer Inst*, 1996 Nov 6;88 (21):1550-9. Comment in: *J Natl Cancer Inst*, 1996 Nov 6;88(21):1513-5; *J Natl Cancer Inst*, 1997 Feb 19;89(4):325-6; and *J Natl Cancer Inst*, 1997 Nov 19;89(22):1722-3.

6 W.A. Weiger, et al., "Advising patients who seek complementary and alternative medical therapies for cancer," *Ann Intern Med*, 2002; 137(11): 889-903. Comment in: *Ann Intern Med*, 2003 Jul 15;139(2):152.

7 Refer to: http://almaproject.dpsk12.org/stories/storyReader$11; http://pages.prodigy.com/GBonline/liquix.htm; and http://www.tdh.state.tx.us/hcqs/ems/MA03Folkmed.htm.

8 Retrieved March 1, 2005 at http://www.fiery-foods.com/dave/capsaicin.asp.

9 Retrieved March 1, 2005 at http:// www.marinol.com.

10 B.R. Cassileth, and C.C. Chapman, "Alternative and complementary cancer therapies," *Cancer*, 1996 Mar 15;77(6):1026-34.

11 Personal communication with Jeanne Wallace, PhD, on Jan 19, 2004; nutritionalsolutions@comcast.net.

12 J.T. Roberstson, et al., "Metabolic Therapy of Malignant Gliomas," *Oncology of the Nervous System*, p. 278, edited by Michael Walker (Boston: Kluwer Academic Pub, 1983). Additionally: P. Gadisseux, et al., "Nutrition and the neurosurgical patient," *J Neurosurg*, 1984;60(2):219-32.

13 Personal communication with Jeanne Wallace, PhD, on January 22, 2004.

14 S. Somasundaram, et al., "Dietary curcumin inhibits chemotherapy-induced apoptosis in models of human breast cancer," *Cancer Res*, 2002 Jul 1;62(13):3868-75.

15 R.H. Mathijssen, J. Verweij, and P. De Bruijn, "Effects of St. John's Wort on Irinotecan Metabolism," *J Natl Cancer Inst*, 2002 Aug 21;94(16):1247-9.

16 E.J. Rousseau, A.J. Davison, and B. Dunn, "Protection by beta-carotene and related compounds against oxygen-mediated cytotoxicity and genotoxicity: implications for carcinogenesis and anticarcinogenesis," *Free Radic Biol Med*, 1992 Oct;13(4):407-33.

17 J.L. Schwartz, and G. Shklar, "Retinoid and carotenoid angiogenesis: a possible explanation for enhanced oral carcinogenesis," *Nutr Cancer*, 1997;27(2):192-9. Erratum in: *Nutr Cancer*, 1997;28(2):218.

18 Verhoef, et al., "Alternative therapy use in neurologic diseases: Use in brain tumor patients," *Neurology*, 1999;52(3):617-622.

19 J. Beuth, et al., "Impact of complementary oral enzyme application on the postoperative treatment results of breast cancer patients--results of an epidemiological multicentre retrospective cohort study," *Cancer Chemother Pharmacol*, 2001 Jul;47 Suppl:S45-54.

20 M. Winking, et al., "Boswellic acids inhibit glioma growth: a new treatment option?" *J Neurooncol*, 2000; 46(2): 97-103.

21 K. Ilc, et al., "Cytotoxic effects of two gamma linoleic salts (lithium gammalinolenate or meglumine gammalinolenate) alone or associated with a nitrosourea: an experimental study on human glioblastoma cell lines," *Anticancer Drugs*, 1999 Apr;10(4):413-7.

22 P. Greenwald P, et al., "Genetic and cellular changes in colorectal cancer: proposed targets of chemopreventive agents," *Cancer Epidemiol Biomarkers Prev*, 1995 Oct-Nov;4(7):691-702. Additionally: P. Greenwald, et al., "Chemoprevention," *CA Cancer J Clin*, 1995 Jan-Feb;45(1): 31-49.

23 A. Cristoni, found in *Natural Medicine—Instructions for Patients*, by L. Pizzorno, J. Pizzorno, Jr., and M. Murray (London: Harcourt Health Sciences, 2002); pp. 374. Additionally: *Fitoterapia*, 2003 Feb;74(1-2):197; and "CAM differentiated," by J.E. Pizzorno, Jr., *Med Anthropol Q.* 2002 Dec;16(4):405-7.

24 F.S. Kenny, et al., "Gamma linolenic acid with tamoxifen as primary therapy in breast cancer," *Int J Cancer*, 2000 Mar 1;85(5):643-8.

25 U.N. Das, V.V. Prasad, and D.R. Reddy, "Local application of gamma-linolenic acid in the treatment of human gliomas," *Cancer Lett*, 1995 Aug 1;94(2):147-55.

26 P. Lissoni, et al., "Increased survival time in brain glioblastomas by a radioneuroendocrine strategy with radiotherapy plus melatonin compared to radiotherapy alone," *Oncology*, 1996 Jan-Feb;53(1):43-6.

27 D. Lenartz, et al., "Survival of glioma patients after complementary treatment with galactoside-specific lectin from mistletoe," *Anticancer Res*, 2000 May-Jun;20(3B):2073-6.

28 H.J. Gabius, et al., "Evidence for stimulation of tumor proliferation in cell lines and histotypic cultures by clinically relevant low doses of the galactoside-binding mistletoe lectin," *Cance Invest*, 2001; 19: 114-126.

29 S. Kurashige, Y. Akuzawa, and F. Endo, "Effects of Lentinus edodes, Grifola frondosa, and Pleurotus Ostreatus administration on cancer outbreak, and activities of macrophages and lymphocytes in mice treated with a carcinogen, N-butyl-n-butanolnitrosoamine," *Immunopharmacology and Immunotoxicology*, 1997, 19(2);175-183.

30 S. Wang S, et al., "The anti-tumor effect of Ganoderma Lucidum is mediated by cytokines released from activated macrophages and T lymphocytes," *Int Journal Cancer*, 1997;70:699-705.

31 H. Nanba, "Activity of Maitake D-fraction to inhibit Carconogenesis and Metastasis," Annals of the New York Academy of Sciences, 1995;768:243-245.

32 Y. Yamada, H. Nanba, and H. Kuroda, "Antitumor effect of orally administered extracts from fruit body of Grifola frondosa (Maitake)," *Chemotherapy*, 1990;38:790-796.

33 M. Torisu, et al., "Significant Prolongation of disease-free period gained by oral polysaccharide K (PSK) administration after curative surgical operation of colorectal cancer," *Cancer Immunol Immunother*, 1990; 31:261-268.

34 J. Zhu, G.M. Halpern, and K. Jones, "The scientific rediscovery of a precious ancient Chinese herbal regimen: Cordyceps Sinesis Part II," *The Journal of Alternative and Complimentary Therapies*, vol. 4; no. 4 (1998), p429-457.

35 C. Xiaoguang, et al., "Cancer chemopreventive and therapeutic activities of red ginseng," *Journal of Ethno Pharmacology*, vol. 60 (1998), p71-78.

36 G. Janssen, et al., "Boswellic acids in the palliative therapy of children with progressive or relapsed brain tumors," *Klin Padiatr*, 2000 Jul-Aug; 212(4): 189-95.

37 Retrieved on March 1, 2005 at http://www.wholehealthmd.com/refshelf/substances_view/ 1,1525,760,00.html.

38 D. Melchart, et al., "Results of five randomized studies on the immunomodulatory activity of preparations of echinacea," *Journal of Alternative and Complementary Medicine*, 1995;1(2):145-159.

39 W. Grimm, "A randomized controlled trial of the effect of fluid extract of echinacea purpura on the incidence of severity of colds and respiratory infections," *The American Journal of Medicine*, 1999;106(2):138-143.

40 O. Hoheisel, "Echinagard treatment shortens the course of the common cold: a double-blind, placebo-controlled clinical trial," *European Journal of Clinical Research*, 1997;9:261-268.

41 J. Snow, "Echinacea (Moench) Spp. Asteraceae," *The Protocol Journal of Botanical Medicine*, Vol 2(2);18-24.

42 J. Buckner, et al., Phase II Study of Antineoplastons A10 (NSC 648539) and AS2-1 (NSC 620261) in Patients With Recurrent Glioma. Mayo Clinic Proceedings,1999 74(2):137-145

43 "Antinoeplastons: a request for phase II trial in CNS malignancies," *CTEP Lett* 1992 May; 10:10.

44 D. Quinn-nance, "A Case History of Glioblastoma," *American Journal of Nursing*, 1999;99(12): 24FF,24HH.

45 Cancer Guide Page By Steve Dunn, © Steve Dunn 1995-2003.

REFERENCES

385

46 Reviewed in L.K. Zeltzer, et al., "A phase I study on the feasibility and acceptability of an acupuncture/hypnosis intervention for chronic pediatric pain," *J Pain Symptom Manage*, 2002 ;24(4):437-46. Additionally: Z.H. Cho, et al., "New findings of the correlation between acupoints and corresponding brain cortices using functional MRI," *Proc Natl Acad Sci*, USA, 1998 ; 95(5): 2670-3.

47 Z.H. Cho, et al., "New findings of the correlation between acupoints and corresponding brain cortices using functional MRI," *Proc Natl Acad Sci*, USA, 1998 ; 95(5): 2670-3.

48 A.J. Vickers, and B.R. Cassileth, "Unconventional therapies for cancer and cancer-related symptoms," *Lancet Oncol*, 2001;2:226.

49 J. Shen, et al., "Electro-acupuncture for control of myeloblative chemotherapy-induced emesis: A randomized controlled trial," *JAMA*, 2000;284:2755.

50 A.J. Vickers, "Can acupuncture have specific effects on health? A systematic review of acupuncture antiemesis trials," *J R Soc Med*, 1996;89:303.

51 J.W. Dundee, et al., "Acupuncture prophylaxis of cancer chemotherapy-induced sickness," *J R Soc Med*, 1989 May;82(5):268-71.

52 D. Melchart, K. Linde, and P. Fischer, "Acupuncture for recurrent headaches: a systematic review of randomized controlled trials," *Cephalalgia*, 1999 Nov;19(9):779-86; discussion 765. Erratum in: *Cephalalgia*, 2000 Oct;20(8):762-3.

53 Comment on Ernst and White, *Pain*, 71 (1997) 123-126. Additionally: S.A. King, *Pain*, 1998 May;76(1-2):267-8.

54 L. Loh, et al., "Acupuncture versus medical treatment for migraine and muscle tension headaches," *J Neurol Neurosurg Psychiatry*, 1984 Apr;47(4):333-7.

55 Vasant Lad, *The Complete Book of Ayurvedic Home Remedies* (Minneapolis: Three Rivers Press, 1999).

56 C.D. Joseph, "Psychological supportive therapy for cancer patients," *Indian Journal of Cancer*, vol.20 (1983), p268-270.

57 S.M. Sellick, and C. Zaza, "Critical review of 5 nonpharmacology strategies for managing cancer pain," *Cancer Prevention and Control*, vol. 2; no.1 (1998), p7-14.

58 S. Wilkinson, "Get the massage," *Nursing Times*, vol. 92; no. 34 (August 21, 1996), p62-64.

59 M.C. Smith, et al., "Outcomes of therapeutic massage for hospitalized cancer patients," *J Nurs Scholarsh*, 2002;34(3):257-62.

60 A.T. Ferrell-Torry, and O.J. Glick, "The use of therapeutic massage as a nursing intervention to modify anxiety and the perception of cancer pain," *Cancer Nursing*, vol. 16; no. 2 (1993), p93-101.

61 M. Villaire, "Healing touch therapy makes a difference in surgery unit," *Crit Care Nurse*, 1999 Feb;19(1):104.

62 S.M. Sellick, and C. Zaza, "Critical review of 5 nonpharmacologic strategies for managing cancer pain," *Cancer Prev Control*, 1998 Feb;2(1):7-14.

63 K. Olson, and J. Hanson, "Using Reiki to manage pain: a preliminary report," *Cancer Prev Control*, (1997) Jun;1(2):108-13.

64 A. Meares, "What can the cancer patient expect from intensive meditation," *Australian Family Physician*, 1980, vol. 9 May p322-325.

65 C.D. Joseph, "Psychological supportive therapy for cancer patients," *Indian Journal of Cancer*, 20 (1983), p268-270.

66 A. Newberg, et al., "The measurement of regional cerebral blood flow during the complex cognitive task of meditation: a preliminary SPECT study," *Psychiatry Res*, 2001 Apr 10;106(2): 113-22.

67 R.J. Davidson, et al., "Alterations in brain and immune function produced by mindfulness meditation," *Psychosom Med*, 2003 Jul-Aug; 65(4): 564-70.

68 K.J. Tracey, "The inflammatory reflex," *Nature*, 2002 Dec 19-26;420(6917):853-9.

69 D.J. Benor, "Prayer study: what about expectancy effects among the researchers themselves?" *Altern Ther Health Med*, 2002 Jan-Feb;8(1):20-1. Additionally: D.J. Benor, "Energy medicine for the internist," *Med Clin North Am*, 2002 Jan;86(1):105-25.

70 P.J. Benson, "Nursing unconquerable hope," *J Pediatr Oncol Nurs*, 1996 Oct;13(4):214-8.

71 J.A. Milton, "A tale of two rivers," *Health Prog*, 1992 Jan-Feb;73(1):87-88.

72 California Pacific Medical Center Research Institute, San Francisco, California, 94115, United States; Recruiting: Andrew Freinkel, M.D., Principal Investigator, 415-600-1294, freinkel@cooper.cpmc.org; Sheila Cahill, LAC (415) 600-1295, scahill@cooper.cpmc.org.

73 M.M. Kogon, et al., "Effects of medical and psychotherapeutic treatment on the survival of women with metastatic breast carcinoma," *Cancer*, 1997 Jul 15;80(2):225-30.

74 L. Zeltzer, and S. LeBaron, "Hypnosis and nonhypnotic techniques for reduction of pain and anxiety during painful procedures in children and adolescents with cancer," *Journal of Pediatrics*, 1982; 101:1032-1035.

75 L. Zeltzer, S. LeBaron, and P.M. Zeltzer, "The effectiveness of behavioral intervention for reducing nausea and vomiting in children and adolescents receiving chemotherapy," *Journal of Clinical Oncology*, 1984;2:683-690.

76 P. Ruzyla-Smith, et al., "Effects of hypnosis on the immune response: B-cells, T-cells, helper and suppressor cells," *Am J Clin Hypn*, 1995 Oct;38(2):71-9.

77 K. Olness, T. Culbert, and D. Uden, "Self-regulation of salivary immunoglobulin A by children," *Pediatrics*, 1989;83(1):66-71.

78 I.G. Finlay, O.L. Jones, "Hypnotherapy in palliative care," *J R Soc Med*, 1996 Sep;89(9):493-6.

79 S.J. Lynn, et al., "Hypnosis as an empirically supported clinical intervention: the state of the evidence and a look to the future," *Int J Clin Exp Hypn*, 2000 Apr;48(2):239-59.

80 E. Farace, and M.E. Shaffrey, "An Intervention with Caregivers Improves QOL for Malignant Brain Tumor Patients," *Neurooncology*, 3 (4). 338, 2001 (Abstract).

81 J.L. Richardson, et al., "The effect of compliance with treatment of survival among patients with hematologic malignancies," *Journal of Clinical Oncology*, vol. 18; (February 1990), p356-364.

82 M.B. Leavitt, S.A. Lamb, and B.S. Voss, "Brain tumor support group: content themes and mechanisms of support," *Oncol Nurs Forum*, 1996 Sep;23(8):1247-56). Retrieved on March 1, 2005 at http://www.ncbi.nlm.nih.gov/entrez/query.fcgi?cmd=Retrieve&db=PubMed&list_uids=8883072&dopt=Abstract

83 C.D. Joseph, "Psychological supportive therapy for cancer patients," *Indian Journal of Cancer*, vol. 20 (1983), 268-270.

84 F.I. Fawzy, et al., "A structured psychiatric intervention for cancer patients. II. Changes over time in immunological measures," *Arch Gen Psychiatry*, 1990 Aug;47(8):729-35.

85 F.I. Fawzy, and N.W. Fawzy, "Group therapy in the cancer setting," *J Psychosom Res*, 1998;45: 191-200.

86 F.I. Fawzy, A.L. Canada, and N.W. Fawzy, "Malignant melanoma: effects of a brief, structured psychiatric intervention on survival and recurrence at 10-year follow-up," *Arch Gen Psychiatry*, 2003 Jan;60(1):100-3.

87 D. Spiegel, et al., "Effect of psychosocial treatment on survival of patients with metastatic breast cancer," *Lancet*, 1989 Oct 14;2(8668):888-91. Comment in: *Lancet*, 1989 Nov 18;2(8673): 1209-10.

88 S. Moorey, et al., «A comparison of adjuvant psychological therapy and supportive counselling in patients with cancer,» *Psychooncology*, 1998 May-Jun;7(3):218-28.

89 R. Sloman, "Relaxation and the relief of cancer pain," *Nurs Clin North Am*, 1995 Dec;30(4):697-709.

90 N.J. Nelson, "Scents or nonsense: aromatherapy's benefits still subject to debate," *J Natl Cancer Inst*, 1997 Sep 17;89(18):1334-6.

91 P.L. Cerrato, "Aromatherapy: Is it for real?" *RN* (June 1998), p51-52.

92 C.E. Sabo, and S.R. Michael, "The influence of personal message with music on anxiety and side effects associated with chemotherapy," *Cancer Nurs*, 1996 Aug;19(4):283-9.

93 S.L. Beck, "The therapeutic use of music for cancer-related pain," *Oncol Nurs Forum*, 1991 Nov-Dec;18(8):1327-37.

94 Ben Williams, *Surviving "Terminal" Cancer* (Minneapolis: Fairview Press, 2002).

95 *Gale Encyclopedia of Alternative Medicine* (Boston: Gale Group, 2001).

CHAPTER 19

1 Paul Zeltzer, *Brain Tumors – Leaving The Garden Of Eden: A Survival Guide To Learning The Basics, Getting Organized & Finding Your Medical Team* (Encino, CA: Shilysca Press, 2004).

2 "To Err Is Human: Building a Safer Health System," edited by Linda T. Kohn, Janet M. Corrigan, and Molla S. Donaldson; Committee on Quality of Health Care in America, Institute of Medicine, Washington DC, 1999. Retrieved on March 2, 2005 at http://www4.nationalacademies.org/news.nsf/isbn/0309068371?OpenDocument

3 "20 Tips to Help Prevent Medical Errors in Children," Patient Fact Sheet, AHRQ Publication No. 02-P034, September 2002. Refer to http://www.ahrq.gov/consumer/20tipkid.htm, Rockville, MD.

4 H.S. Friedman, et al., "Irinotecan therapy in adults with recurrent or progressive malignant glioma," *J Clin Oncol*, 1999 May; 17(5):1516-25.

5 C.L. Bennett, et al., "Thalidomide-associated deep vein thrombosis and pulmonary embolism," *American Journal of Medicine*, 2002;113:603-606.

6 V.A. Levin, et al., "Phase III randomized study of post-radiotherapy chemotherapy with combination alpha-difluoromethylorni-thine PCV versus PCV for anaplastic gliomas," *Clin Cancer Res*, 2003;9(3):981-90.

7 G. Cairncross, et al., "Chemotherapy for anaplastic oligodendroglioma," National Cancer Institute of Canada Clinical Trials Group, *J Clin Oncol*, 1994 Oct;12(10):2013-21.

8 D.F. Lehmann, et al., "Anticonvulsant usage is associated with an increased risk of procarbazine hypersensitivity reactions in patients with brain tumors," *Clin Pharmacol Ther*, 1997; 62: 225-9.

9 Retrieved on March 2, 2005 at http://www.medformation.com/ac/mm_qdis.nsf/qd/nd2007g.htm.

10 Retrieved on March 2, 2005 at http://virtualtrials.com/pcvdiet.cfm.

11 E.S. Newlands, T. Foster, and S. Zaknoen, "Phase I study of temozolamide (TMZ) combined with procarbazine (PCB) in patients with gliomas," *Br J Cancer*, 2003 Jul 21;89(2):248-51.

12 R.B. Khan, et al., "A phase II study of extended low-dose temozolomide in recurrent malignant gliomas," *Neuro-oncol*, 2002 Jan;4(1):39-43.

13 Retrieved on March 2, 2005 at http://www.virtualtrials.com/tamoxifen4.cfm.

14 M. Westphal, et al., "A phase 3 trial of local chemotherapy with biodegradable carmustine (BCNU)wafers (Gliadel wafers) in patients with primary malignant glioma," *Neuro-oncol*, 2003: 5(2):79-88.

15 L. Kim, M.J. Glantz, "Neoplastic meningitis," *Curr Treat Options Oncol*, 2001 Dec;2(6):517-27.

16 M.C. Chamberlain, P.A. Kormanik, and D. Barba, "Complications associated with intraventricular chemotherapy in patients with leptomeningeal metastases," *J Neurosurg*, 1997 Nov;87(5): 694-9.

17 J.L. Gabrilove, et al., "Clinical evaluation of once-weekly dosing of epoetin alfa in chemotherapy patients: improvements in hemoglobin and quality of life are similar to three-times-weekly dosing," *J Clin Oncol*, 2001 Jun 1;19(11):2875-82.

18 G.D. Demetri, et al., "Quality-of-life benefit in chemotherapy patients treated with epoetin alfa is independent of disease response or tumor type: results from a prospective community oncology study," *J Clin Oncol*, 1998 Oct;16(10):3412-25.

19 P.L. Mitchell, B. Morland, and M.C. Stevens, "Granulocyte colony-stimulating factor in established febrile neutropenia: a randomized study of pediatric patients," *J Clin Oncol*, 1997 Mar;15(3):1163-70.

20 E.J. Yeoh, et al., "Topotecan-filgrastim combination is an effective regimen for mobilizing peripheral blood stem cells," *Bone Marrow Transplant*, 2001 Sep;28(6):563-71.

21 R.I. Jakacki, et al., "Dose-intensive, time-compressed procarbazine, CCNU, vincristine (PCV) with peripheral blood stem cell support and concurrent radiation in patients with newly diagnosed high-grade gliomas," *J Neurooncol*, 1999 Aug;44(1):77-83.

22 "American Society of Clinical Oncology guidelines for the use of hematopoietic colony-stimulating factors," *Curr Opin Hematol*, 1996 Jan; 3(1):3-10.

23 R. Garcia-Carbonero, et al., "Granulocyte colony-stimulating factor in the treatment of high-risk febrile neutropenia: a multicenter randomized trial," *J Natl Cancer Inst*, 2001 Jan 3;93(1):31-8.

24 J. Crawford, and M.A. O'Rourke, "Vinorelbine (Navelbine)/carboplatin combination therapy: dose intensification with granulocyte colony-stimulating factor," *Semin Oncol*, 1994 Oct;21(5 Suppl 10):73-8.

25 I. Tepler, L. Elias, and J.W. Smith, "A randomized placebo-controlled trial of recombinant human interleukin-11 in cancer patients with severe thrombocytopenia due to chemotherapy," *Blood*, 1996 May 1;87(9):3607-14.

26 J.W. Smith, "Tolerability and side effect profile of rhIL-11," *Oncology* (Huntingt), 2000 Sep;14 (9 Suppl 8):41-7.

Chapter 20

1 Paul Zeltzer, *Brain Tumors – Leaving The Garden Of Eden: A Survival Guide To Learning The Basics, Getting Organized & Finding Your Medical Team* (Encino, CA: Shilysca Press, 2004).

2 Retrieved on March 4, 2005 at http://www.chiroweb.com/archives/13/14/05.html.

3 Christina A. Meyers and Anne E. Kayl, in Chapter 26, "Neurocognitive Function" in *Cancer in The Nervous System*, 2nd Edition, edited by Victor A. Levin, M.D. (New York: Oxford University Press, 2002).

4 P. Ganz, UCLA Mann Center Lecture, Dec 2001. Retrieved on March 4, 2005 at http://cancerresources.mednet.ucla.edu/5_info/5c_archive_lec/2001/late_effects_survivor.htm

5 Retrieved on March 4, 2005 at http://www.cancer.org/docroot/NWS/content/NWS_1_1x_Researchers_Verify_%E2%80%98Chemo_Brain%E2%80%99_in_Cancer_Survivors.asp.

6 E.T. Viscosi, et al., «Quality of life (QOL) and sexual function in brain tumor (BT) patients,» 38th ASCO Annual Meeting, Orlando, FL, May 18-21, 2002 (Abstract No. 291).

7 W. Arlt, et al., «Frequent and frequently overlooked: treatment-induced endocrine dysfunction in adult long-term survivors of primary brain tumors,» *Neurology*, 1997 Aug;49(2):498-506.

8 Retrieved on March 4, 2005 at http://www.virtualtrials.com/faq\Sex.cfm.

9 L.R. Kleinberg, et al., "Clinical course and pathologic findings after Gliadel and radiotherapy for newly diagnosed malignant glioma: implications for patient management," *Cancer Invest*, 2004;22(1):1-9. Comment on: *Cancer Invest*. 2004;22(1):169.

10 G. Berg, E. Blomquist, and E. Cavallin-Stahl, "A systematic overview of radiation therapy effects in brain tumours," *Acta Oncol*, 2003;42(5-6):582-8.

11 A.A. Brandes, and S. Monfardini, "The treatment of elderly patients with high-grade gliomas," *Semin Oncol*, 2003 Dec;30(6 Suppl 19):58-62.

12 L. Recht, et al., "Quantitative measurement of quality outcome in malignant glioma patients using an independent living score (ILS). Assessment of a retrospective cohort," *J Neurooncol*, 2003 Jan;61(2):127-36.

13 M. Glantz, et al., "Temozolomide as an alternative to irradiation for elderly patients with newly diagnosed malignant gliomas," *Cancer*, 97; 2262-66, 2003.

14 Retrieved on March 4, 2005 at http://www.braintrust.org/forums/General/posts/207.html.

15 Thanks to Teresea Kenzig. Used with permission, 2003.

CHAPTER 21

1 R.L. Comis, et al., "Public attitudes toward participation in cancer clinical trials," *J Clin Oncol*, 2003 Mar 1;21(5):830-5.

2 D.D. Von Hoff, "The Future of Cancer Research," *Oncology Issues* 17(6):38-40, 2002.

3 M. Agrawal, and E.J. Emanuel, "Ethics of phase 1 oncology studies: reexamining the arguments and data," *JAMA*, 2003;290(8) :1075-82.

4 Paul Zeltzer, *Brain Tumors – Leaving The Garden Of Eden: A Survival Guide To Learning The Basics, Getting Organized & Finding Your Medical Team* (Encino, CA: Shilysca Press, 2004).

5 Retrieved on February 18, 2005 at http://virtualtrials.com/karnofsky.cfm.

6 Retrieved on February 18, 2005 at http://www.cdc.gov/nchstp/od/tuskegee/time.htm.

7 Retrieved on February 18, 2005 at http://www.hhs.gov/ohrp/humansubjects/guidance/belmont.htm.

8 Retrieved on February 18, 2005 at http://www.hhs.gov/ohrp/humansubjects/guidance/45cfr46.htm

9 Retrieved on February 18, 2005 at http://www.med.umich.edu/irbmed/FederalDocuments/hhs/HHS45CFR46.html

10 Robert Finn, *Cancer Clinical Trials: Experimental Treatments & How They Can Help You*, 1st Edition (Sebastopol, CA: O'Reilly Press, 1999). Additionally: Retrieved on February 18, 2005 at http://www.oreilly.com/catalog/cancerct.

11 A.A. Brandes, et al., "A prospective study on glioblastoma in the elderly," *Cancer*, 2003 Feb 1;97(3):657-62.

12 Clinical Trial Web Sites: A Promising Tool to Foster Informed Consent, May 2002. Office Of Inspector General, Washington DC; OEI-01-97-00198. Retrieved on February 18, 2005 at http://oig.hhs.gov/oei/reports/oei-01-97-00198.pdf.

13 BBC News Front Page, Tuesday, 29 July 2003. Retrieved on February 18, 2005 at http://news.bbc.co.uk/1/hi/england/hampshire/dorset/3107805.stm.

14 Retrieved on February 18, 2005 at http://www.fda.gov/orphan/progovw.htm.

CHAPTER 22A

1 T. Shiminski-Maher, Patsy Cullen, and M. Sansalone, *Childhood Brain & Spinal Cord Tumors: A Guide for Families, Friends, & Caregivers* (Sebastapol, CA: O'Reilly & Associates, 2002).

2 National Children's Cancer Foundation, 2004. Retrieved at http://www.nccf.org/childhoodcancer/facts.asp.

3 W.A. Bleyer, "The impact of childhood cancer on the United States and the world," *Cancer -Journal for Clinicians*, 1990; 40, 355-367.

4 N.S. Kadan-Lottick, et al., "Childhood cancer survivors' knowledge about their past diagnosis and treatment: Childhood Cancer Survivor Study," *JAMA*, 2002 Apr 10;287(14):1832-9.

5 F.D. Armstrong, and M. Horn, "Educational issues in childhood cancer," *School Psychology Quarterly*, 1995; 10, 292-304.

6 Paul Zeltzer, *Brain Tumors – Leaving The Garden Of Eden: A Survival Guide To Learning The Basics, Getting Organized & Finding Your Medical Team* (Encino, CA: Shilysca Press, 2004).

7 D.P. Frush, L.F. Donnelly, and N.S. Rosen, "Computed tomography and radiation risks: what pediatric health care providers should know," *Pediatrics*, 2003 Oct;112(4):951-7. Comment in: *Pediatrics*, 2003 Oct;112(4):971-2.

8 W.A. Bleyer, et al., "Reduction in central nervous system leukemia with a pharmacokinetically derived intrathecal methotrexate dosage regimen," *J Clin Oncol*, 1983 May;1(5):317-25.

9 Retrieved on February 16, 2005 at http://www.globalrph.com/bsa.cgi.

10 A.L. Albright, et al., "Correlation of neurosurgical subspecialization with outcomes in children with malignant brain tumors," *Neurosurgery*, 2000 Oct;47(4):879-85; discussion 885-7.

11 L. Harisiadis, and C.H. Chang, "Medulloblastoma in children: a correlation between staging and results of treatment," *Int J Radiat Oncol Biol Phys*, 1977 Sep-Oct;2(9-10):833-41.

12 P.M. Zeltzer, et al., "Metastasis stage, adjuvant treatment, and residual tumor are prognostic factors for medulloblastoma in children: conclusions from the Children's Cancer Group 921 randomized phase III study," *J Clin Oncol*, 1999 Mar;17(3):832-45.

13 S. Kramer, et al., "Influence of place of treatment on diagnosis, treatment, and survival in three pediatric solid tumors," *J Clin Oncol*, 1984 Aug;2(8):917-23.

14 Retrieved on February 16, 2005 at http://www.nccf.org/childhoodcancer/clinicaltrial.asp.

15 J.R. Geyer, et al., "Survival of infants with primitive neuroectodermal tumors or malignant ependymomas of the CNS treated with eight drugs in 1 day: a report from the Children's Cancer Group," *J Clin Oncol*, 1994 Aug;12(8):1607-15.

16 R.K. Mulhern, "Neuropsychological late effects," as found in D.J. Bearison & R.K. Mulhern (Eds.), *Pediatric Psychooncology: Psychological Perspectives on Children with Cancer* (Oxford University Press, 1994) pp. 99-121.

17 R. T. Brown, and A. Madan-Swain, "Cognitive, neuropsychological, and academic sequelae in children with leukemia," *Journal of Learning Disabilities*, 1993; 26, 74-90.

18 S. LeBaron, et al., "Assessment of quality of survival in children with medulloblastoma and cerebellar astrocytoma," *Cancer*, 1988 Sep 15;62(6):1215-22.

19 F.D. Armstrong, and M. Horn, "Educational issues in childhood cancer," *School Psychology Quarterly*, 1995; 10, 292-304.

20 R.T. Brown, et al., "A 3-year follow-up of the intellectual and academic functioning of children receiving central nervous system prophylactic chemotherapy for leukemia," *Developmental and Behavioral Pediatrics*, 1996; 17, 392-398.

21 Retrieved on February 16, 2005 at http://www.childhoodbraintumor.org/02cerebellarmutisml oice.htm.

22 P. Steinbok, et al., "Mutism after posterior fossa tumour resection in children: incomplete recovery on long-term follow-up," *Pediatr Neurosurg*, 2003 Oct; 39(4): 179-83.

23 J.G. Gurney, et al., "Endocrine and cardiovascular late effects among adult survivors of childhood brain tumors: Childhood Cancer Survivor Study," *Cancer*, 2003 Feb 1; 97(3): 663-73.

REFERENCES

CHAPTER 22B

1 A.E. Kazak, "Implications of survival: Pediatric oncology patients and their families," as found in D.J. Bearison & R.K. Mulhern (Eds.), *Pediatric Psychooncology: Psychological Perspectives on Children with Cancer* (Oxford University Press, 1994) pp. 171-193.

2 E.R. Katz, M.J. Dolgin, and J.W. Varni, "Cancer in children and adolescents," as found in A.M. Gross & R.S. Drabman (Eds.), *Handbook of Clinical Behavioral Pediatrics: Applied Clinical Psychology* (Plenum US, 1990) pp.129-146.

3 J.S. Pendley, L.M. Dahlquist, and Z. Dreyer, "Body image and psychosocial adjustment in adolescent cancer survivors," *Journal of Pediatric Psychology*, 1997; 22, 29-43.

4 J.W. Varni, et al., "Perceived physical appearance and adjustment of children with newly diagnosed cancer: A path analytic model," *Journal of Behavioral Medicine*, 1995; 18, 261-278.

5 J.W. Varni, et al., "Perceived social support and adjustment of children with newly diagnosed cancer," *Developmental and Behavioral Pediatrics*, 1994; 15, 20-26.

6 S. Shetsky, address at Florida Brain Tumor Association meeting, 2003.

7 N.S. Kadan-Lottick, et al., "Childhood Cancer Survivors' Knowledge About Their Past Diagnosis and Treatment: Childhood Cancer Survivor Study," *JAMA*, 2003; 287: 1832-1839.

8 M.M. Hudson, et al., "Health status of adult long-term survivors of childhood cancer: a report from the Childhood Cancer Survivor Study," *JAMA*, 2003 Sep 24;290(12):1583-92.

9 B.J. Zebrack, et al., "Psychological outcomes in long-term survivors of childhood brain cancer: a report from the childhood cancer survivor study," *J Clin Oncol*, 2004 Mar 15;22(6):999-1006.

10 M. Stuber, et al., "Stress responses after pediatric bone marrow transplantation: Preliminary results of a prospective longitudinal study," *Journal of the American Academy of Child and Adolescent Psychiatry*, 30, 952-957, (1991).

11 M.M. Stevens, and J.C. Dunsmore, "Adolescents who are living with a life-threatening illness," as found in C.A. Corr & D.E. Balk (Eds.), *Handbook of Adolescent Death and Bereavement* (Springer Publishing Company, 1996) pp. 107-135.

12 S.C. Carpentieri, et al., "Behavioral resiliency among children surviving brain tumors: A longitudinal study," *Journal of Clinical Child Psychology*, 22, 236-246, (1993).

13 M. Macedoni-Luksic, B. Jereb, and L. Todorovski, "Long-term sequelae in children treated for brain tumors: impairments, disability, and handicap," *Pediatr Hematol Oncol*, 2003 Mar; 20(2): 89-101.

14 Y. Kitajima, et al., "Successful twin pregnancy in panhypopituitarism caused by suprasellar germinoma," *Obstet Gynecol*, 2003 Nov; 102(5 Pt 2): 1205-7.

15 T. Petterson, et al., "Hyperprolactinaemia and infertility following cranial irradiation for brain tumours: successful treatment with bromocriptine," *Br J Neurosurg*, 1993; 7(5): 571-4.

16 P. Steinbok, et al., "Mutism after posterior fossa tumour resection in children: incomplete recovery on long-term follow-up," *Pediatr Neurosurg*, 2003 Oct; 39(4): 179-83.

17 Retrieved on February 18, 2005 at http://www.curesearch.org/patients/endtreatment/.

18 A.E. Kazak, et al., "Young adolescent cancer survivors and their parents: Adjustment, learning problems, and gender," *Journal of Family Psychology*, 1994; 8, 74-84.

19 R. Mulhern, et al., "Social competence and behavioral adjustment of children who are long-term survivors of cancer," *Pediatrics*, 1989; 83, 18-25.

20 J.S. Pendley, L.M. Dahlquist, and Z. Dreyer, "Body image and psychosocial adjustment in adolescent cancer survivors," *Journal of Pediatric Psychology*, 1997; 22, 29-43.

21 J.W. Varni, et al., "The impact of social skills training on the adjustment of children with newly diagnosed cancer," *Journal of Pediatric Psychology*, 1993; 18, p. 753.

22 Retrieved on February 18, 2005 at http://www.wrightslaw.com/info/section504.ada.peer.htm.

23 S.B. Lansky, M.A. List, and C. Ritter-Sterr, "Psychological consequences of cure," *Cancer*, 1986; 58, 529-533.

24 E.R. Katz, "Illness impact and social reintegration," as found in J. Kellerman (Ed.), *Psychological Aspects of Childhood Cancer* (Springfield, IL: Charles C. Thomas, 1980).

25 S.B. Lansky, et al., "School attendance among children with cancer: A report from two centers," *Journal of Psychosocial Oncology*, 1983; 1, 75-82.

26 S.B. Lansky, et al., "School phobia in children with malignant neoplasms," *American Journal of Disabilities in Children*, 1975; 129, 42-46.

27 Adapted, in part, from Sarah McDougal, Indiana University, December 11, 1997. Retrieved on February 16, 2005 at http://www.acor.org/ped-onc/cfissues/backtoschool/cwc.html.

28 S.B. Sexson, and A. Madan-Swain, "School reentry for the child with chronic illness," *Journal of Learning Disabilities*, 1993; 26, 115-125.

29 J.J. Spinetta, and P. Deasy-Spinetta, "The patient's socialization in the community and school during therapy," *Cancer*, 1986; 58, 512-518.

30 P. Deasy-Spinetta, and J. Spinetta, "The child with cancer in school," *American Journal of Pediatric Hematology and Oncology*, 1980; 2, 89-92.

31 S. Nessim, and E.R. Katz, "A model for school and social reintegration of children with chronic illness," Los Angeles, California: Children's Center for Cancer and Blood Diseases, 1995.

32 A. Goodell, "Peer education in schools for children with cancer," *Issues in Comprehensive Pediatric Nursing*, 1984; 7, 101-106.

33 E.R. Katz, M.J. Dolgin, and J.W. Varni, "Cancer in children and adolescents," as found in A.M. Gross & R.S. Drabman (Eds.), *Handbook of Clinical Behavioral Pediatrics: Applied Clinical Psychology* (Plenum US, 1990) pp.129-146.

34 J. Henning, and G.K. Fritz, "School reentry in childhood cancer," *Psychosomatics*, 1983; 24, 261-269.

35 J. Chekryn, M. Deegan, and J. Reid, "Normalizing the return to school of the child with cancer," *Journal of the Association of Pediatric Oncology Nurses*, 1986; 3, 20-24.

36 E.R. Katz, et al., "School and social reintegration of children with cancer," *Journal of Psychosocial Oncology*, 1988; 6, 123-140.

37 J. Chekryn, M. Deegan, and J. Reid, "Impact on teachers when a child with cancer returns to school," *Children's Health Care*, 1987; 15, 161-165.

38 L.L. Fryer, et al., "Helping the child with cancer: What school personnel want to know," *Psychological Reports*, 1989; 65, 563-566.

39 A.M. LaGreca, "Social consequences of pediatric conditions: Fertile area for future investigation and intervention," *Journal of Pediatric Psychology*, 1990; 15, 285-307.

40 P.A. Mabe, W.T. Riley, and F.A. Treiber, "Cancer knowledge and acceptance of children with cancer," *J Sch Health*, 1987 Feb;57(2):59-63.

41 R. Mulhern, et al., "Social competence and behavioral adjustment of children who are long-term survivors of cancer," *Pediatrics*, 1989; 83, 18-25.

42 V.C. Peckham, "Children with cancer in the classroom," Teaching Exceptional Children, 26, 1993, pp 26-32.

43 A.E. Kazak, et al., "Young adolescent cancer survivors and their parents: Adjustment, learning problems, and gender," *Journal of Family Psychology*, 1994; 8, 74-84.

44 P. Deasy-Spinetta, "The school and the child with cancer," as found in J. Spinetta & P. Deasy-Spinetta (Eds.), *Living with Childhood Cancer* (Mosby-Year Book, 1981) pp. 153-168.

45 E.R. Katz, et al., "Teacher, parent, and child evaluative ratings of a school reintegration intervention for children with newly diagnosed with cancer," *Children's Health Care*, 21, 69-75. 1992.

46 L.K. Zeltzer LK, and C.B. Schlank, *Conquering Your Child's Chronic Pain* (New York: HarperResource, 2005), pp 162-172.

47 Retrieved on February 16, 2005 at http://www.campronaldmcdonald.org/goodtimes/index2.htm and http://www.coca-intl.org.

48 Retrieved on February 16, 2005 at http://www.holeinthewallgang.org and http://www.hitwgcamps.org.

49 J.D. Dockerty, D.C.G. Skegg, and S.M. Williams, "Economic effects of childhood cancer on families," *Journal of Paediatrics and Child Health*, 2003; 39 (4), 254-258.

50 A.E. Kazak, et al., "Posttraumatic stress, family functioning, and social support in survivors of childhood leukemia and their mothers and fathers," *Journal of Consulting and Clinical Psychology*, 1997; 65, 120-129.

51 J.E. VanDongen-Melman, et al., "Late psychosocial consequences for parents of children who survived cancer," *Journal of Pediatric Psychology*, 1995; 20 567-586.

52 P.M. Zeltzer, et al., "Utilization of Medical Facility Support by European Children with Brain Tumors (CBT) at Barretstown: A Summer Therapeutic Recreation Camp," Abstract. Societe Internacionale Oncologie Pediatrie (SIOP Sept 2002), in *Med Ped Oncol* Sept. 2002.

53 B. Zebrack, "Reflections of a cancer survivor/research scientist," *Cancer*, 2003 Jun 1;97(11):2707-9.

54 U. Kreicbergs, et al., "Talking about death with children who have severe malignant disease," *N Engl J Med*, 2004 Sep 16;351:1175-86.

55 U. Kreicbergs, et al., "A population-based nationwide study of parents' perceptions of a questionnaire on their child's death due to cancer," *Lancet*, 2004 Aug 28;364(9436):787-9.

CHAPTER 23A

1 Brain Tumor Survival Guide, Brain Tumor Foundation of New York Web site, retrieved Dec 11, 2001.

2 Paul Zeltzer, *Brain Tumors – Leaving The Garden Of Eden: A Survival Guide To Learning The Basics, Getting Organized & Finding Your Medical Team* (Encino, CA: Shilysca Press, 2004).
   * See Glossary at end of chapter

3 Bush Administration proposal: "Medicare Drug Benefit May Cost $1.2 Trillion Estimate Dwarfs Bush's Original Price Tag," by Ceci Connolly and Mike Allen, Washington *Post* Staff Writers, Wednesday, February 9, 2005; Page A01.

4 "Prescription Drug Coverage for Medicare Beneficiaries: A Summary of the Medicare Prescription Drug, Improvement, and Modernization Act of 2003," Henry J. Kaiser Family Foundation 10 Dec 2003.

5 Adapted, in part, from "Checkup on Health Insurance Choices," AHCPR Publication No. 93-0018, December 1992. Agency for Health Care Policy and Research, Rockville, MD. Retrieved on February 12, 2005 at http://www.ahrq.gov/consumer/insuranc.htm.

6 Adapted, in part, from Danial Fortuno and Keren Stronach, MPH, Manager, Cancer Resource Center of the University of California, San Francisco, Comprehensive Cancer Center. Retrieved on February 12, 2005 at http://cc.ucsf.edu/crc/insurance per cent 5Fnotes.html.

CHAPTER 23B

1 Stella Chang, et al., "Estimating the Cost of Cancer: Results on the Basis of Claims Data Analyses for Cancer Patients Diagnosed with Seven Types of Cancer During 1999 to 2000," *J Clin Oncol*, 2004:22, pp. 3524-353.

2 Retrieved on February 12, 2005 at http://www.braintumorfoundation.org/hmos.htm.

3 Chapter 6, Paul Zeltzer, *Brain Tumors – Leaving The Garden Of Eden: A Survival Guide To Learning The Basics, Getting Organized & Finding Your Medical Team* (Encino, CA: Shilysca Press, 2004).

4 I am indebted to Ted Schreck, Chief Exec. Officer, University of Southern California University Hospital, for this advice on the manuscript.

5 *Oncology News International*, Volume 11, issue 11, Nov. 2002.

6 Paul Zeltzer, *Brain Tumors – Leaving The Garden Of Eden: A Survival Guide To Learning The Basics, Getting Organized & Finding Your Medical Team* (Encino, CA: Shilysca Press, 2004).

CHAPTER 24

1 S. Preston-Martin, "Epidemiology of primary CNS neoplasms," *Neurol Clin*, 1996 May;14(2):273-90.

2 Retrieved on March 9, 2005 at http://www.accessexcellence.org/AB/GG/dna.html.

3 B.P. O'Neill, et al., "Risk of cancer among relatives of patients with glioma," *Cancer, Epidemiol Biomarkers Prev*, 2002 Sep;11(9):921-4.

4 S. Baba, "Molecular biological background of FAP and HNPCC, and treatment strategies of both diseases depend upon genetic information," *Nippon Geka Gakkai Zasshi*, 1998 Jun;99(6):336-44.

5 J.G. Cairncross, et al., "Specific genetic predictors of chemotherapeutic response and survival in patients with anaplastic oligodendrogliomas," *J Natl Cancer Inst*, 1998 Oct 7;90(19):1473-9.

6 S.L. Pomeroy, "Prediction of central nervous system embryonal tumour outcome based on gene expression," *Nature*, January 24, 2002, Vol. 415, pp. 436-442.

7 I.F. Pollack, et. al., "Expression of p53 and prognosis in children with malignant gliomas," *The New England Journal of Medicine*, February 7, 2002, Vol. 346, No. 6, pp. 420-427.

8 2 Marylebone Road, London, NW1 4DF, phone: 020 7770 7000

9 "Hands-Free Kits Cut Exposure to Mobile Phone Radiation," by Dominic Evans, London, Aug 9, 2000 (Reuters). Additionally: "Earpieces Cut Mobile Phone Radiation Risk," Canberra, Aug 7 (Reuters); "Hands-free mobile phone kits can reduce the effects of electromagnetic radiation," Retrieved on March 9, 2005 at http://www.mercola.com/2000/nov/26/mobile_phones.htm.

10 J.E. Muscat JE, et al., "Handheld cellular telephones and risk of acoustic neuroma," *Neurology*, 2002 Apr 23;58(8):1304-6.

11 A. Stang, et al., "The possible role of radiofrequency radiation in the development of uvealm melanoma," *Epidemiology*, 2001 Jan;12(1):7-12. Comment in: *Epidemiology*, 2001 Jan;12(1):1-4.

12 L.I. Kheifets, et al., "Occupational electric and magnetic field exposure and brain cancer: a meta-analysis," *J Occup Environ Med*, 1995 Dec;37(12):1327-41.

13 P.D. Inskip, "Multiple primary tumors involving cancer of the brain and central nervous system as the first or subsequent cancer," *Cancer*, 2003 Aug 1;98(3):562-70.

14 S.A. Khuder, A.B. Mutgi, and E.A. Schaub, "Meta-analyses of brain cancer and farming," *Am J Ind Med*, 1998 ;34(3):252-60.

15 M.P. Little, et al., "Variations with time and age in the risks of solid cancer incidence after radiation exposure in childhood," *Stat Med*, 1998 Jun 30;17(12):1341-55.

16 J.M. Pogoda, and S. Preston-Martin, "Maternal cured meat consumption during pregnancy and risk of paediatric brain tumour in offspring: potentially harmful levels of intake," *Public Health Nutr*, 2001 Apr;4(2):183-9. Comment in: *Public Health Nutr*, 2001 Dec;4(6):1303-5.

17 T. Zheng, K.P. Cantor, and Y. Zhang, "Occupational risk factors for brain cancer: a population-based case-control study in Iowa," *J Occup Environ Med,* 2001 Apr;43(4):317-24.

18 F. Menegoz, et al., "Contacts with animals and humans as risk factors for adult brain tumours. An international case-control study," *Eur J Cancer,* 2002 Mar;38(5):696-704.

19 E.A. Holly, et al., "Farm and animal exposures and pediatric brain tumors: results from the United States West Coast Childhood Brain Tumor Study," *Cancer Epidemiol Biomarkers Prev,* 1998 Sep;7(9):797-802.

20 J.M. Pogoda, and S. Preston-Martin, "Household pesticides and risk of pediatric brain tumors," *Environ Health Perspect,* 1997 Nov;105(11):1214-20.

21 M.A. Norman, E.A. Holly, and S. Preston-Martin, "Childhood brain tumors and exposure to tobacco smoke," *Cancer Epidemiol Biomarkers Prev,* 1996 Feb;5(2):85-91.

22 R.E. Patterson, et al., "Vitamin supplements and cancer risk: the epidemiologic evidence," *Cancer Causes Control,* 1997 Sep;8(5):786-802. Comment in: *Cancer Causes Control,* 1997 Sep;8(5): 685-7.

23 G.S. Omenn, et al., "Risk factors for lung cancer and for intervention effects in CARET, the Beta-Carotene and Retinol Efficacy Trial," *J Natl Cancer Inst,* 1996 Nov 6;88(21):1550-9. Comment in: *J Natl Cancer Inst,* 1996 Nov 6;88(21):1513-5; *J Natl Cancer Inst,* 1997;89(4):325-6; and *J Natl Cancer Inst.,*1997 Nov 9;89(22):1722-3.

24 A. Bendich, "From 1989 to 2001: what have we learned about the 'Biological Actions of Beta-Carotene'?" *J Nutr,* 2004 Jan;134(1):225S-30S.

25 C. Eng, "Genetics of Cowden syndrome: through the looking glass of oncology," *Int J Oncol,* 1998 Mar;12(3):701-10.

CHAPTER 25

1 Bauby, Jean Dominique, *The Butterfly and the Diving Bell* (New York: Alfred Knopf, 1997).

2 Arthur Frank, *The Wounded Storyteller: Body, Illness and Ethics* (Chicago: University of Chicago Press, 1995).

3 Pablo Picasso to Henri Matisse (1950's). Tate Modern Museum exhibit (2003). London, England.

4 Catherine Garrett, "Weal and Woe: Suffering, Sociology and the Emotions of Julian of Norwich," *Pastoral Psychology,* 2001; 49 (3): 187-203.

5 Retrieved on March 9, 2005 at http://www.savvypatients.com/braincancer.htm.

6 Retrieved on March 9, 2005 at http://home.earthlink.net/~sdepesa/.

7 R. Becchetti R, *Oncology Issues,* 18 (1) 36-39, 2003. Retrieved on March 9, 2005 at http://66.102.7.104/search?q=cache:hBIEvY2xWugJ:www.accc-cancer.org/publications/journalmay02/Meeting.pdf+Becchetti+R.++Oncology+Issues:&hl=en.

8 Retrieved on March 9, 2005 at http://www.standardlegal.net/Merchant2/merchant.mv?Affiliate=noel&Screen=PROD&Store_Code=SLN&Product_Code=SLS514.

9 Retrieved on March 9, 2005 at http://money.cnn.com/2003/10/24/pf/living_will.

10 C.C. Earle, et al., "Trends in the aggressiveness of cancer care near the end of life," *J Clin Oncol,* 2004 Jan 15; 22(2): 315-21.

11 C. Saunders, "Patient care: an Introduction," as found in D.W. Vere (Ed.), *Topics in Therapeutics 4* (London: Pitman Medical, 1978).

12 Retrieved on March 9, 2005 at http://www.hospicenet.org.

13 C. Saunders, "Patient care: an Introduction," as found in D.W. Vere (Ed.), *Topics in Therapeutics 4* (London: Pitman Medical, 1978).

14 Dr. David Clark at http://www.ampainsoc.org/pub/bulletin/jul00/hist1.htm. Retrieved on March 9, 2005.

Index

INDEX

SYMBOLS

1p/ 19q chromosome deletion *310*
504 plan *223*

A

ABTA *57*
Accutane *43*
Acoustic neuroma *33, 190, 318*
 trials *180*
ACTH *77*
Activities of daily living *181*
Acupuncture *53, 61, 76*
 effectiveness *77*
ADHD *210*
Advance directives *328*
Advil *108*
Advocate-Representative *278*
After-effects of treatments
 questions *135*
Albert Finney *325*
Allergies with procarbazine *114*
Alleviation of suffering *58*
Alternative
 medical systems *53, 91*
 medicine *52*
 therapy *53, 62*
Amifostine *115*
Amygdalin *68*
ANC *106, 123*
Anemia *108*
Angioma *319*
Anti-angiogenesis agents *46*
Anti-emetics *99, 100*
 medication *101*

Anti-oncogene, p53 *311*
Anti-oxidant *69*
Antibiotics *126*
 combinations *127*
Antineoplaston *53, 74, 75, 89*
 treatment *73*
Anxiety *31, 220*
Anzmet *99*
APC gene *307*
Apoptosis *55*
Appetite *61, 145*
Ara-C *44*
Arachnoiditis *120*
Aromatherapy *87, 91*
 psychological effects *87*
Arteriovenous malformations *33*
Aspirin *108*
Assessing *81*
Association of Hole in the Wall Camps
232
Astrocytomas *114, 317, 318*
 anaplastic *112*
Ayurveda *77*
Ayurvedic medicine *58, 77, 79*
 institutes *91*
 techniques *78*

B

Bach flower remedy *61*
Bactrim *127*
Barretstown gang camp *231, 233*
BCNU *42, 43, 113*
Behavior problems *220*
Belmont report
 ethical principles and guidelines *173*
Beta-carotene *66*
Bill of rights *192*
Biofeedback *83*

INDEX

INDEX

What Leading Brain Tumor Specialists Are Saying About These Books

...a remarkable effort aimed at educating, inspiring, and preparing brain tumor patients and their caregivers at facing the arduous road with such a diagnosis. Ray Sawaya, M.D., Chairman of Neuro Surgery, MD Anderson Hospital and Clinics

...empowering...can help patients and families articulate questions they may not have known to ask. Dr. Henry Friedman & Bebe Guill, Tug Mcgraw Neuro-Oncology Quality Of Life Center, Duke University

The book is an "owners' manual". Steven Brem, M.D. H. Lee Moffitt Cancer Center

...an extraordinarily useful tool for patients and families to navigate the confusing & frightening brain tumor experience. The index and glossary make the information easily accessible. Joseph V. Simone, MD, Chair, National Cancer Policy Board, Institute of Medicine

...provides a road map for the complex route that patients must navigate after they are diagnosed with a brain tumor. Reid Thompson M.D. Director of Neurosurgical Oncology, Vanderbilt University

"Meaty" and practical" –the antidote for patients who...become paralyzed with fear and indecision. Dr Jonathan Finlay MD, Children's Hospital, Los Angeles, CA

...an excellent resource for brain tumor patients in North America...valuable to health care professionals with a special interest in brain tumors...adds significantly to the current available literature. Dr. Rolando Del Maestro, Clinical Director, Brain Tumour Research Centre, Montreal, Canada

This is a must read for anyone...trying to cope with a brain tumor. It should be read as soon as the diagnosis is made or even suspected. Al Musella, DPM, President, Musella Foundation For Brain Tumor Research & Information, Inc www.virtualtrials.com

...an excellent resource for brain tumor patients in North America... valuable to health care professionals with a special interest in brain tumors...adds significantly to the current available literature. Dr. Rolando Del Maestro, Clinical Director, Brain Tumour Research Centre, Montreal, Canada

...an important resource for patients. Keith Black M.D., Director, Maxine Dunitz Neurosurgical Institute, Los Angeles, CA